GREAT RETREATS
YOGA

EDITED & COMPILED BY ANGELIKA TASCHEN   TEXT BY KRISTIN RÜBESAMEN

GREAT RETREATS
YOGA

TASCHEN

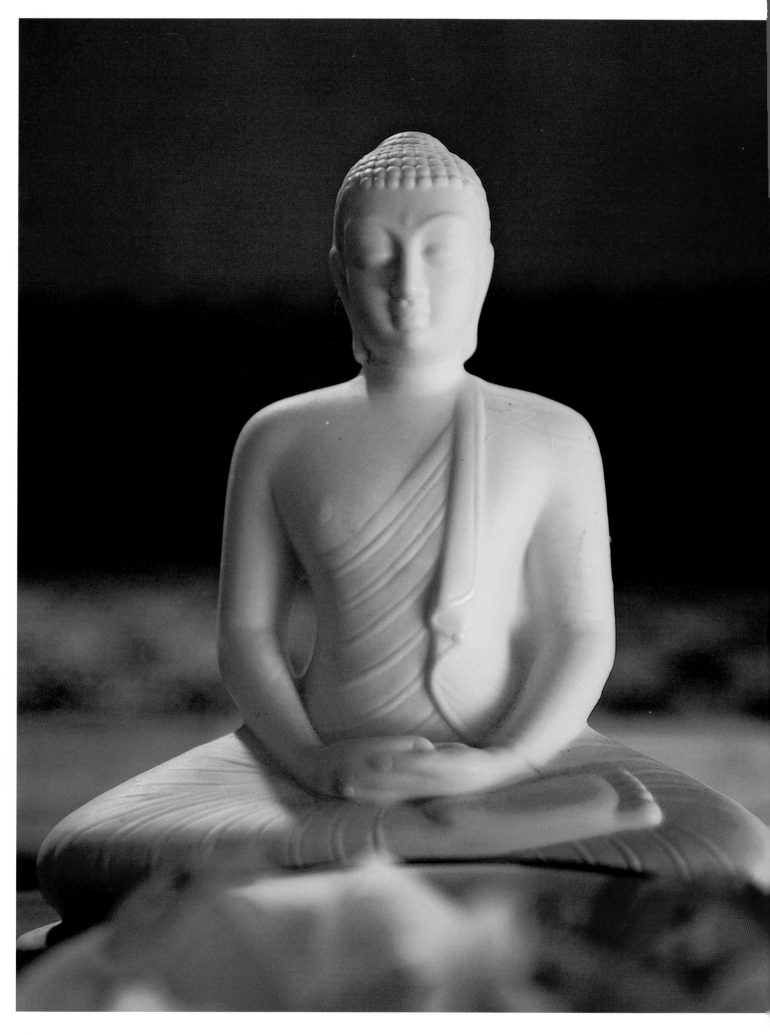

योग (yō′gə) is one of the six schools of Indian philosophy; it has its roots in Hinduism and Buddhism. Originally yoga was a purely spiritual path to enlightenment through meditation. The asanas (body poses) were only meant to prepare for meditation posture.

Yoga ist eine der sechs Schulen der indischen Philosophie; ihre Wurzeln liegen in Hinduismus und Buddhismus. Ursprünglich war Yoga ein rein spiritueller Weg zur Erleuchtung durch Meditation. Die Asanas (Körperhaltungen) sollten zunächst nur auf die Meditationshaltung vorbereiten.

Le yoga est une des six écoles de la philosophie indienne ; elle plonge ses racines dans l'hindouisme et le bouddhisme. À l'origine, le yoga était un moyen spirituel de parvenir à l'illumination par la méditation. Les asanas (postures corporelles) ne servaient qu'à préparer le corps à la posture de méditation.

Why Yoga? by Angelika Taschen

After more than 12 years of intensive yoga practice, I plan not only my day around the daily yoga session but also my holidays around yoga retreats.

Constant overstimulation, unhealthy food, insufficient sleep—life in the digital age can be very stressful. A couple of yoga sessions per week are sometimes not enough to outbalance the toll this takes on our bodies and minds. That's where a yoga retreat comes in: above and beyond the daily yoga classes, it welcomes visitors with healthy, mostly vegetarian cuisine, total relaxation and inspiring natural surroundings (yogis tend to know a thing or two about real beauty). All this helps us to recharge our batteries and gain a fresh perspective in next to no time.

For this book, I have selected the world's most special places where instruction is provided by the very best yoga teachers. According to need and experience, you can choose either a spiritually oriented ashram, small hotels with basic comforts and convivial atmosphere, or a five-star resort that offers daily yoga sessions.

I am absolutely confident that yoga has a big future. All around the world, awareness of the spiritual as well as the need for counteracting day-to-day stress are on the rise. Much more than just some kind of gymnastics to strengthen the back and maintain general flexibility, yoga is a comprehensive way of living that embraces body, spirit and soul in equal measure. Namasté!

Seit über zwölf Jahren praktiziere ich Yoga und plane nicht nur meinen Alltag um tägliche Yogastunden herum, sondern inzwischen auch oft meine Reisen um Retreats.

Ständige Reizüberflutung, ungesundes Essen, zu wenig Schlaf: Das Leben im digitalen Zeitalter kann anstrengend sein. Einige Yogastunden pro Woche reichen oft nicht, um all das auszugleichen. Es ist kein Zufall, dass sich unsere Batterien in einem Yoga-Retreat besonders gründlich aufladen: Neben täglichen Yogastunden gibt es gesundes, meist vegetarisches Essen, die Chance zu völliger Entspannung und die Inspiration durch die umgebende Natur (Yogis sind Experten, wenn es um wahre Schönheit geht). Das alles verhilft in kurzer Zeit zu frischer Energie und einer neuen Perspektive.

Für dieses Buch habe ich wunderbare Orte in aller Welt ausfindig gemacht, an denen die besten Yogalehrer unterrichten – von spirituell ausgerichteten Ashrams und kleinen Hotels mit gemeinschaftlicher Atmosphäre bis hin zu Fünf-Sterne-Resorts, die tägliche Yoga-Sessions anbieten.

Ich bin überzeugt, dass Yoga eine große Zukunft hat. Der Wunsch nach mehr Spiritualität und die Erkenntnis, dass unser Alltagsstress ein Gegengewicht braucht, nehmen weltweit zu. Yoga ist nicht nur eine Gymnastik, die den Rücken stärkt und uns beweglich hält, sondern ein umfassender Lebensstil, der auf Körper, Geist und Seele positiv einwirkt. Namasté!

Aujourd'hui, après plus de douze années de pratique intensive du yoga, non seulement j'organise mes journées autour des séances de yoga, mais je programme aussi mes vacances dans des centres de yoga.

Trop-plein de sollicitations permanentes, alimentation malsaine, manque de sommeil : la vie à l'ère numérique peut être épuisante. Souvent, quelques heures de yoga par semaine ne suffisent pas à compenser tout ce stress. Ce n'est pas un hasard si nos batteries se rechargent dans une retraite de yoga : en plus de séances quotidiennes de yoga sont proposés une alimentation saine, en général végétarienne, la possibilité d'une détente totale et l'inspiration émanant de la nature environnante (les yogis savent ce qu'est la vraie beauté). Tout ceci contribue en peu de temps à un regain d'énergie et offre une perspective nouvelle.

Pour cet ouvrage j'ai déniché à travers le monde des lieux fabuleux où enseignent les meilleurs professeurs de yoga. Selon vos besoins, vous pouvez choisir entre les ashrams d'orientation spirituelle, les petites sites à l'atmosphère conviviale et les hôtels cinq étoiles, qui proposent chaque jour des séances de yoga.

Je suis certaine que le yoga a un grand avenir devant lui. La quête de spiritualité et la nécessité d'un équilibre réel face au stress quotidien s'amplifient dans le monde entier. Le yoga n'est pas seulement un type de gymnastique destiné à fortifier le dos et assouplir le corps, il est un mode de vie complet, impliquant à la fois le corps, l'esprit et l'âme. Namasté!

Contents Inhalt Sommaire

Contents   Inhalt   Sommaire

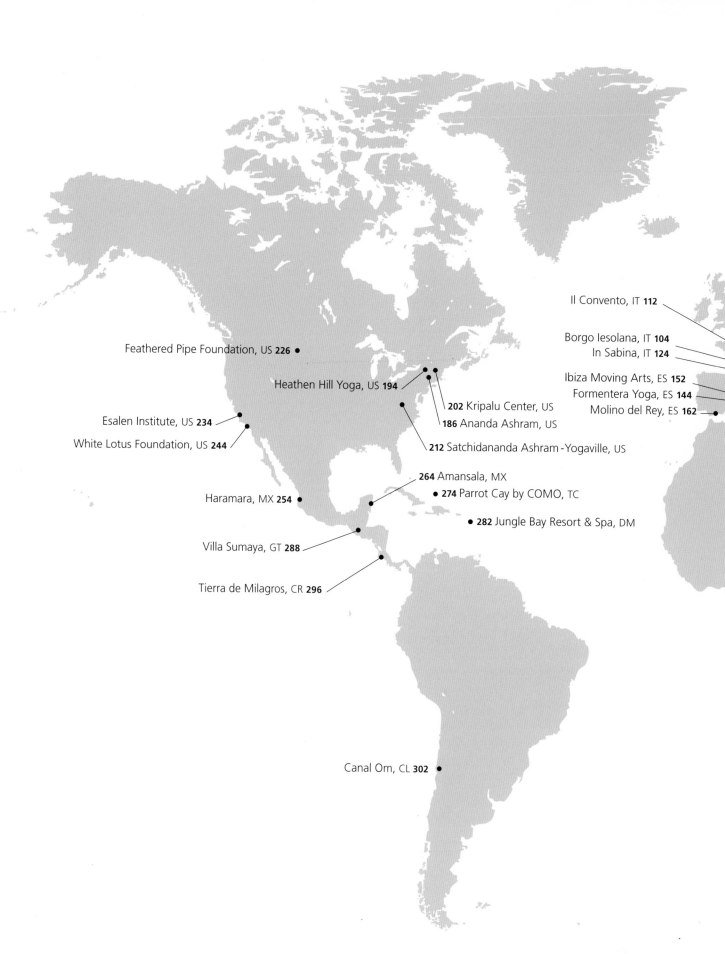

Il Convento, IT **112**

Borgo Iesolana, IT **104**
In Sabina, IT **124**

Ibiza Moving Arts, ES **152**
Formentera Yoga, ES **144**
Molino del Rey, ES **162**

Feathered Pipe Foundation, US **226** ●

Heathen Hill Yoga, US **194**

202 Kripalu Center, US

186 Ananda Ashram, US

Esalen Institute, US **234**

White Lotus Foundation, US **244**

212 Satchidananda Ashram - Yogaville, US

264 Amansala, MX

Haramara, MX **254** ●

● **274** Parrot Cay by COMO, TC

● **282** Jungle Bay Resort & Spa, DM

Villa Sumaya, GT **288**

Tierra de Milagros, CR **296**

Canal Om, CL **302** ●

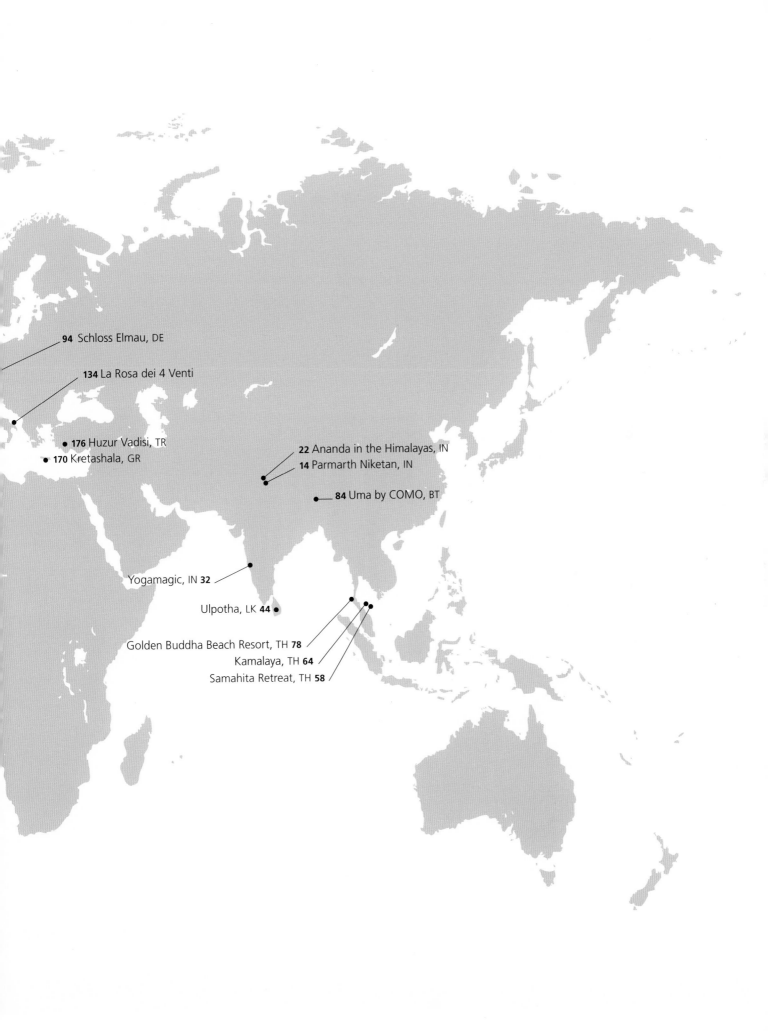

94 Schloss Elmau, DE

134 La Rosa dei 4 Venti

● **176** Huzur Vadisi, TR
● **170** Kretashala, GR

22 Ananda in the Himalayas, IN
14 Parmarth Niketan, IN

84 Uma by COMO, BT

Yogamagic, IN **32**

Ulpotha, LK **44** ●

Golden Buddha Beach Resort, TH **78**

Kamalaya, TH **64**

Samahita Retreat, TH **58**

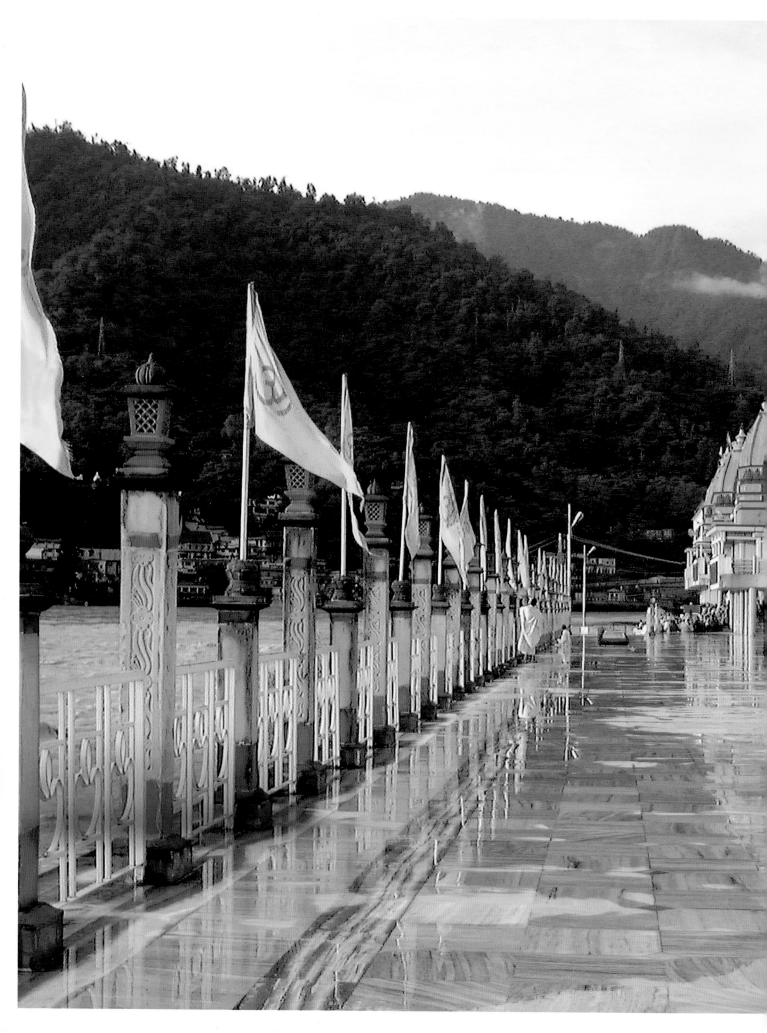

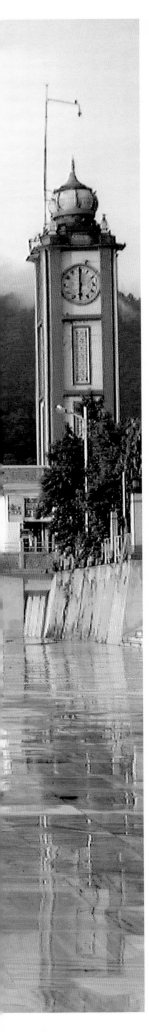

The simple rooms in the ashram are clean and well swept, the day's agenda clearly organised; in fact, the management of the whole place is surprisingly disciplined in view of the fact that this, the birthplace of yoga, is in India, in Rishikesh. Of the countless yoga schools in Rishikesh the instructions given in the Parmarth Niketan are among the best, which is why many students register for the twice-yearly teacher-training course. As soon as the sun rises, the first of them begin to do their sun salutations and to meditate. Universal prayers, Asana classes and readings on philosophy follow, and the day continues with asanas until the evening. Then, with great spectacle, the president and spiritual head of the ashram, Swami Chidanand Saraswatiji, conducts Ganga Aarti, the evening lighting ceremony. Swamiji doesn't just have strikingly beautiful eyes and a hotline to God; he is also a man deeply involved in serving humanity. Every year at the beginning of March he organises an impressive international yoga festival in the ashram, at which the best-known Indian yoga teachers and spiritual leaders as well as those from the West assemble. He was invited by the United Nations to speak on the subject of religion, and he has founded several orphanages in which Indian orphans, in addition to receiving a school education, learn yoga and Sanskrit and study the Vedas. When, in the evening, happy and close to a state of bliss, they start to sing while huddled up on cushions on the floor of the steps at the river, you understand why Indian families from all over the world return every year to support the ashram. Even Ringo Starr would have liked it here—in his youth, he once only left Rishikesh because his supply of baked beans had run out.

Books to pack: "The Bhagavad Gita" (2 volumes) by Paramahansa Yogananda and "Siddhartha" by Hermann Hesse

Parmarth Niketan Ashram

P.O. Swargashram
Rishikesh (Himalayas)
Uttaranchal 249304
India
Tel. +91 135 244 0011
Fax +91 135 244 0066
parmarth@parmarth.com
www.parmarth.com

Directions	Located on the bank of the Ganges, south of the Ram Jhula Bridge. 30 min from Jolly Grant Airport in Rishikesh/Dehradun. By train from Delhi to Haridwar, continuing by taxi or bus to Rishikesh
Yoga	Traditional Hatha, Kriya Yoga, Yoga Nidra
Teachers	Swami Ramdevji, Swami Veda Bharati, Swami Yoganandaji, Manouso Manos, Gurmukh Kaur Khlsa and Gabriela Bozic come to the International Yoga Festival
Rooms	Over 1000 rooms that accommodate 2–4 people each
Food	Indian vegetarian, without onions or garlic
Treatments	Ayurveda
Leisure	Trekking, whitewater rafting

Sauber und gefegt sind die einfachen Zimmer im Ashram, klar organisiert die Tagesordnung, überraschend diszipliniert der ganze Betrieb angesichts der Tatsache, dass man sich in Rishikesh in Indien befindet, und zwar an der Geburtsstätte des Yoga. Unter den unzähligen Yogaschulen in Rishikesh gehört Parmarth Niketan dank des Unterrichts zu den besten, weshalb sich viele Schüler zur zweimal jährlich stattfindenden Lehrerausbildung anmelden. Sobald die Sonne aufgeht, beginnen die Ersten, ihre Sonnengrüße zu machen und zu meditieren. Universelle Gebete, Asana-Klassen und Vorlesungen über Philosophie folgen, und weiter geht es mit Asanas bis zum Abend. Dann führt in großer Inszenierung der Präsident und das spirituelle Oberhaupt des Ashrams, Swami Chidanand Saraswatiji, die Lichterzeremonie Ganga Aarti am Ganges durch. Swamiji hat nicht nur auffallend schöne Augen und einen heißen Draht zu Gott, er ist auch ein Mann, der sich zutiefst dem Wohl der Menschheit verpflichtet fühlt. Er organisiert im Ashram jährlich Anfang März ein beeindruckendes internationales Yoga-Festival, an dem außer den bekanntesten indischen auch westliche Yogalehrer und -meister teilnehmen. Er wurde von den United Nations als Redner zum Thema Religion eingeladen und hat mehrere Waisenhäuser gegründet, in denen indische Waisenjungen zusätzlich zu einer Schulbildung Yoga und Sanskrit lernen und die Veden studieren. Wenn sie abends vergnügt und geradezu selig auf den Stufen am Fluss auf Kissen gekauert zu singen beginnen, versteht man, warum Inderfamilien aus der ganzen Welt jedes Jahr wiederkommen, um den Ashram zu unterstützen. Hier hätte es sogar Ringo Starr gefallen, der damals aus Rishikesh abreisen musste – ihm waren die mitgebrachten Dosen mit Baked Beans ausgegangen.

Reisebegleiter: »Die Bhagavad Gita« (2 Bände) von Paramahansa Yogananda und »Siddhartha« von Hermann Hesse

Dans l'âshram, les chambres simples sont propres et nettes, l'emploi du temps clairement organisé, la maison tout entière étonnamment disciplinée vu que nous nous trouvons en Inde et à Rishikesh, berceau du yoga. Parmi les innombrables écoles de yoga de Rishikesh, l'enseignement donné au Parmarth Niketan compte parmi les meilleurs, raison pour laquelle nombre d'élèves s'inscrivent à la formation de professeurs qui se tient deux fois par an. A peine le soleil levé, les premiers commencent leurs saluts du matin et leurs méditations. Ensuite ont lieu les prières universelles, les classes d'Âsanas et les cours magistraux, suivis d'exercices d'Âsanas jusqu'au soir. Puis, dans une mise en scène grandiose, Swami Chidanand Saraswatiji, Ganga Aarti, président et chef spirituel, procède à la cérémonie du feu. En excellents termes avec Dieu, Swamiji n'a pas seulement des yeux magnifiques, c'est aussi un homme du monde. Chaque année, il organise début mars un brillant festival de yoga international auquel, outre les plus grandes célébrités indiennes, participent aussi des stars occidentales. Il est invité par les Nations Unies pour parler de la religion, dans l'âshram même il a fondé un orphelinat où les garçons, en plus de leur formation scolaire, apprennent le yoga, le sanskrit et étudient les Védas. Lorsque, le soir venu, sur le sol de l'autel de pierre au bord du fleuve, ils se mettent à chanter dans une joyeuse béatitude, accroupis sur des coussins, on comprend pourquoi de riches familles indiennes de Londres reviennent chaque année apporter leur soutien à l'âshram. Même Ringo Starr s'est senti à l'aise ici ; à l'époque il avait dû quitter Rishikesh – sa réserve de boîtes de baked beans était épuisée.

Livres à emporter : « La Bhagavad Gîtâ » de Swami Chinmayananda et « Siddhartha » de Hermann Hesse

Anreise	Am Ganges, südlich der Brücke Ram Jhula gelegen, 30 min vom Jolly Grant Airport in Rishikesh/Dehradun entfernt. Mit dem Zug von Delhi nach Haridwar, weiter per Taxi oder Bus
Yoga	Traditional Hatha, Kriya Yoga, Yoga Nidra
Lehrer	Zum International Yoga Festival kommen Swami Ramdevji, Swami Veda Bharati, Swami Yoganandaji, Manouso Manos, Gurmukh Kaur Khalsa, Gabriela Bozic
Zimmer	Über 1000 Zimmer für je 2–4 Personen
Küche	Indisch-vegetarisch, ohne Zwiebeln oder Knoblauch
Anwendungen	Ayurveda
Aktivitäten	Trekking, Wildwasser-Rafting

Accès	Situé au bord du Gange, au sud du pont Ram Jhula. A 30 min de l'aéroport Jolly Grant de Rishikesh/Dehradun. Trajet en train de Dehli à Haridwar, puis en taxi ou bus à Rishikesh
Yoga	Traditional Hatha, Kriya Yoga, Yoga nidra
Professeurs	Participent au Festival international de yoga Swami Ramdevji, Swami Veda Bharati, Swami Yoganandaji, Manouso Manos, Gurmukh Kaur Khalsa, Gabriela Bozic
Chambres	Plus de 1000 chambres de 2 à 4 personnes
Restauration	Cuisine indienne et végétarienne, sans oignon ni ail
Traitements	Ayurveda
Activités	Trekking, rafting en eau vive

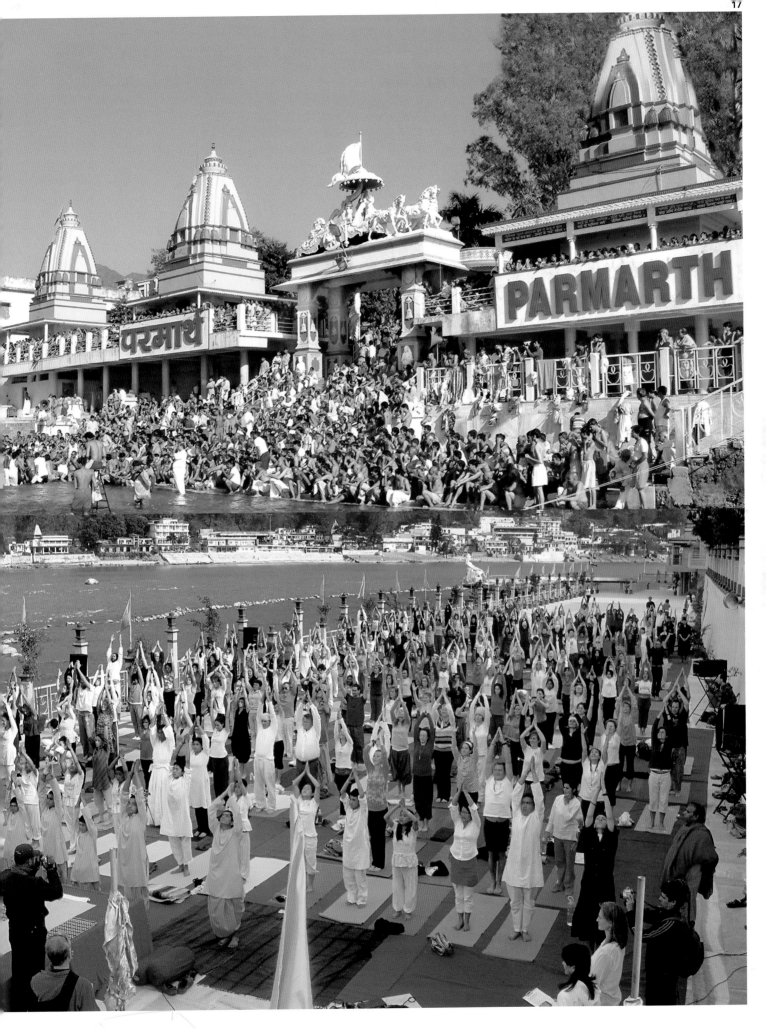

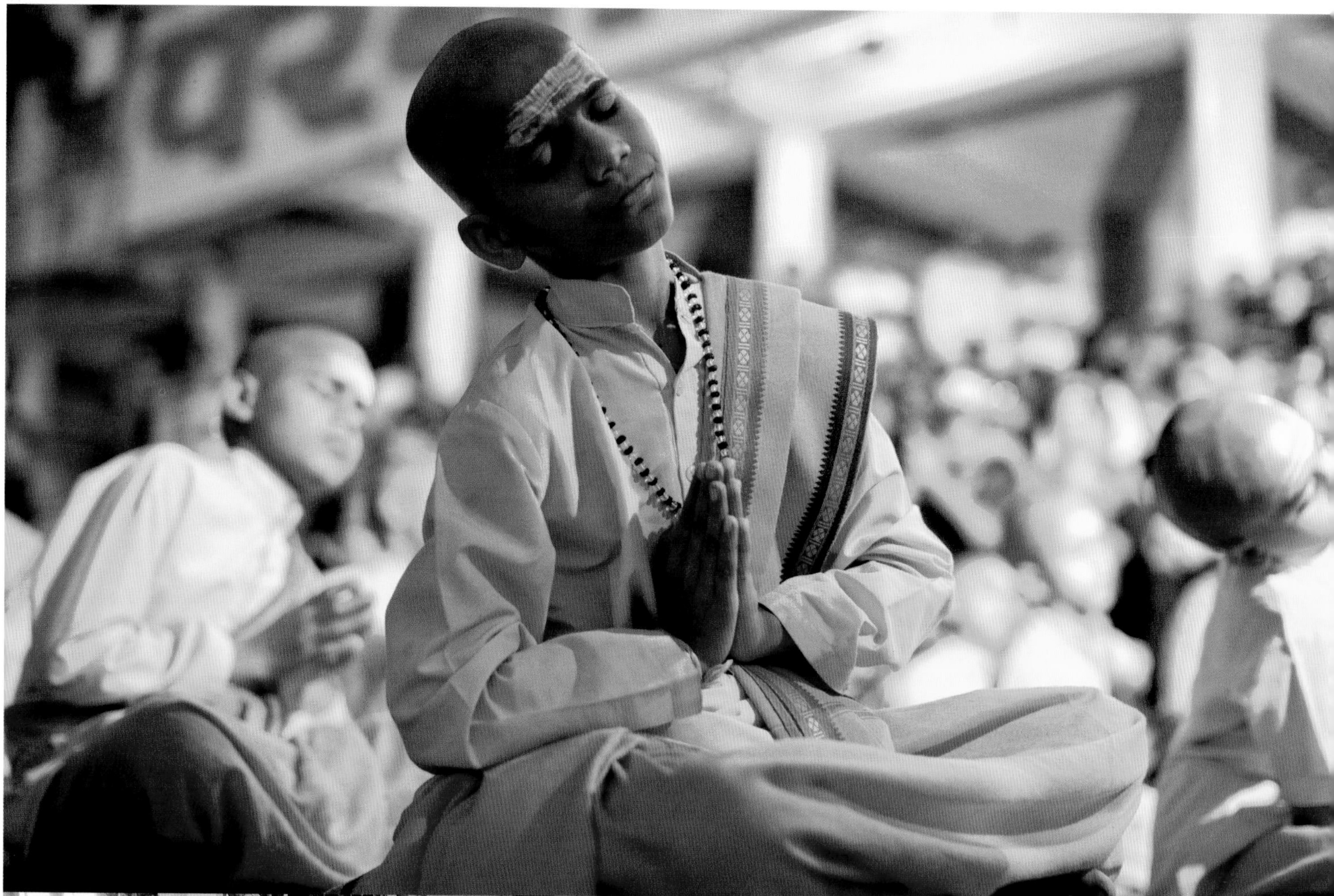

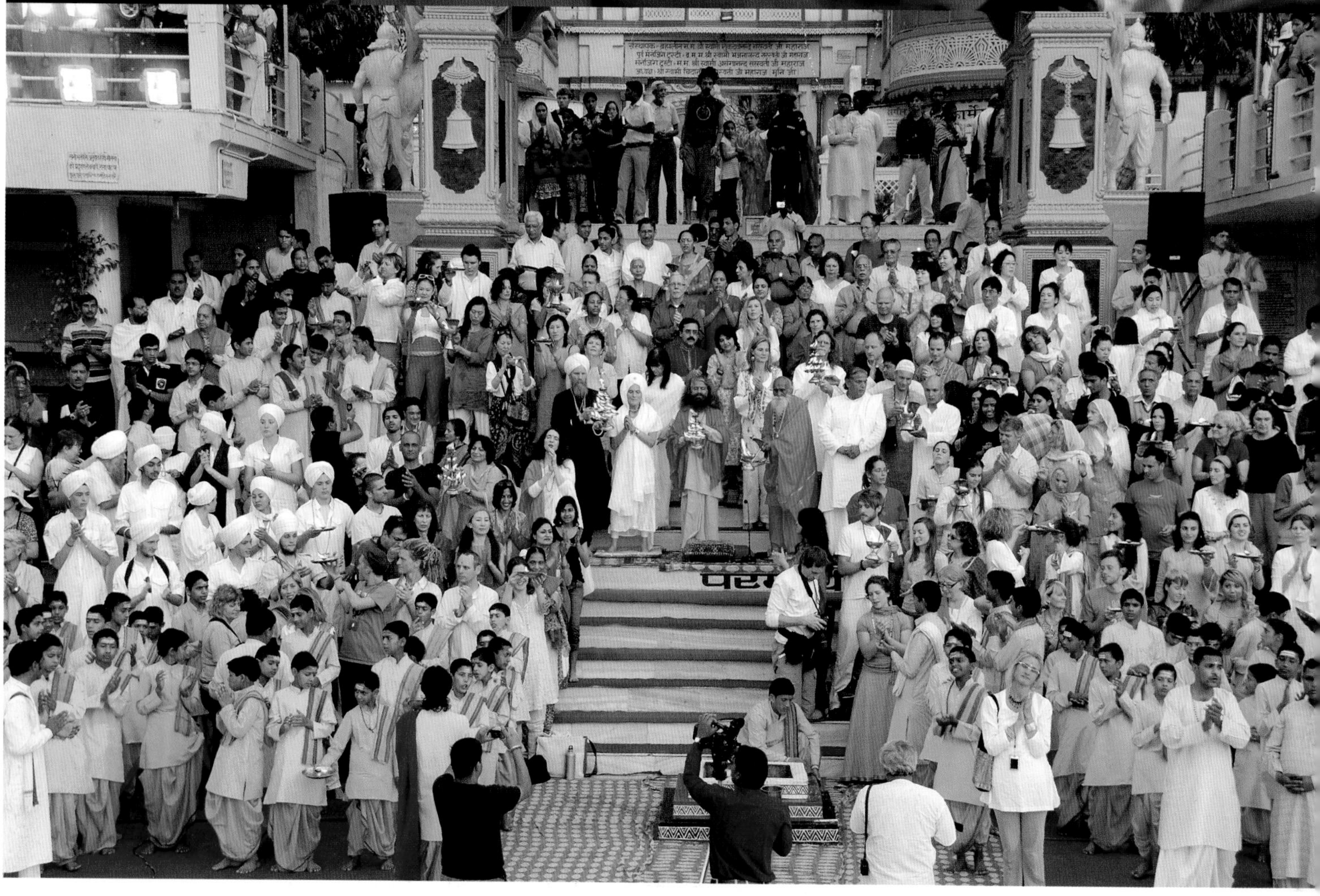

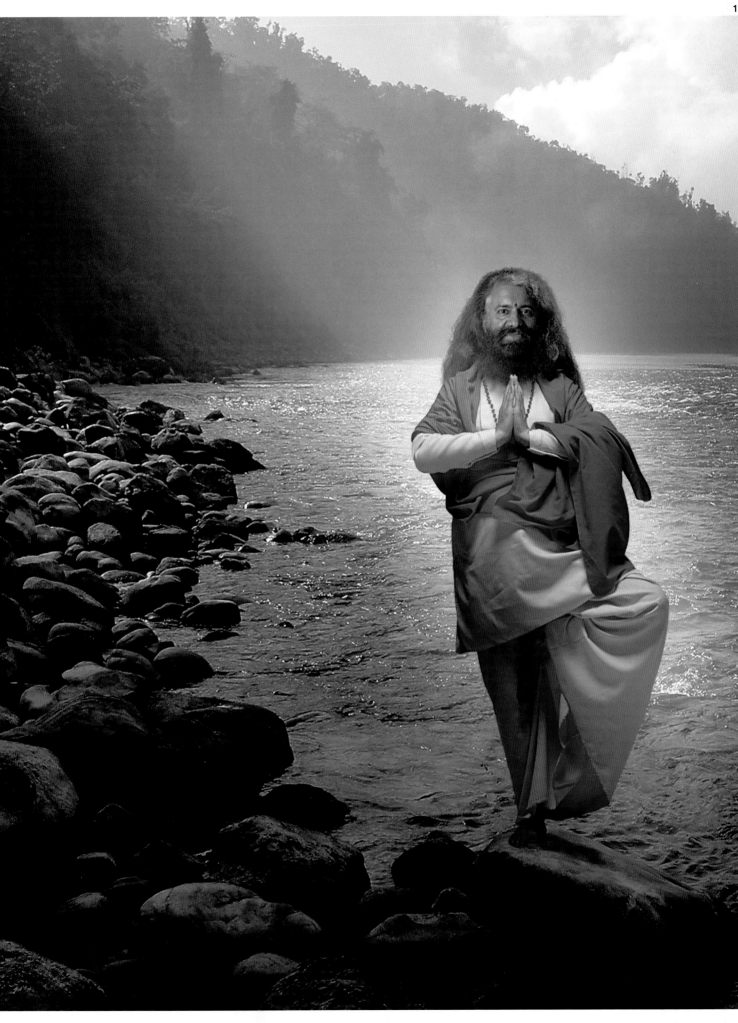

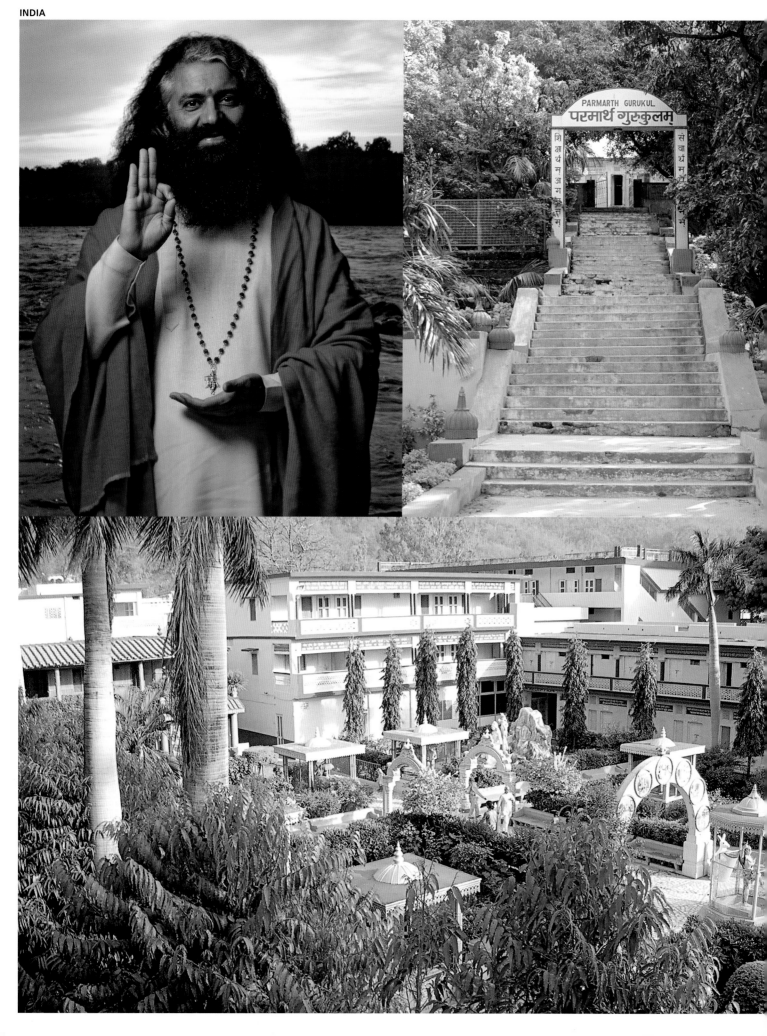

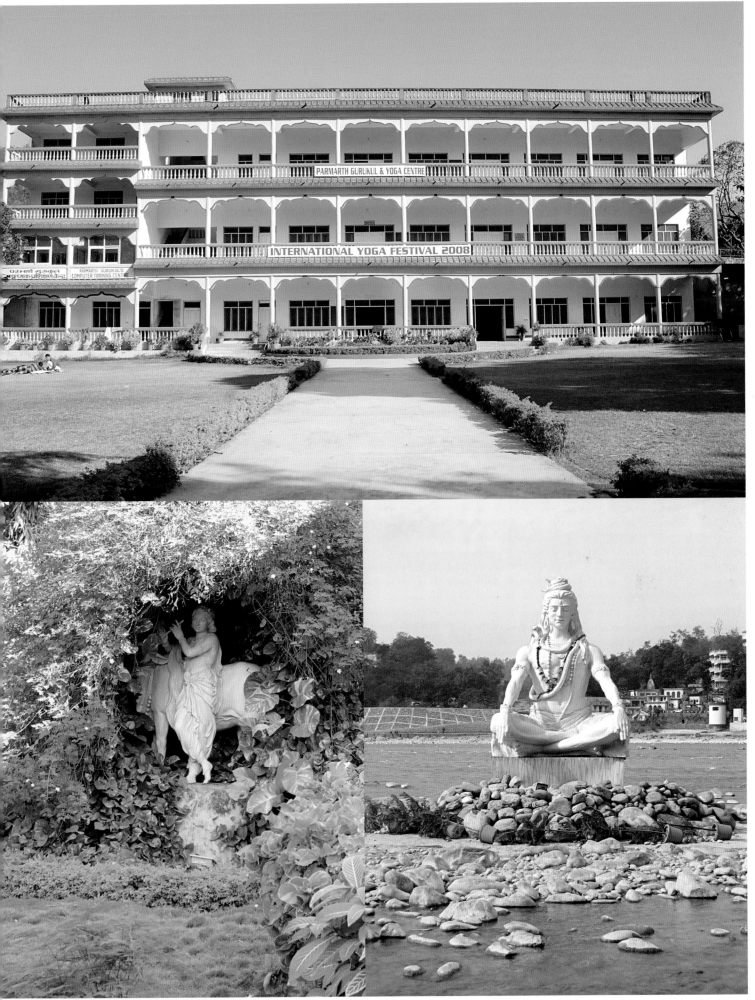

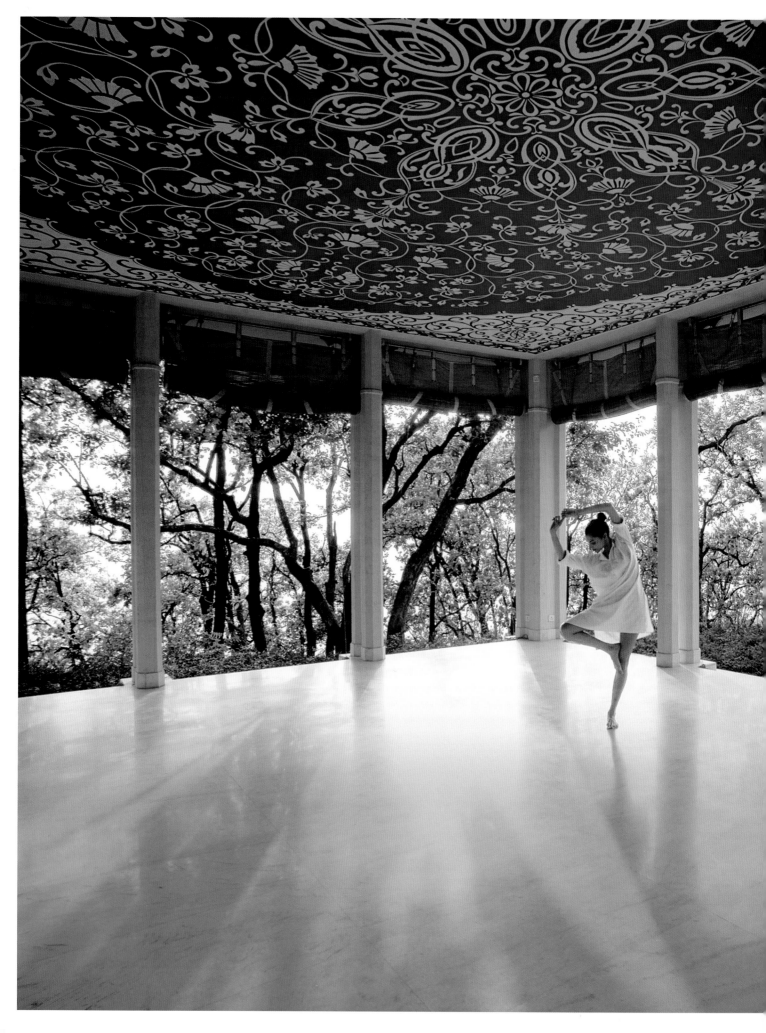

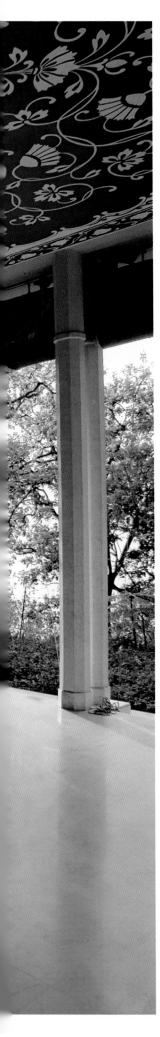

The palace lies high up in the mist. From the whitish veil of light, green hills emerge, more and more of them—the foothills of the Himalayas. Down in the valley the broad, turquoise Ganges winds southwards through the countryside. Up here you live like they did in the time of the maharajas, or would do if the stress that brings the guests to Ananda weren't so modern. Sirodhara treatments (hot oil poured onto the forehead) lasting for hours, sesame oil massages, a soothingly babbling waterfall, the scent of sandalwood and ginger tea await the guest after the yoga sessions, which take place at least twice daily—in the palace, in the pavilion or in the amphitheatre in the marvellous park. The teachers who offer instruction here did not qualify with a mere weekend seminar. As a rule, they hail from nearby Rishikesh, the birthplace of yoga, and teach a gentle Hatha yoga in as natural a way as it has been passed down through the generations. Private tuition is available. Ananda is the Sanskrit word for "bliss"—which sets in easily after the morning's meditation and yoga, even before you have been served your sweet toast, made of chickpea flour, with roasted melon seeds and fresh mango compote on the terrace built like a tree house into the ancient Sal trees.

Books to pack: "Life in Freedom" by Jiddu Krishnamurti and "Into Thin Air" by Jon Krakauer

Ananda in the Himalayas

The Palace Estate
Narendra Nagar, Tehri-Garhwai
Uttaranchal 249175
India
Tel. +91 1378 227 500
Fax +91 1378 227 550
sales@anandaspa.com
www.anandaspa.com

Directions	162 miles north of New Delhi, 45-min flight to Jolly Grant Airport in Rishikesh/Dehradun, 5-hr train journey from Delhi to Haridwar, transfer by arrangement
Yoga	Hatha, Kriya, Raja Yoga
Teacher	Bhavini Kalan
Rooms	70 deluxe rooms, 5 deluxe suites, 3 separate luxury villas
Food	Indian, Asian and Western organic cuisine. Vata, Pitta and Kapha meals
Treatments	Over 79 different traditional Ayurveda treatments, detox, anti-aging, weight & inch loss, aromatherapy
Leisure	Courses in Vedanta, swimming, temple trekking, whitewater rafting, safaris, billiards, golf, cooking

Hoch oben im Nebel liegt der Palast. Aus dem weißlichen Schleier aus Licht tauchen grüne Hügel auf, immer mehr, die Ausläufer des Himalajas. Unten im Tal windet sich der Ganges breit und türkis durchs Land nach Süden. Hier oben lebt man wie zu Zeiten der Maharadschas, wäre der Stress, der die Gäste herbringt, nicht so modern. Stundenlange Stirngüsse, Sesamölmassagen, ein beruhigend plätschernder Wasserfall, der Geruch nach Sandelholz und Ingwertee erwarten den Gast nach den Yogastunden, die mindestens zweimal täglich stattfinden, im Palast, im Pavillon oder im Amphitheater des herrlichen Parks. Die Lehrer, die hier unterrichten, haben sich nicht nur mit einem Wochenend-seminar qualifiziert. Sie kommen in der Regel aus dem nahe gelegenen Rishikesh, dem Geburtsort von Yoga, und unter-richten ein sanftes Hatha Yoga so selbstverständlich, wie es von Generation zu Generation weitergegeben wurde, auf Wunsch auch im Einzelunterricht. Ananda heißt auf Sans-krit »Seligkeit«. Diese stellt sich leicht ein nach Morgen-meditation und Yoga, noch bevor einem auf der Terrasse, die wie ein Baumhaus in die uralten Sal-Bäume gebaut ist, süßer Toast aus Kichererbsenmehl mit gerösteten Melonen-samen und frischem Mangokompott serviert wird.

Reisebegleiter: »Vollkommene Freiheit« von Jiddu Krishnamurti und »In eisige Höhen« von Jon Krakauer

Bien au-dessus des brumes resplendit le palais. Emergeant du voile blanchâtre de lumière, apparaissent de plus en plus nombreuses les collines vertes, contreforts de l'Himalaya. En bas, dans la vallée, le Gange traverse le pays en larges méandres turquoise en direction du sud. Dans les hauteurs on vit comme au temps des maharadjas, si ce n'était le stress moderne qui fait affluer les visiteurs. De longues affusions du front, des massages à l'huile de sésame, une cascade qui clapote doucement, l'odeur du bois de santal et une tisane au gingembre attendent le visiteur après les séances de yoga, qui se tiennent au moins deux fois par jour dans le palais, le pavillon ou l'amphithéâtre du magnifique parc. Les profes-seurs enseignant ici n'ont pas acquis leur qualification dans un séminaire de week-end. Le plus souvent, ils viennent de Rishikesh, berceau du yoga situé à proximité, et enseignent le Hatha-yoga doux avec le même naturel qu'on le leur a appris de génération en génération, en cours particulier sur demande. En sanskrit, ananda signifie béatitude ; celle-ci vous envahit agréablement après la méditation du matin et le yoga, avant même que l'on vous serve, sur la terrasse construite comme une maison-arbre dans les sals ancestraux, un toast sucré de farine de pois chiches aux graines de melon grillées, accompagné de compote de mangue fraîche.

Livres à emporter : « De la liberté » de Jiddu Krishnamurti et « Tragédie à l'Everest » de Jon Krakauer

Anreise	260 km nördlich von Delhi, 45 min Flug zum Jolly Grant Airport in Rishikesh/Dehradun, 5 Std. Zug von Delhi nach Haridwar. Transfer nach Absprache
Yoga	Hatha, Kriya, Raja Yoga
Lehrer	Bhavini Kalan
Zimmer	70 Deluxe-Zimmer, 5 Suiten, 3 separate Villen
Küche	Indisch-, asiatisch oder westlich-organisch. Vata-, Pitta- und Kapha-Mahlzeiten.
Anwendungen	Über 79 verschiedene Ayurveda-Anwendungen, Detox, Anti-Aging, Weight & Inch Loss, Aromatherapie
Aktivitäten	Unterricht in Vedanta, Schwimmen, Tempel-Trekking, Wildwasser-Rafting, Safari, Billard, Golf, Kochkurse

Accès	Situé à 260 km au nord de Delhi, à 45 min de vol du Jolly Grant Airport à Rishikesh/Dehradun, à 5 h de train de Delhi à Haridwar, transfert peut être organisé
Yoga	Hatha, Kriya, Raja Yoga
Professeur	Bhavini Kalan
Chambres	70 chambres de luxe, 5 suites, 3 villas de luxe
Restauration	Cuisine organique indienne, asiatique, occidentale. Repas de types Vata, Pitta et Kapha.
Traitements	Plus de 79 traitements de l'Ayurveda, détox, anti-âge, weight & inch loss, aromathérapie
Activités	Cours en védânta, natation, temple trekking, rafting en eau vive, safari, billard, golf, cours de cuisine

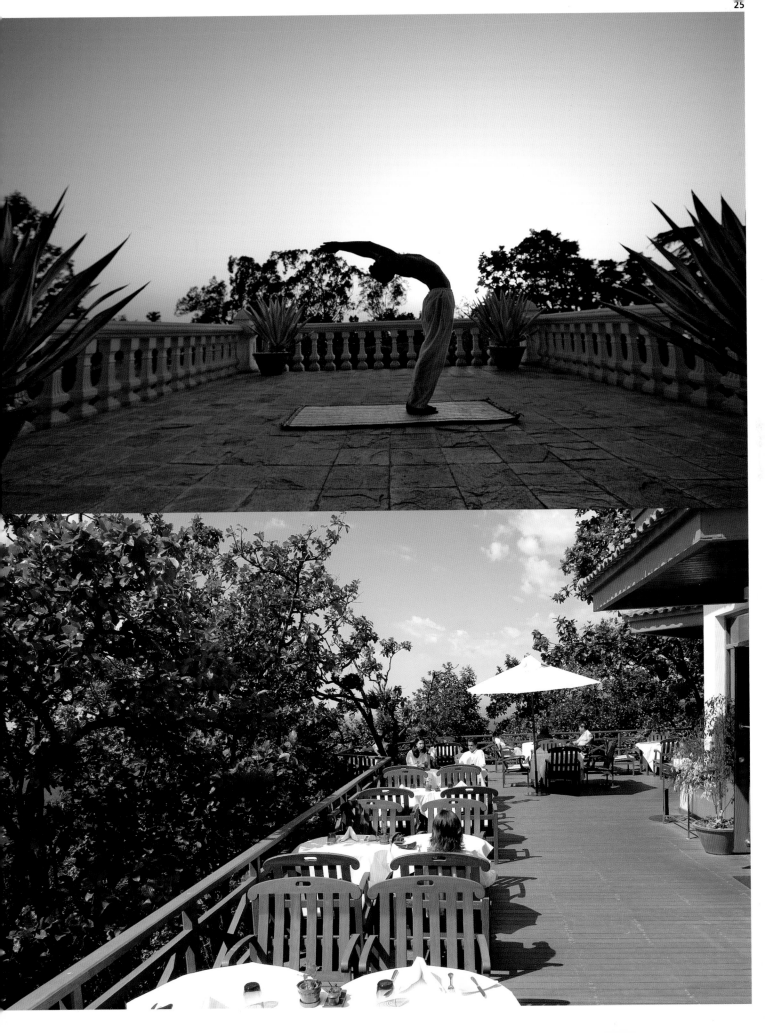

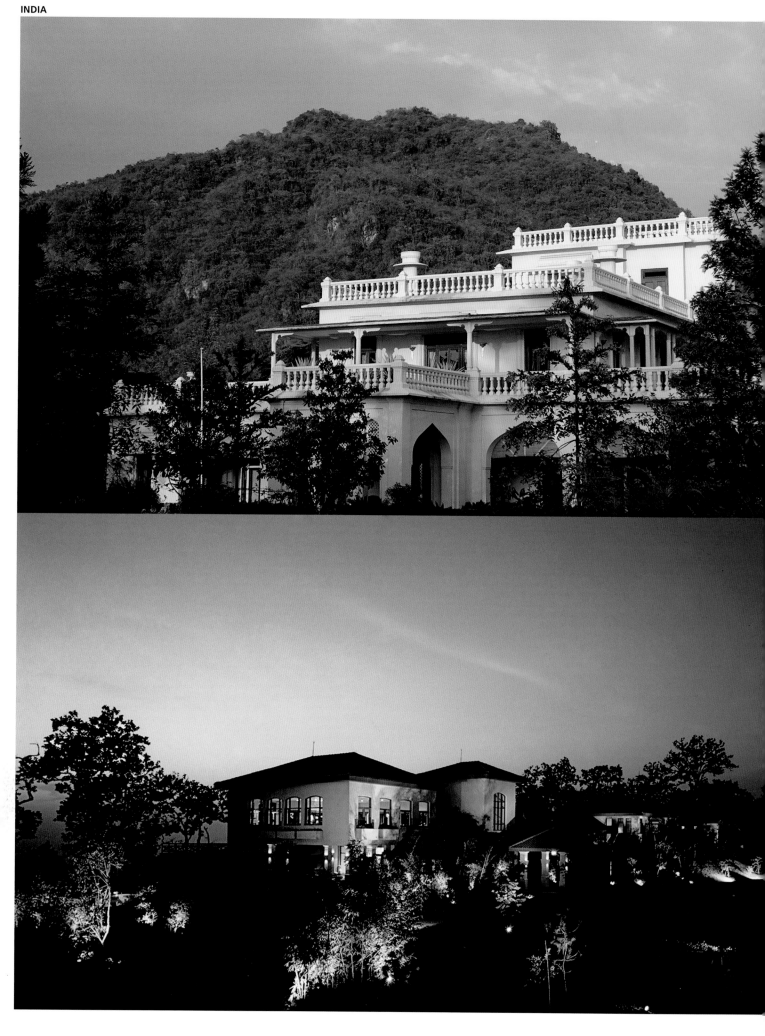

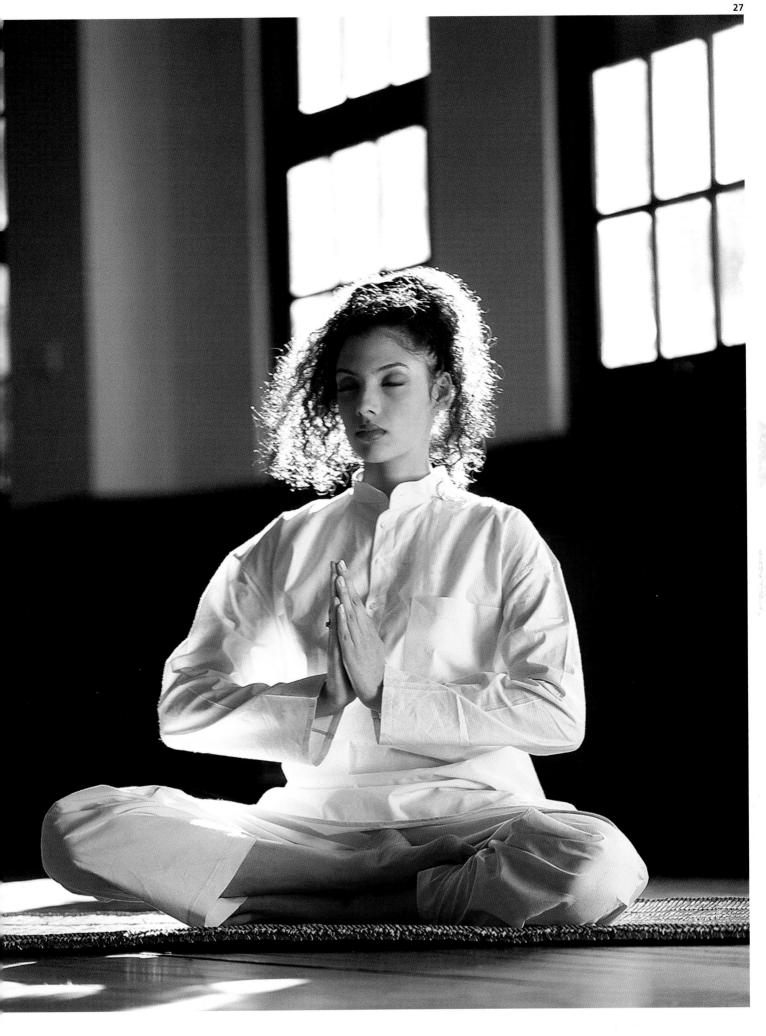

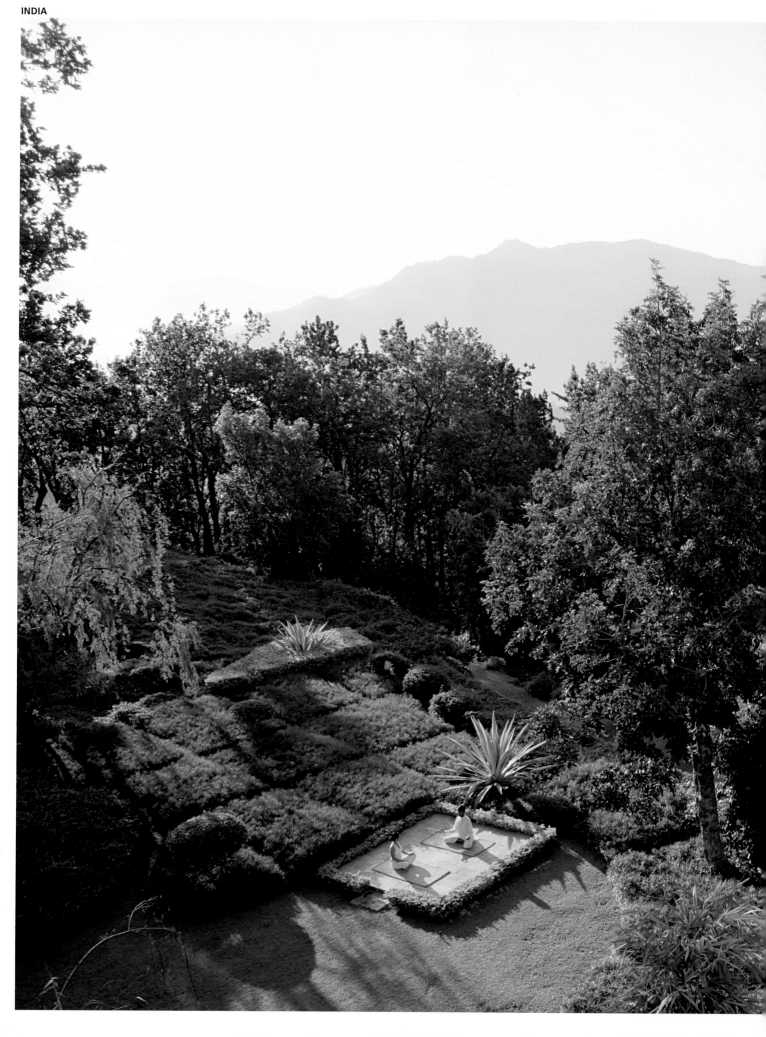

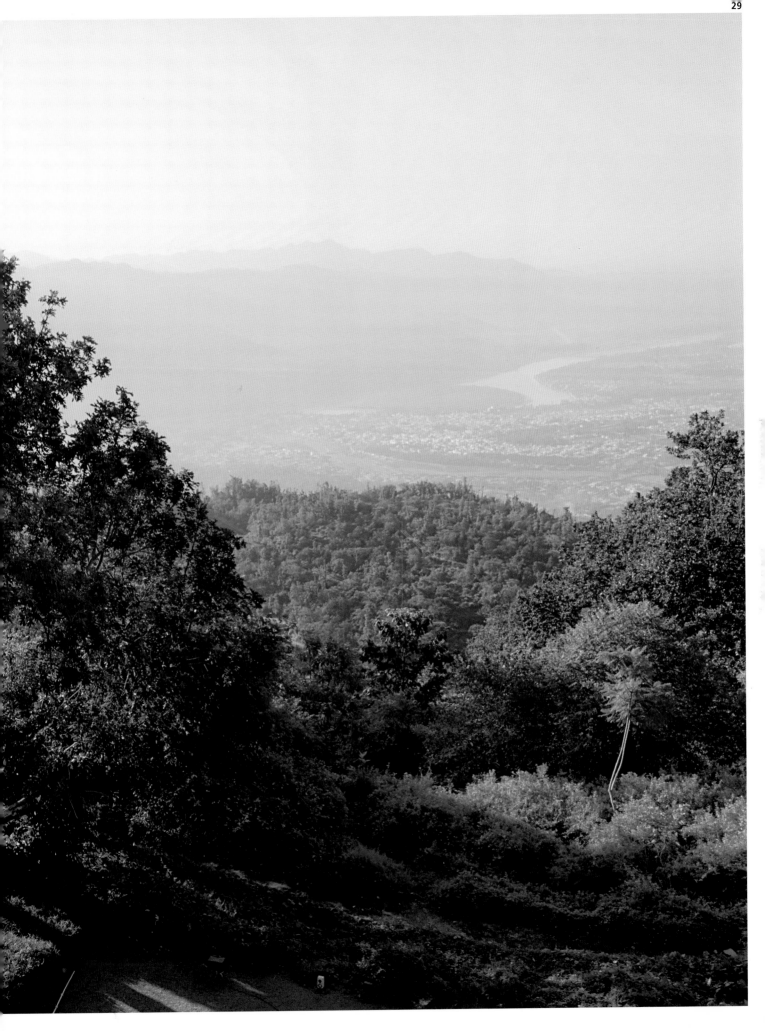

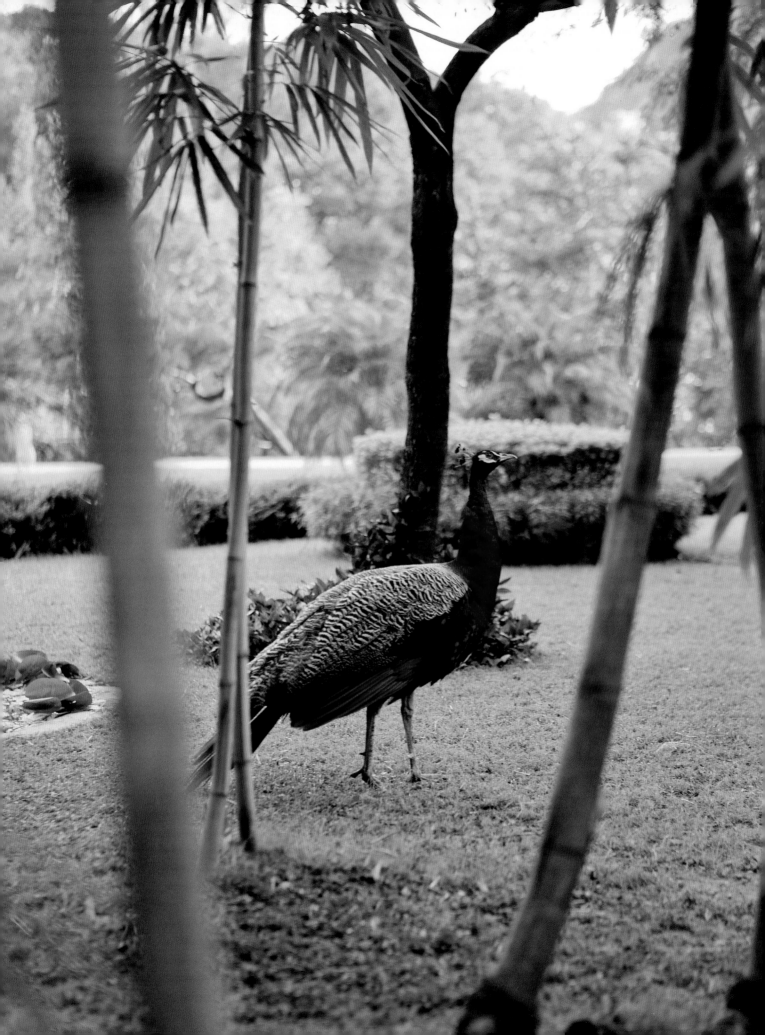

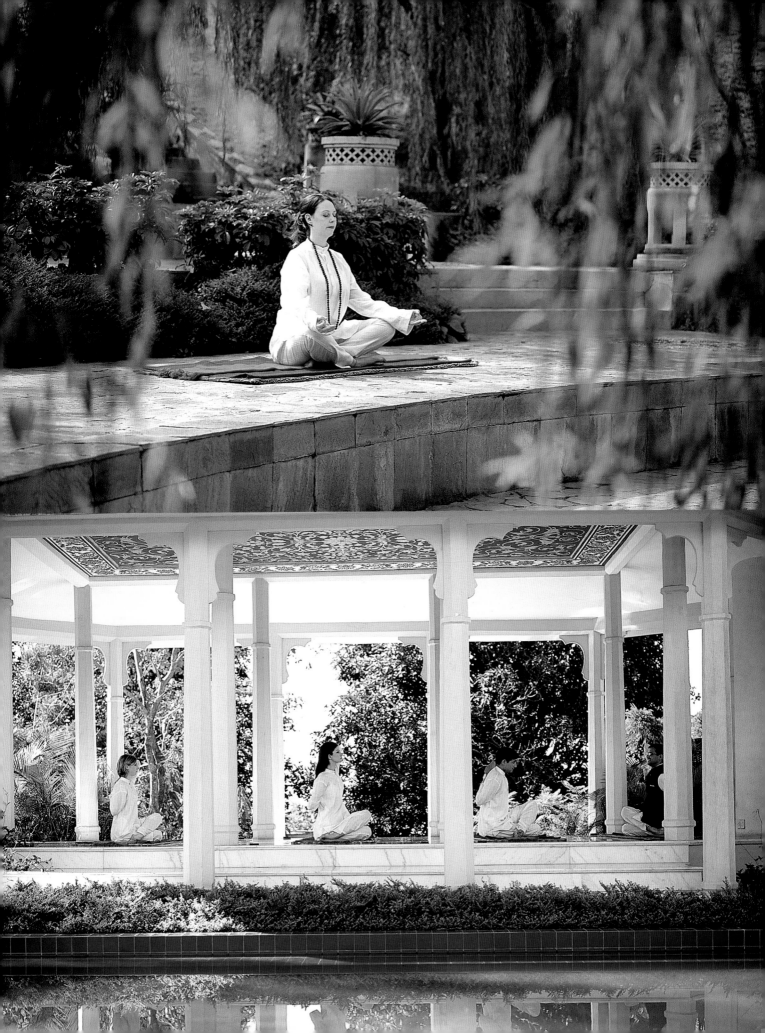

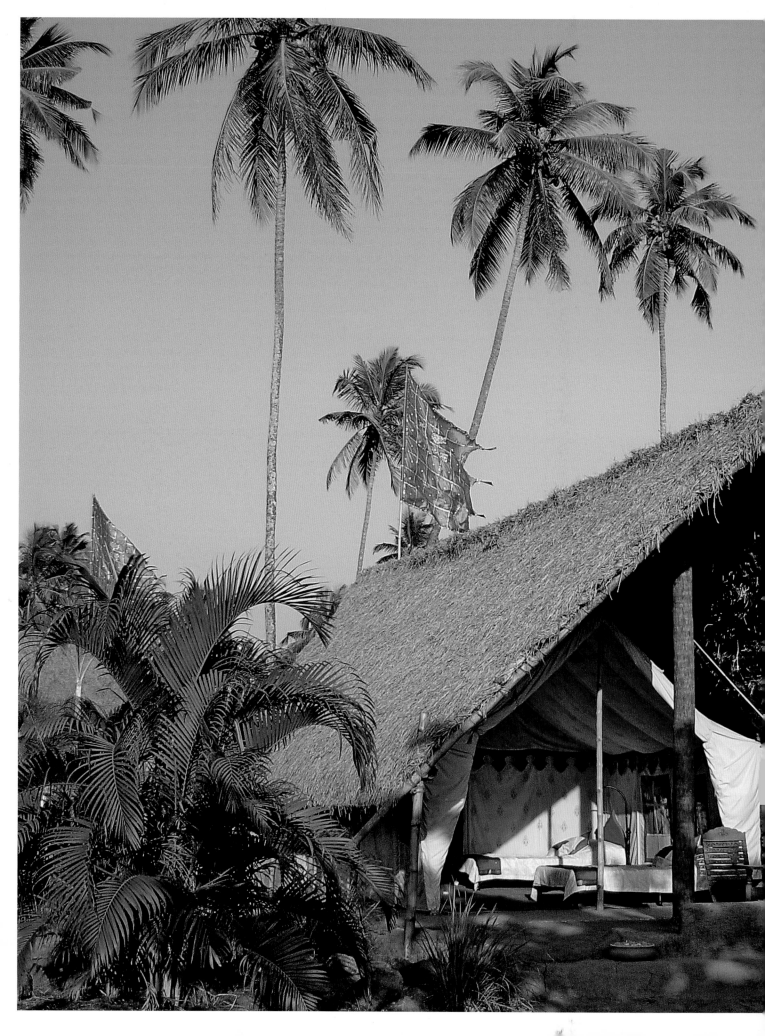

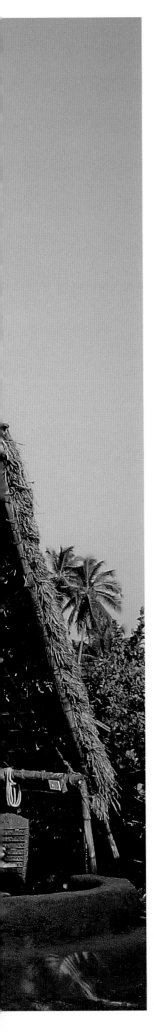

Rice fields and rainforest in the hinterland, whitewashed Catholic churches in the villages, enchanted 17th-century manor houses, endless white beaches on the Arabian Sea: no wonder that Goa was declared a paradise of free love by the hippies in the 1960s. The former Portuguese colony only survived the onslaught of stoned dropouts in a rather tarnished state. But beyond the party beaches, insiders' tips such as yogamagic serve as reminders of the unmistakable appeal India's smallest state has always had for its visitors. Half an hour from the sea and built in a coconut grove, the magic of this eco resort comes purely from its natural resources. Those who, at the end of the morning yoga session, lie on the floor of the yoga temple, which has been conjured up using dried mud, cow dung and clay, and look up into the high roof made of bamboo and palm leaves will experience a fully legal trip. And if that's not enough, try Vishnu, the legendary masseur from Pune, to help you relax, or the delicious chai, served at sunrise on the veranda of the solar-powered luxury tents.

Books to pack: "Be Here Now" by Ram Dass, "A Son of the Circus" by John Irving and "The God of Small Things" by Arundhati Roy

Yogamagic Eco Retreat

1586/1 Grand Chinvar
Anjuna, Bardez
403509 North Goa
India
Tel. +91 832 652 3796
info@yogamagic.net
www.yogamagic.net

Directions	25 miles north of Dabolim Airport; just over a mile away from Anjuna Beach
Yoga	Ashtanga, Vinyasa Flow, Scaravelli, Sivananda, Kundalini, Iyengar
Rooms	7 tents for 2–3 people, 2 suites for 2–3 people
Food	Organic tropical vegetarian cuisine. Especially delicious: caramelised pumpkin couscous
Treatments	Ayurvedic massage, Reiki, Indian head massage, foot massage, nutritional advice
Leisure	Ayurvedic massage courses, swimming, art and music sessions

Reisfelder und Regenwald im Hinterland, weiß getünchte katholische Kirchen in den Dörfern, verwunschene Herrensitze aus dem 17. Jahrhundert, endlose weiße Strände an der Arabischen See – kein Wunder, dass die ehemalige portugiesische Kolonie von den Hippies in den 1960ern zum Paradies der freien Liebe erklärt wurde und den jahrelangen Ansturm bekiffter Aussteiger nur ziemlich angeschlagen überlebte. Doch jenseits der Partystrände erinnern Geheimtipps wie Yogamagic daran, welchen unverwechselbaren Reiz der kleinste Bundesstaat Indiens seit jeher auf seine Besucher hat. Eine halbe Stunde vom Meer, in einen Kokospalmenhain gebaut, gewinnt dieses Öko-Resort seinen Zauber ganz aus natürlichen Ressourcen. Wer am Schluss der morgendlichen Yogastunde auf dem aus Schlamm, Lehm und Kuhdung gestampften Boden des Yoga-Tempels liegt und den Blick zum hohen lichten Dach aus Bambus und Palmblättern hebt, erlebt einen völlig legalen Trip. Wem das nicht genügt, dem hilft Vishnu, der legendäre Masseur aus Pune, bei der Entspannung. Und natürlich der köstliche Chai, der bei Sonnenaufgang auf der Veranda der mit Solarenergie versorgten Luxuszelte serviert wird.

Reisebegleiter: »Sei jetzt hier« von Ram Dass, »Zirkuskind« von John Irving und »Der Gott der kleinen Dinge« von Arundhati Roy

Rizières et forêts vierges dans l'arrière-pays, églises catholiques aux murs blanchis dans les villages, manoirs féeriques datant du 17e siècle, plages blanches longeant à l'infini la mer d'Arabie : quoi d'étonnant si l'ancienne colonie portugaise fut instituée paradis de l'amour libre par les hippies dans les années 1960 et sortit bien éprouvée de la longue invasion de ces fumeurs de hasch en quête d'aventure. Pourtant, au-delà des plages festives, des endroits cachés, comme le Yogamagic, rappellent le charme incomparable que le plus petit Etat indien exerce depuis toujours sur ses visiteurs. Situé à une demi-heure de la mer au cœur d'un petit bois de cocotiers, ce site écologique tire toute sa magie de ressources naturelles. Celui qui, après une séance matinale, est étendu sur le sol du temple de yoga, mélange de terre battue, de boue séchée, de bouse de vache et d'argile, et qui lève très haut les yeux vers le toit aéré fait de bambous et de feuilles de palmiers, vit un trip entièrement légal. Celui qui recherche davantage s'adresse pour sa relaxation à Vishnu, le masseur légendaire de Pune ou déguste le succulent Chai, servi au lever du soleil sur la véranda d'une des luxueuses tentes chauffées à l'énergie solaire.

Livres à emporter : « Vieillir en pleine conscience » de Ram Dass, « Un enfant de la balle » de John Irving et « Le Dieu des petits riens » d'Arundhati Roy

Anreise	40 km nördlich vom Flughafen Dabolim, etwa 2 km von Anjuna Beach entfernt
Yoga	Ashtanga, Vinyasa Flow, Scaravelli, Sivananda, Kundalini, Iyengar
Zimmer	7 Zelte für 2–3 Personen, 2 Suiten für 2–3 Personen
Küche	Organisch-vegetarisch-tropisch. Besonders köstlich: karamellisierter Kürbis-Couscous
Anwendungen	Ayurvedische Massage, Reiki, indische Kopfmassage, Fußmassage, Ernährungsberatung
Aktivitäten	Ayurvedische Massagekurse, Schwimmen, Kunst- und Musiksessions

Accès	Situé à 40 km au nord de l'aéroport de Dabolim, à environ 2 km d'Anjuna Beach
Yoga	Ashtânga, Vinyasa Flow, Scaravelli, Shivananda, Kundalinî, Iyengar
Chambres	7 tentes pour 2–3 personnes, 2 suites pour 2–3 personnes
Restauration	Cuisine tropicale organique et végétarienne. Couscous caramélisé au potiron absolument délicieux
Traitements	Massage ayurvédique, reiki, massage crânien de tradition indienne, massage des pieds, conseils de diététique
Activités	Cours de massage ayurvédique, natation, sessions artistiques et musicales

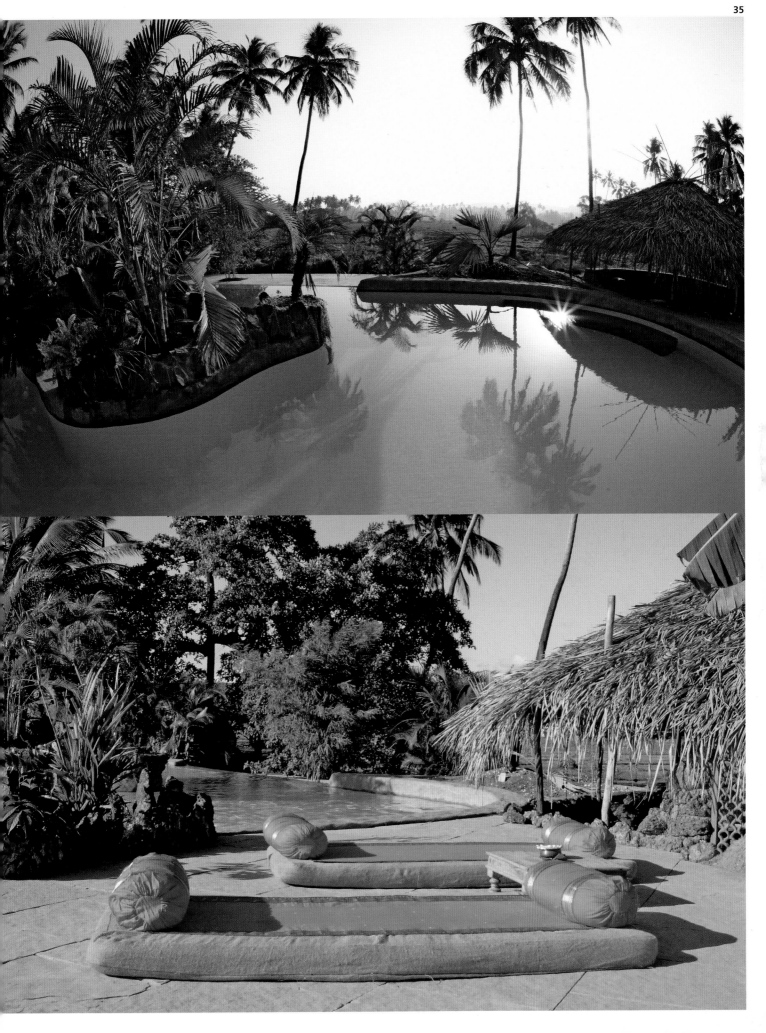

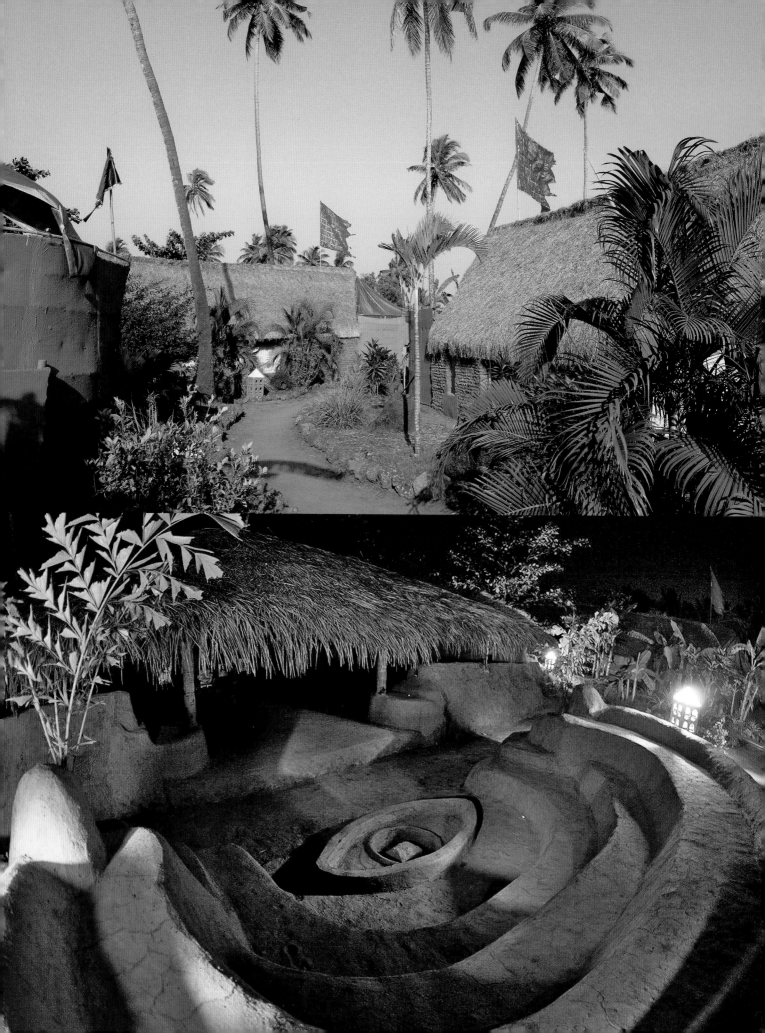

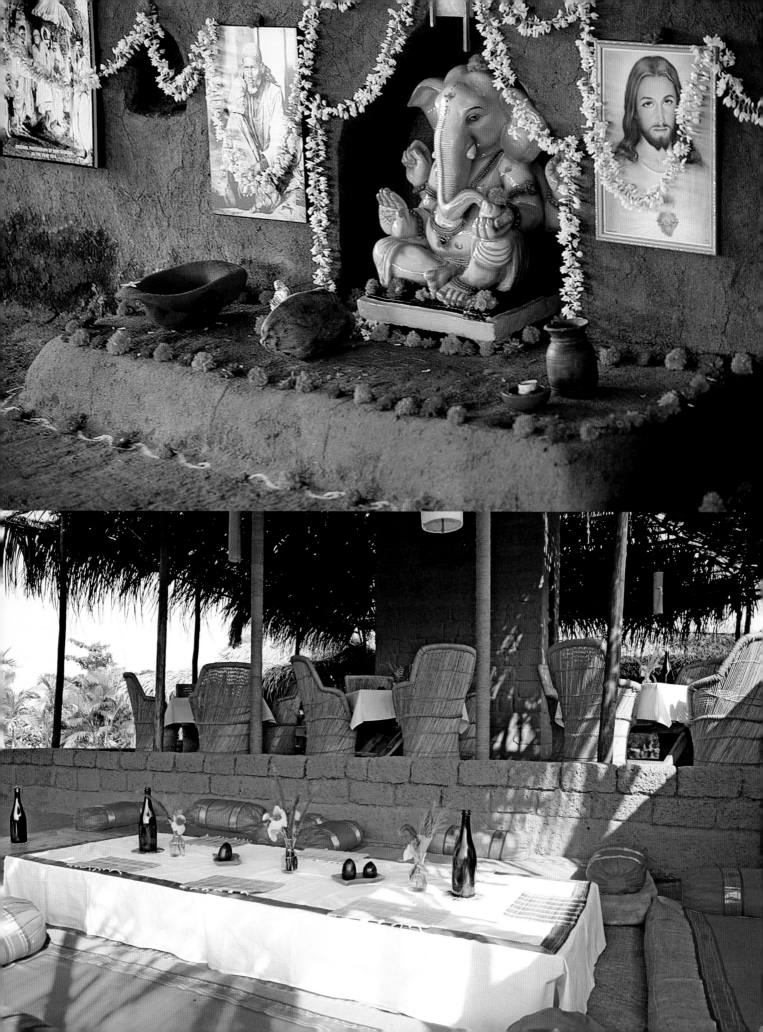

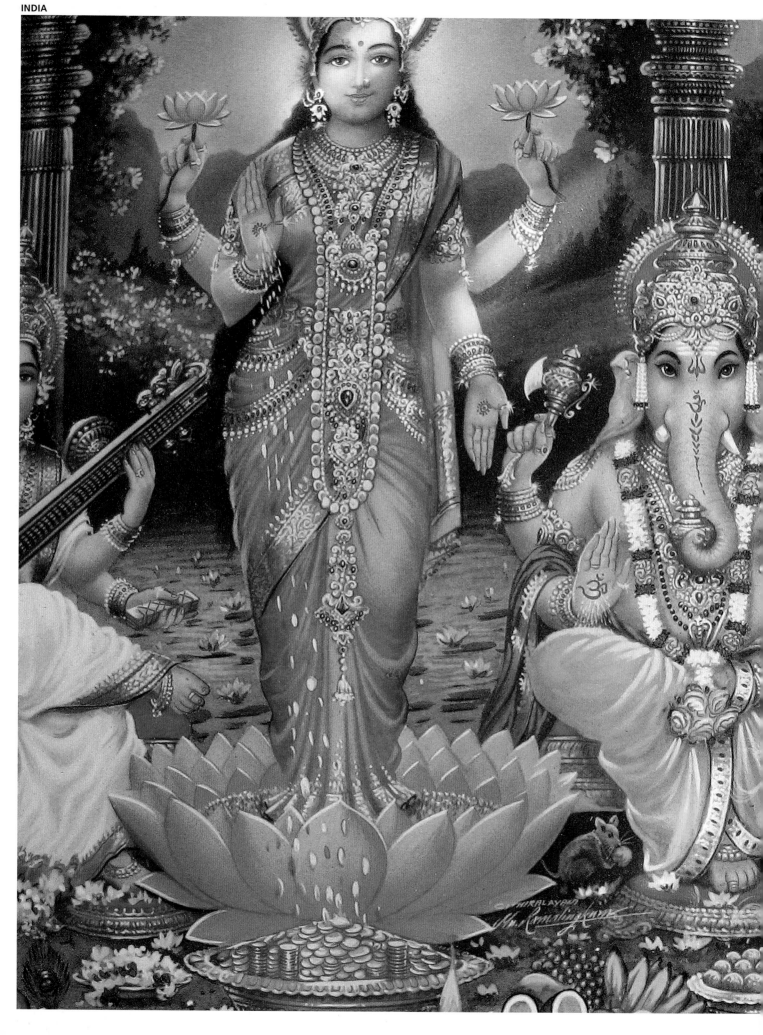

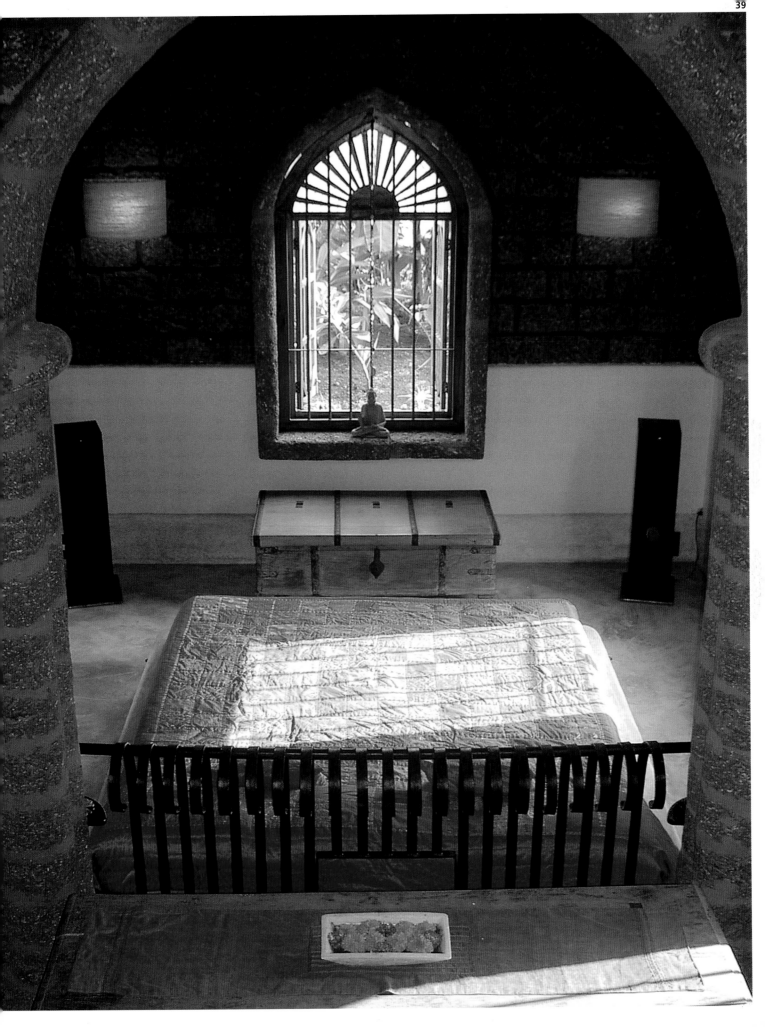

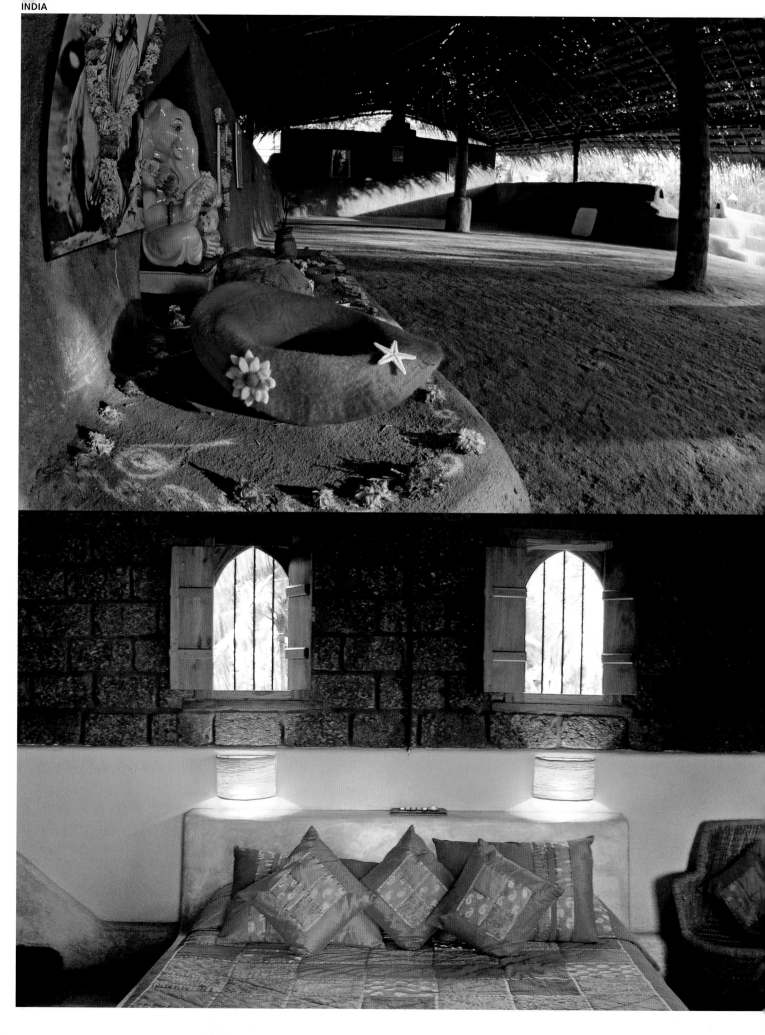

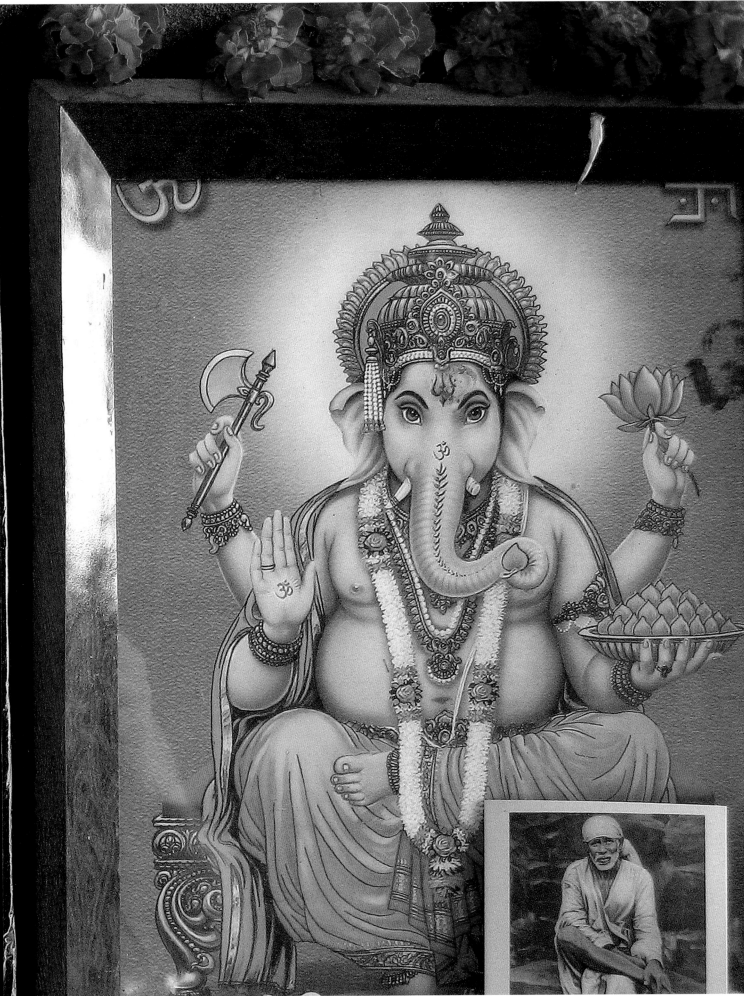

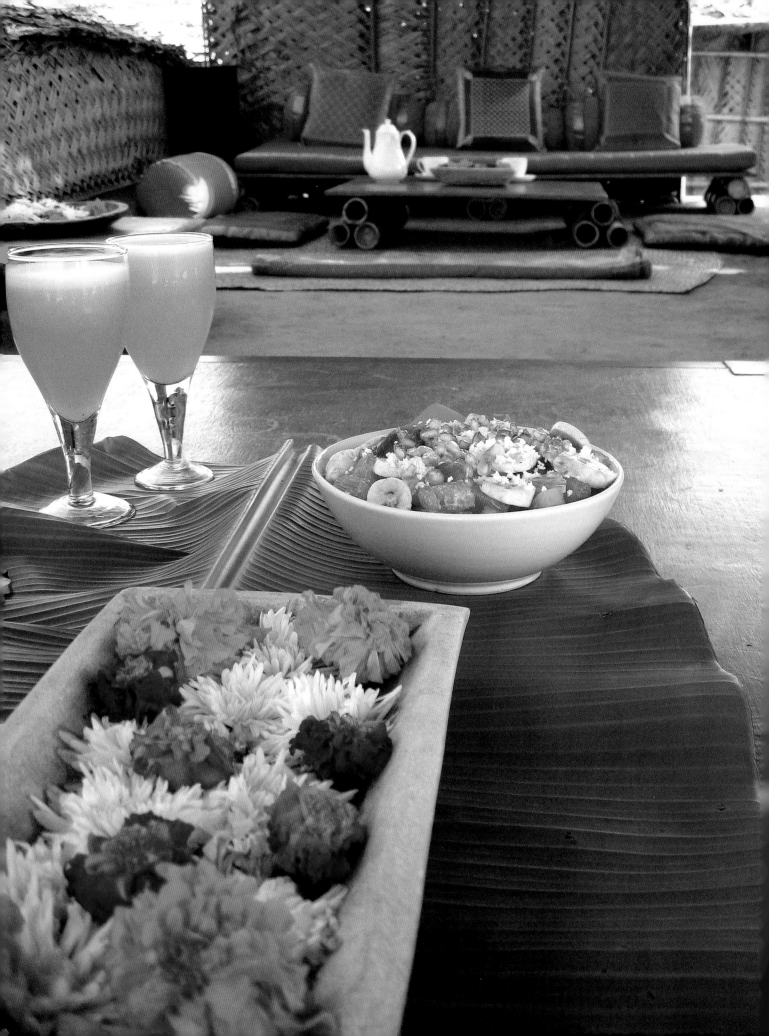

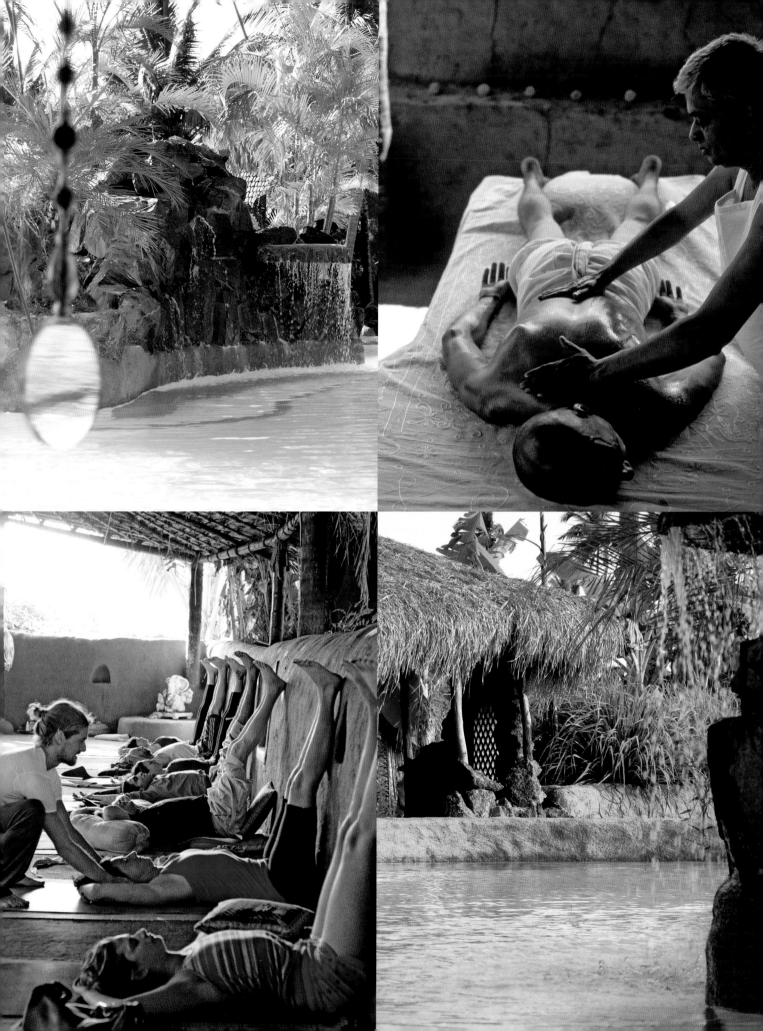

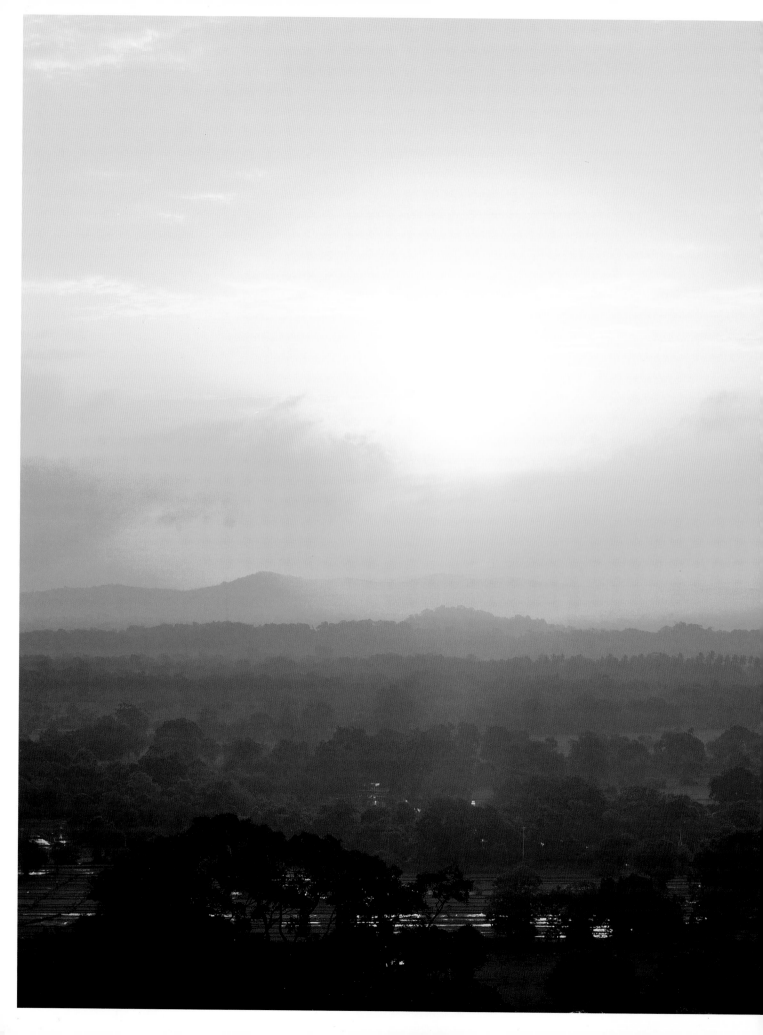

One of Asia's most extraordinary ecotourism projects came into being at the place where elephant paths crossed, Shiva's son had a shrine built and a prince fled with his legendarily beautiful but poor lover. Rebuilt as a traditional farming village, Ulpotha lies in the middle of former Ceylon's deepest jungle next to a small lake, surrounded by seven hills in which ascetics and shamans still meditate in their caves. But Ulpotha is by no means withdrawn. The Ayurveda treatments in the eco lodge, a treasure trove of centuries-old remedies, are considered an insiders' tip and are included in the price. With no electricity and limited mobile phone reception, Ulpotha's luxury consists in making contact with nature: ambling between hibiscus plants along the sandy paths to the lake, observing how lizards stretch out in the sun, swimming among the water lilies, or taking a stroll in the surrounding hills at sunset. Typical British understatement in outstanding surroundings.

Books to pack: "Yoga and Ayurveda: Self-Healing and Self-Realization" by David Frawley and "Running in the Family" by Michael Ondaatje

Ulpotha

Embogama
Kurunegala District
Sri Lanka
Tel. +44 208 123 3603
info@ulpotha.com
www.ulpotha.com

Directions	Located in central Sri Lanka. Some 3 hrs away from Colombo Airport, airport transfer by arrangement
Yoga	Hatha, Ashtanga, Sivananda, Iyengar, Anusara, Vinyasa
Teachers	Stephen Thomas, Angus Ford Robertson, Mika, Wade Gotwals, Lara Baumann, Nigel Gilderson, Daniela Schmid (each teacher gives instruction for a period of 14 days)
Rooms	11 cottages, max. 23 people
Food	Strictly organic vegetarian food with produce grown on site and locally, e.g. green mango curry with coconut milk
Treatments	Ayurveda therapy, massages, sauna, herbal baths, detox and rejuvenation cures, Shiatsu
Leisure	Swimming, hiking, biking

Wo sich Elefantenwege kreuzten, Shivas Sohn einen Schrein errichten ließ und wohin ein Prinz mit seiner legendär schönen, aber armen Geliebten floh, dort entstand eines der außergewöhnlichsten Ökotourismus-Projekte Asiens. Wieder aufgebaut als traditionelles Bauerndorf, liegt Ulpotha mitten im tiefsten Dschungel des ehemaligen Ceylon an einem kleinen See, umringt von sieben Hügeln, in denen noch immer Asketen und Schamanen in ihren Höhlen meditieren. Doch Ulpotha ist alles andere als weltabgewandt. Als Schatzkammer jahrhundertealter Heilmittel gelten die Ayurveda-Behandlungen in der Öko-Lodge als Geheimtipp und sind im Preis inbegriffen. Ohne Strom und nur teilweisem Handyempfang besteht der Luxus von Ulpotha darin, Kontakt zur Natur aufzunehmen – auf den sandigen Wegen zwischen Hibiskuspflanzen zum See zu schlendern, zuzusehen, wie sich Eidechsen in der Sonne räkeln, zwischen den Wasserlilien zu schwimmen oder bei Sonnenuntergang eine Wanderung auf die umliegenden Hügel zu machen. Typisch britisches Understatement in herausragender Umgebung.

Reisebegleiter: »Das große Handbuch des Yoga und Ayurveda« von David Frawley und »Es liegt in der Familie« von Michael Ondaatje

Là où les routes des éléphants se croisaient, où le fils de Shiva fit ériger un sanctuaire et où un prince vint se réfugier avec sa bien-aimée, une très belle mais très pauvre jeune fille, a vu le jour un des projets les plus extraordinaires d'éco-tourisme en Asie. Ulpotha, reconstruit comme village de paysans traditionnel, est implanté au fin fond de la jungle, dans l'ancien territoire du Ceylan, au bord d'un petit lac entouré de sept collines, dans les grottes desquelles méditent, aujourd'hui encore, les ascètes et les chamans. Toutefois, Ulpotha est tout sauf isolé du monde. Trésors de remèdes séculaires, les traitements d'Ayurveda pratiqués dans l'éco-village sont une référence incontournable et sont inclus dans le prix. Sans électricité et avec réception de portable limitée, le luxe d'Ulpotha consiste à prendre contact avec la nature : sur les chemins sableux entre les plants d'hibiscus, flâner vers le lac, observer les lézards qui s'étirent au soleil, nager parmi les fleurs de lotus ou, au coucher du soleil, faire une promenade dans les collines environnantes. Discrétion toute britannique dans un cadre grandiose.

Livres à emporter : « Yoga et Ayurvéda : Autoguérison et Réalisation de Soi » de David Frawley et « Un air de famille » de Michael Ondaatje

Anreise	Mitten in Sri Lanka gelegen. Etwa 3 Std. vom Flughafen Colombo entfernt, Flughafentransfer nach Absprache
Yoga	Hatha, Ashtanga, Sivananda, Iyengar, Anusara, Vinyasa
Lehrer	Stephan Thomas, Angus Ford Robertson, Mika, Wade Gotwals, Lara Baumann, Nigel Gilderson, Daniela Schmid (jeder Lehrer unterrichtet jeweils 14 Tage)
Zimmer	11 Cottages, max. 23 Personen
Küche	Streng organisch-vegetarisch mit Produkten aus eigenem oder lokalem Anbau, zum Beispiel grünes Mangocurry mit Kokosnussmilch
Anwendungen	Ayurveda, Massagen, Kräuterbad, Detox- und Verjüngungskuren, Shiatsu
Aktivitäten	Schwimmen, Wandern, Radfahren

Accès	Situé au cœur du Sri Lanka à 3 h environ de l'aéroport de Colombo, transfert de l'aéroport sur demande
Yoga	Hatha, Ashtânga, Shivananda, Iyengar, Anusara, Vinyasa
Professeurs	Stephan Thomas, Angus Ford Robertson, Mika, Wade Gotwals, Lara Baumann, Nigel Gilderson, Daniela Schmid (chaque professeur invité enseigne pendant 14 jours)
Chambres	11 cottages, pour 23 personnes max.
Restauration	Cuisine organique et végétarienne stricte avec des produits récoltés sur place ou dans la région, comme le curry vert à la mangue et au lait de coco
Traitements	Thérapie ayurvédique, massages, bains d'herbes, cures de détox et de rajeunissement, shiatsu
Activités	Natation, randonnées, vélo

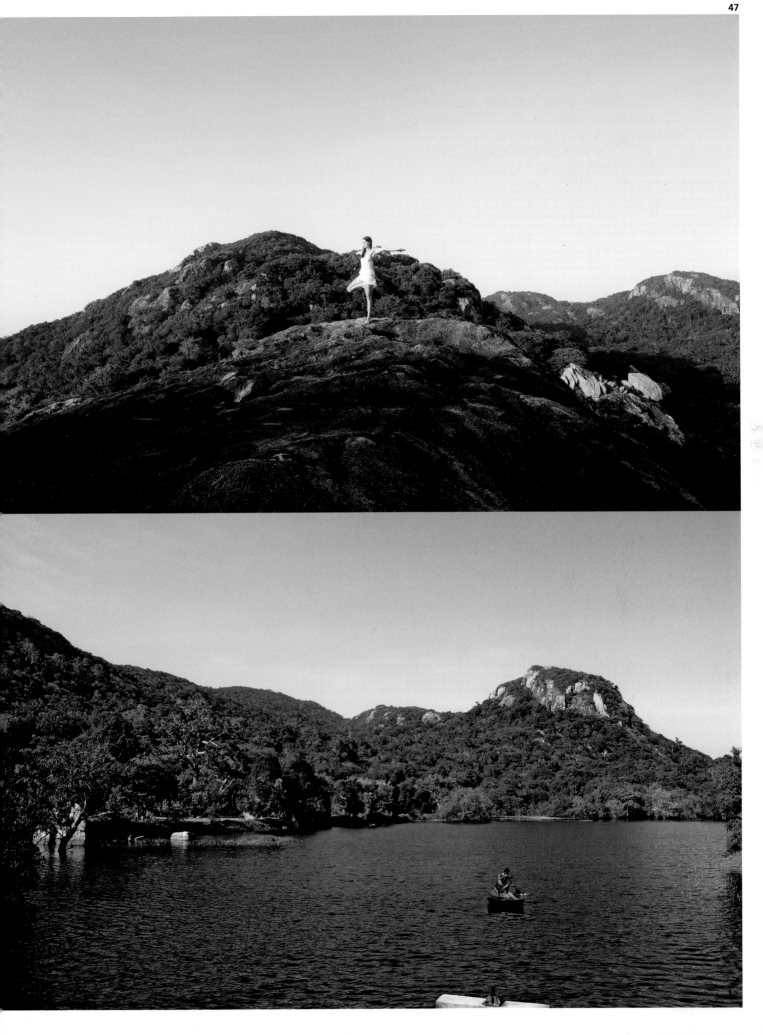

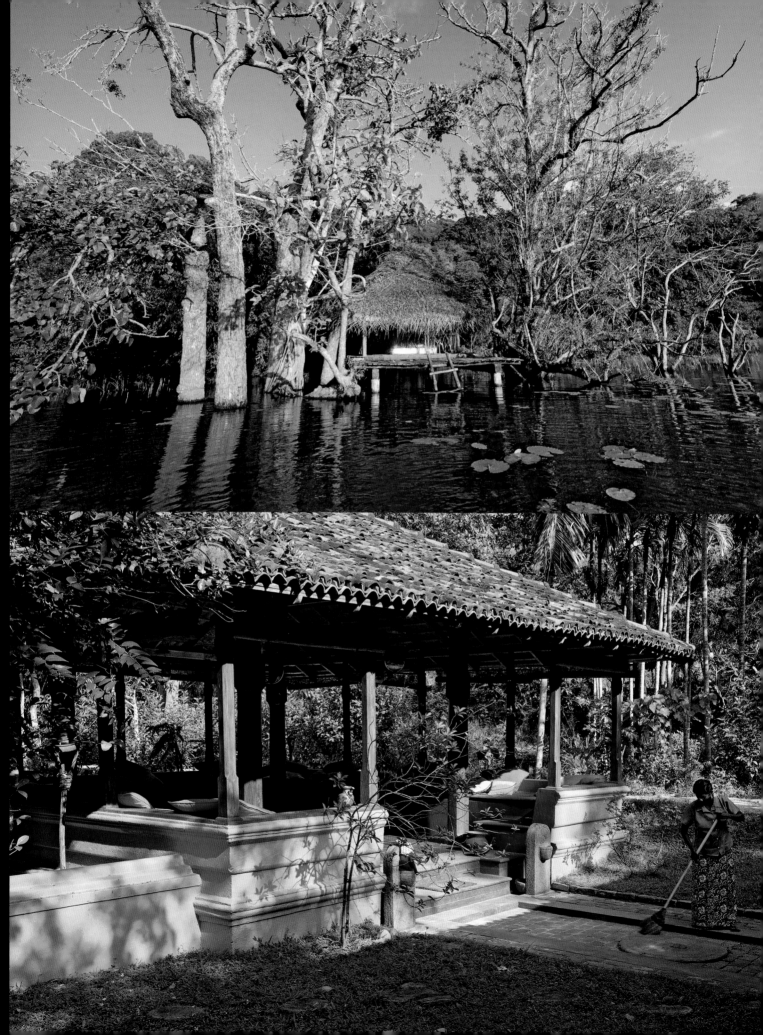

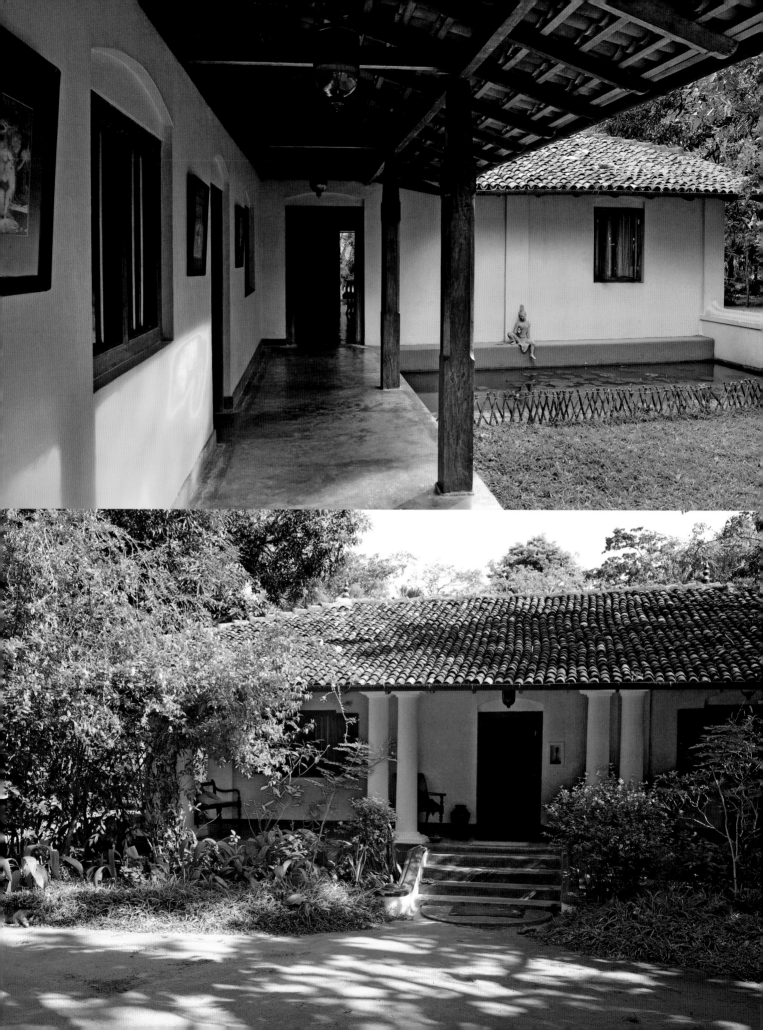

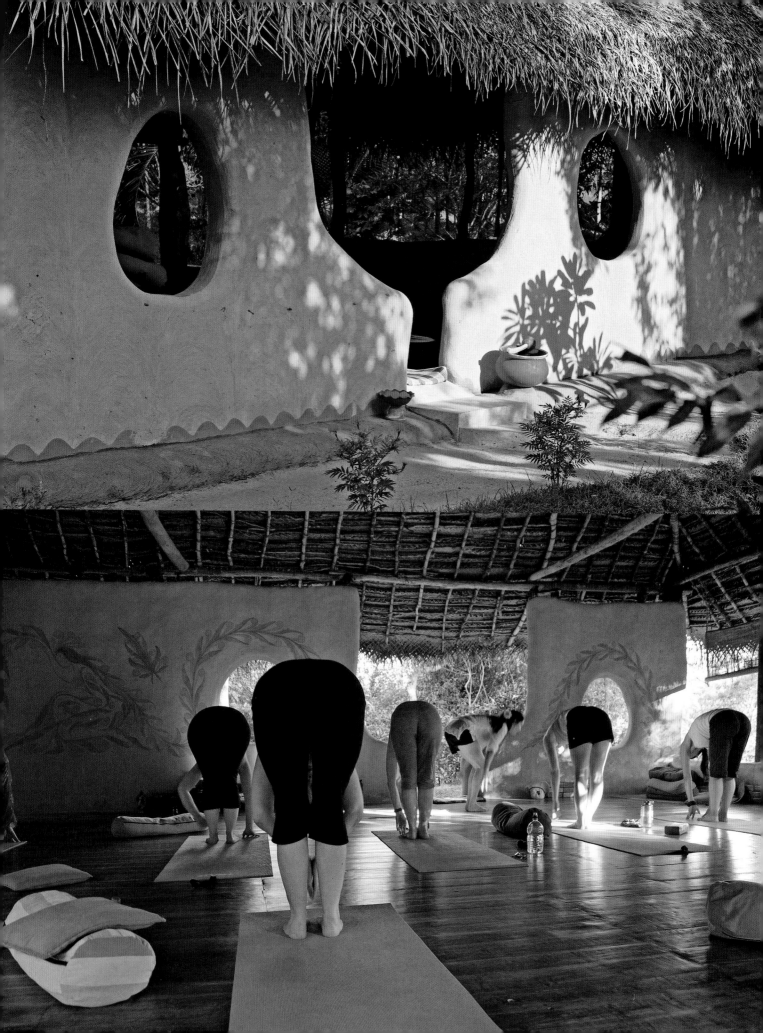

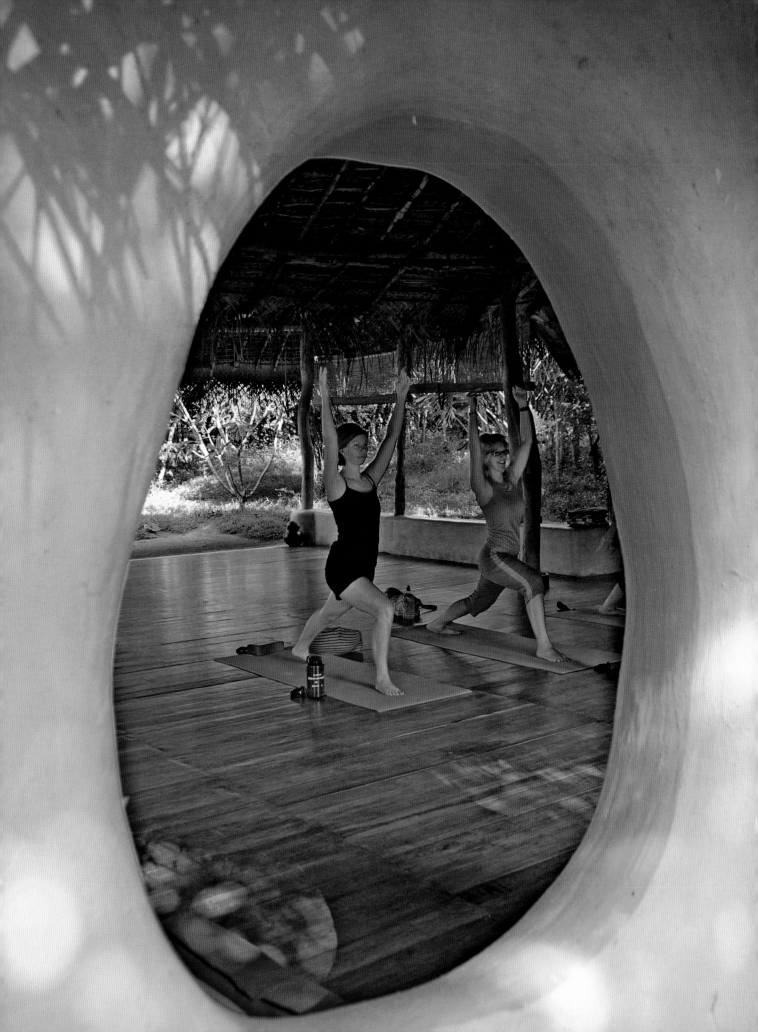

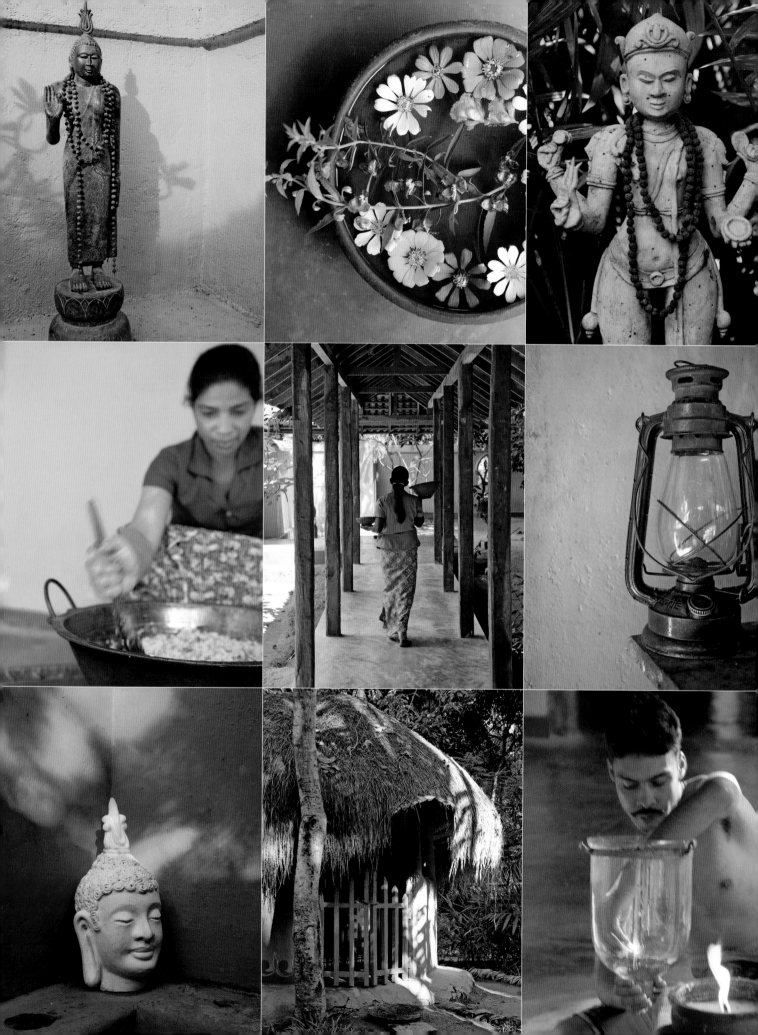

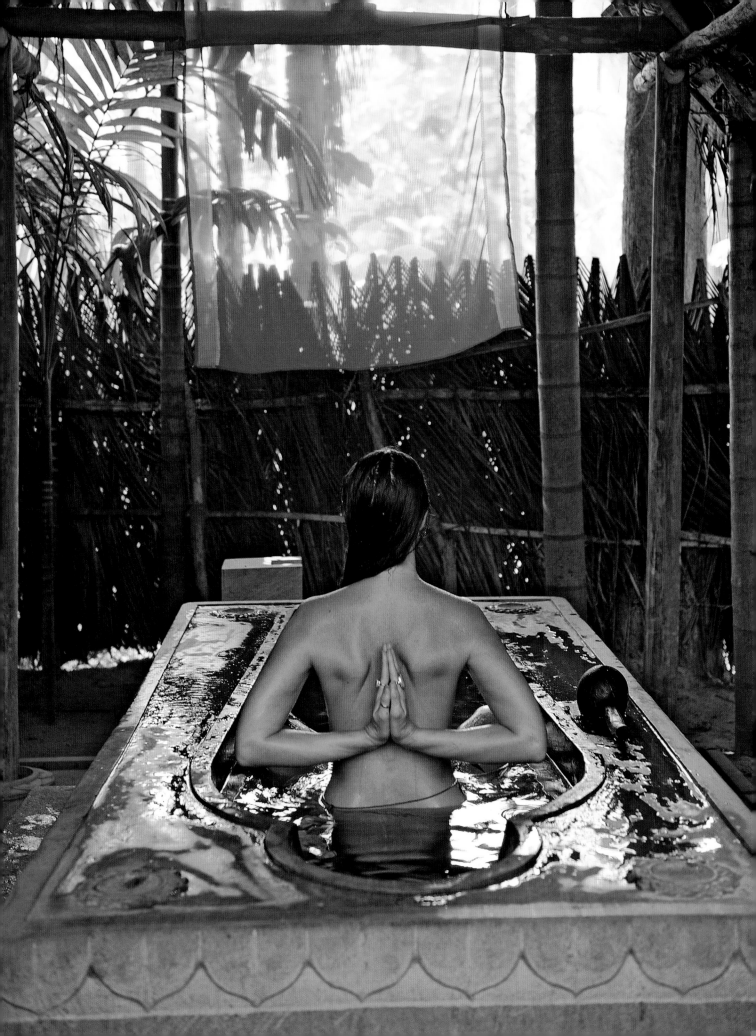

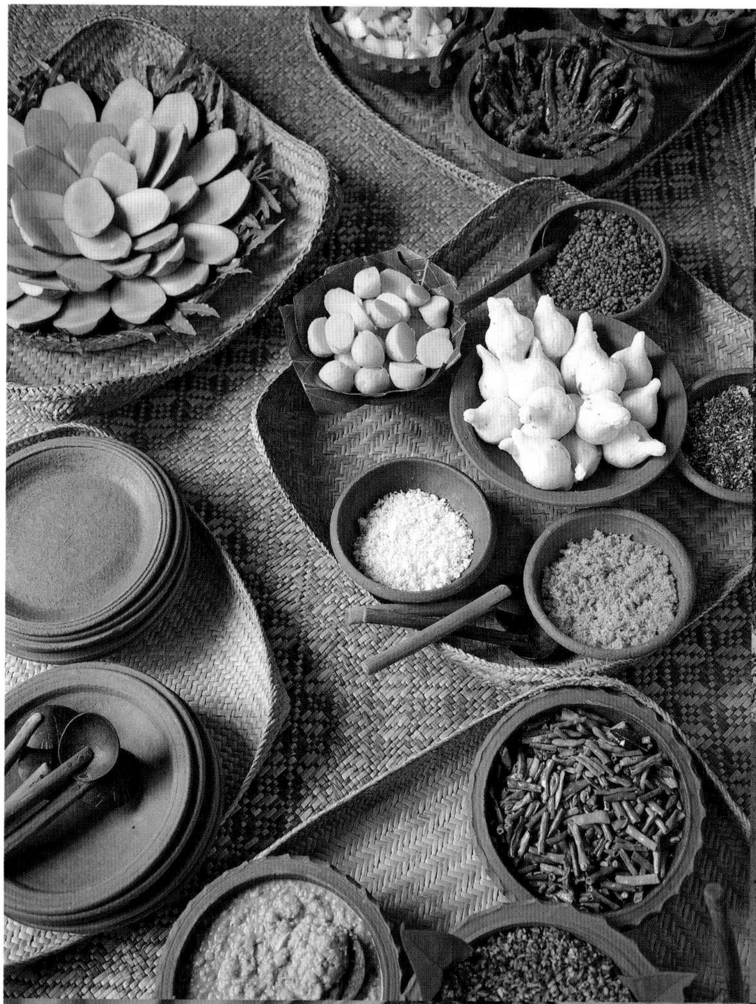

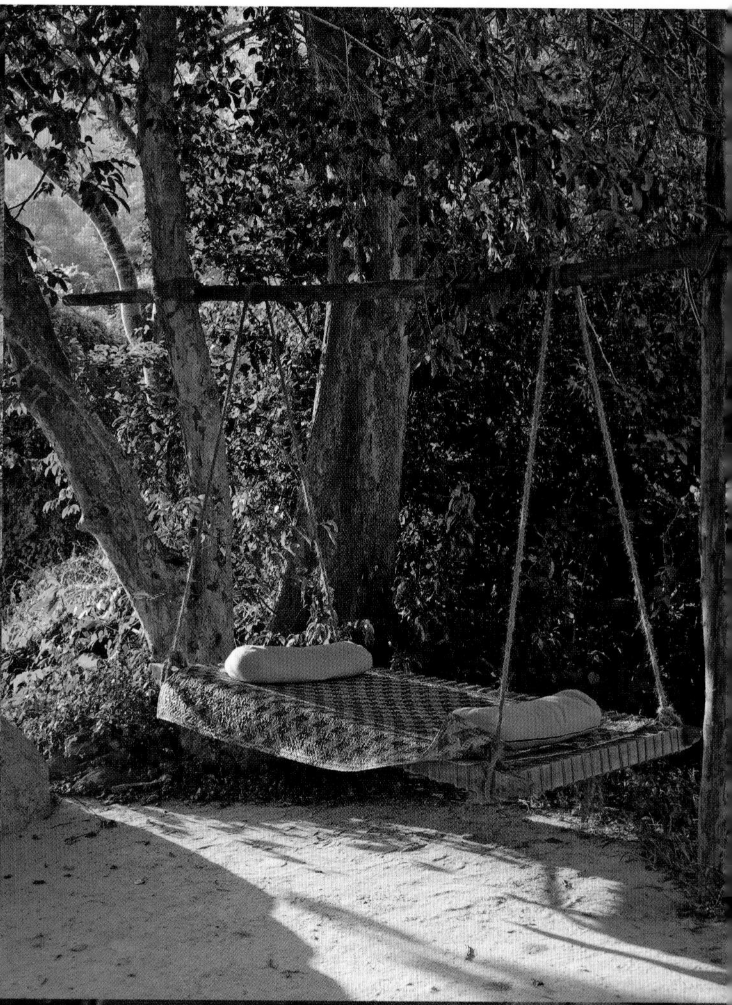

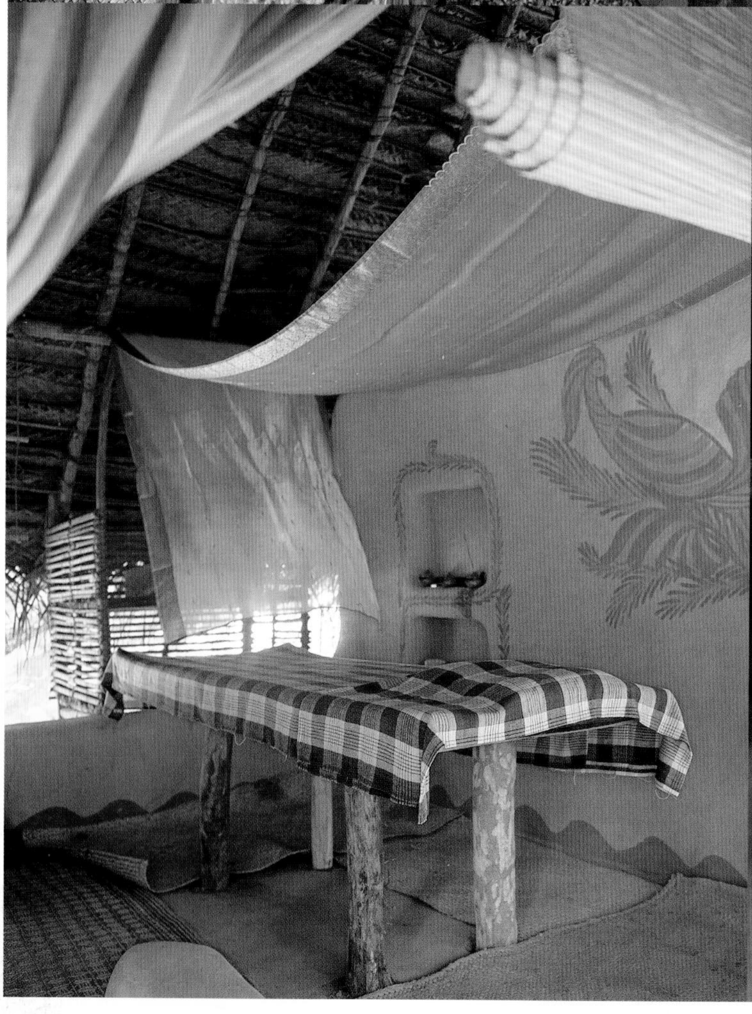

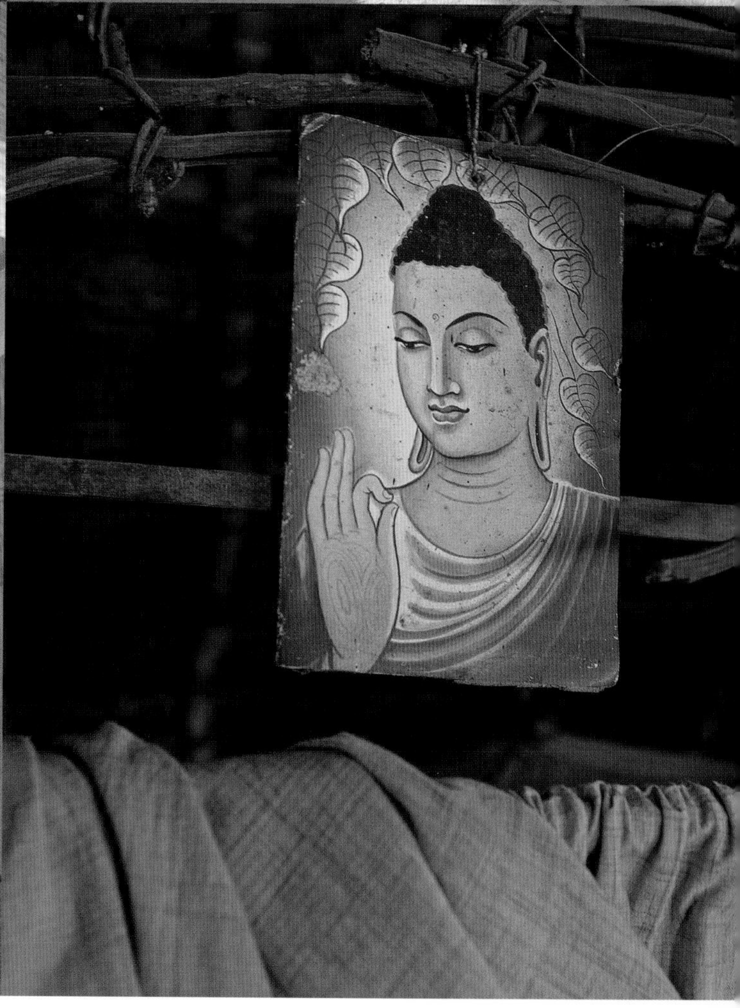

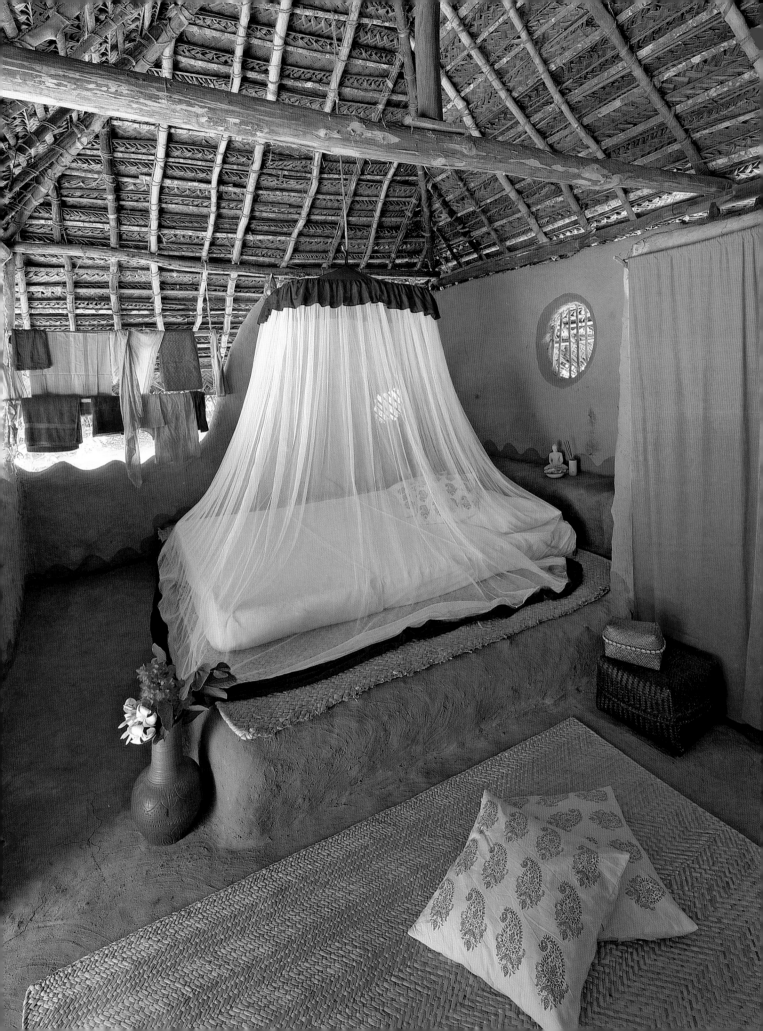

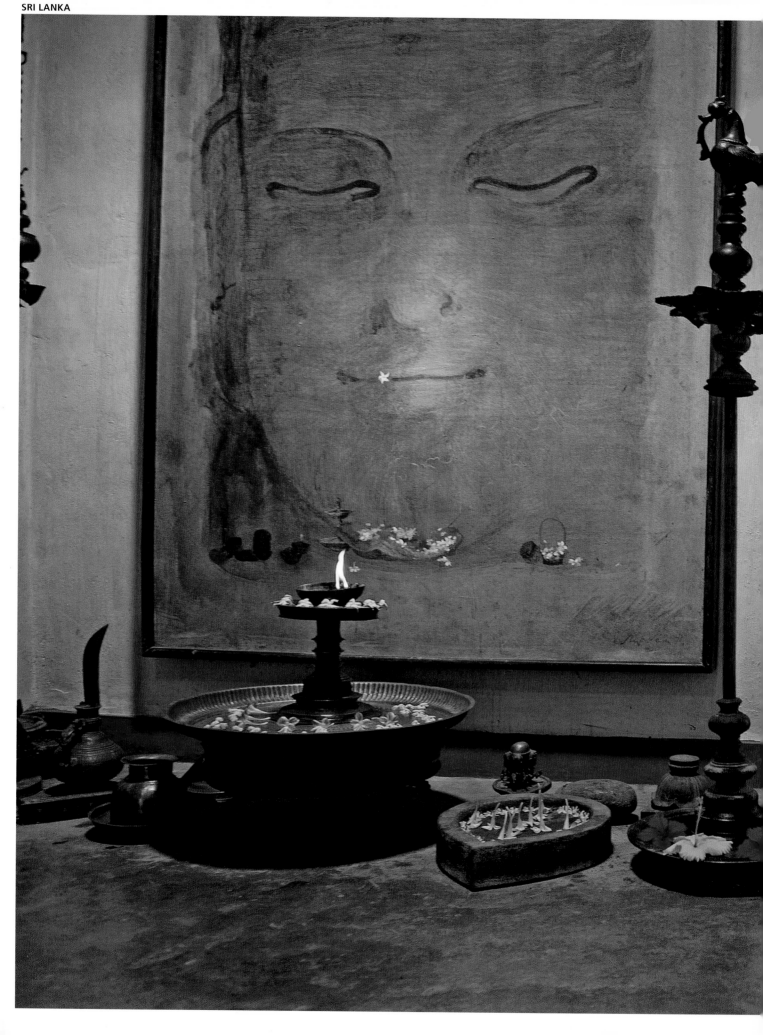

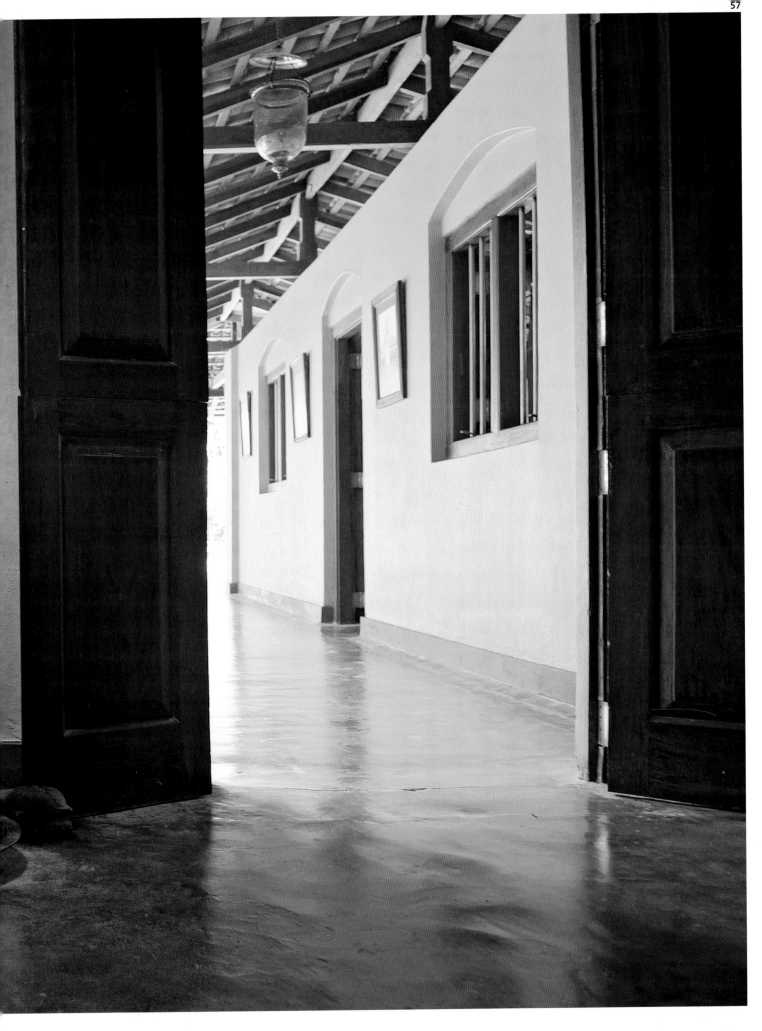

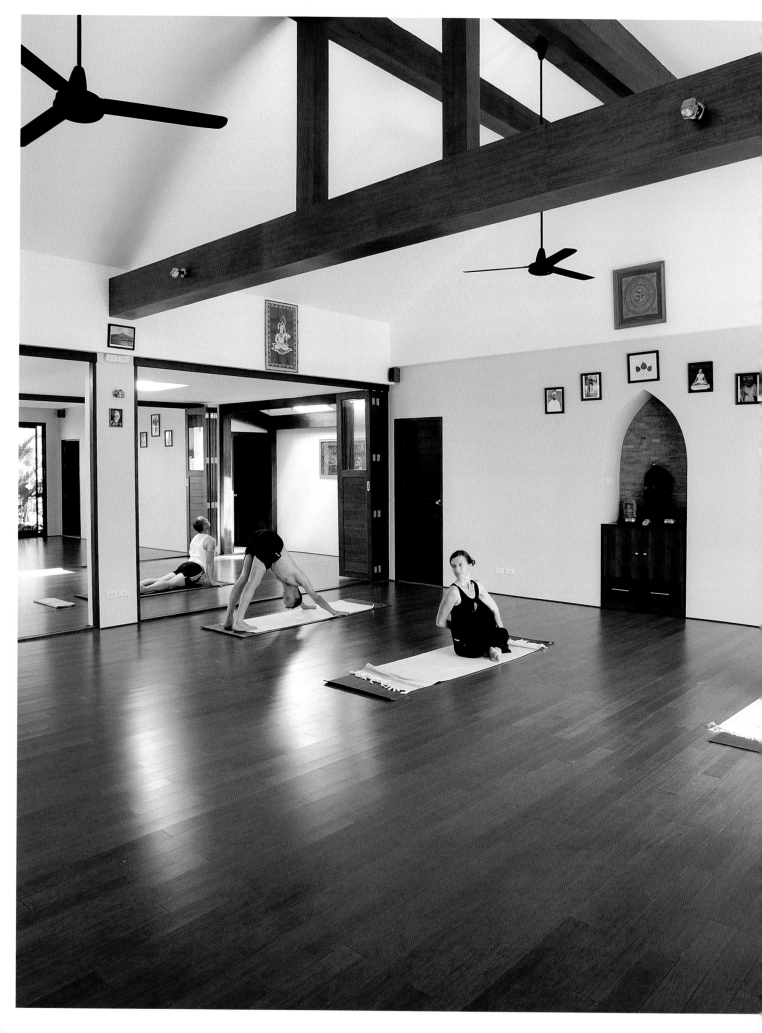

When in 2001, with modest savings, Paul and Jutima squinted at the light at the end of the Lincoln Tunnel, they were leaving not only New York but also their early years in training as yoga teachers behind them. Their next stop was Los Angeles, their destination Bangkok, Jutima's place of birth. Before they founded yoga Thailand, they travelled to India in order to study in Mysore with their teacher Pattabhi Jois and his grandson Sharath. The respect and the seriousness that are the features of the constant practice of the couple are also present in every detail of this beautiful resort, which has expanded to offer a fully holistic wellness centre. From the light Yoga Shala—on whose bamboo floor sweating bodies raise themselves into a handstand, the excellent equipment including props such as Iyengar belts hanging from the ceiling and the wall—to the delightful meditation garden, the saltwater pool and on to the inviting lounge: lucidity and a cool head, deference to the masters and silent contentment are the goal. yoga is everywhere. As Pattabhi Jois said: "Practise. And the rest will follow."

Books to pack: "The Yoga Sutras of Patanjali" by Sri Swami Satchidananda and "Shantaram" by Gregory David Roberts

Samahita Retreat

55/20–24 Moo 4,
T. Namuang, Koh Samui
Suratthani 84140
Thailand
Tel. +66 77 920 090 and +66 77 920 091
info@yoga-thailand.com
www.yoga-thailand.com

Directions	Located on the south coast of Koh Samui at Laem Sor Beach, 45 min from the airport
Yoga	Ashtanga, Pranayama, Prenatal, Restorative, Yin, Yoga Anatomy, teacher training
Teachers	Paul Dallaghan, Richard Freeman, Sri O.P. Tiwari, Simon Low, Claudia Jones, Elonne Stockton, Stephen Thomas, Kino MacGregor
Rooms	28 rooms
Food	Asian-European freshly prepared using local produce, occasionally fish and eggs, juice bar, raw food
Treatments	Ayurvedic detox, wellness and weight loss, bodywork, massages, infra-red sauna, steam bath, colon hydrotherapy
Leisure	Saltwater pool, walks along the beach, healthy cooking classes

Als Paul und Jutima mit wenig Erspartem 2001 in das Licht am Ende des Lincoln-Tunnels blinzelten, ließen sie nicht nur New York, sondern auch ihre frühen Lehrjahre als Yogalehrer hinter sich. Ihr nächster Halt war Los Angeles, das Ziel Bangkok, Jutimas Geburtsort. Bevor sie Yoga Thailand gründeten, reisten sie nach Indien, um in Mysore bei ihrem Lehrer Pattabhi Jois und dessen Enkel Sharath zu studieren. Der Respekt und die Ernsthaftigkeit, die das beständige Üben der beiden auszeichnen, steckt auch in jedem Detail dieses wunderschönen Resorts, das auch mit einem komplett ganzheitlichen Gesundheitszentrum aufwarten kann. Von der lichten Yoga-Shala, auf deren Bambusboden sich schwitzend die Körper in den Handstand heben, und der ausgezeichneten Ausstattung mit Hilfsmitteln inklusive Iyengar-Gurten, die von der Decke und der Wand hängen, über den lieblichen Meditationsgarten, den Salzwasserpool, bis zur einladenden Lounge: Hier geht es um Transparenz und einen kühlen Kopf, Verneigung vor den Meistern und stille Fröhlichkeit. Yoga ist überall. Wie Pattabhi Jois sagte: »Übe. Der Rest ergibt sich.«

Reisebegleiter: »The Yoga Sutras of Patanjali« von Sri Swami Satchidananda und »Shantaram« von Gregory David Roberts

Lorsqu'en 2001 Paul et Jutima, quelques économies en poche, voient le bout du tunnel Lincoln, ils laissent New York derrière eux, mais aussi leurs années de formation comme professeurs de yoga. Direction Los Angeles, puis Bangkok, ville natale de Jutima. Avant de fonder le Yoga Thailand, ils vont en Inde, à Mysore, pour s'instruire auprès de leur professeur Pattabhi Jois et de son petit-fils Sharath. Le respect et le sérieux qui caractérisent l'entraînement constant auquel ils s'adonnent sont présents dans chaque détail de ce merveilleux site, qui a récemment étendu ses activités pour proposer un centre de bien-être holistique. De la yoga-shala très aérienne au plancher de bambou sur lequel les corps en sueur font le poirier, à l'excellent équipement avec des accessoires comme la ceinture Iyengar, accrochés au plafond et sur le mur, en passant par l'exquis jardin de méditation, la piscine d'eau salée jusqu'à l'attrayant salon : transparence et idées claires, déférence pour les maîtres et joie sereine sont la finalité. Le yoga est omniprésent. Comme Pattabhi Jois a dit : « Entraînez-vous et le reste suivra. »

Livres à emporter : « The Yoga Sutras of Patanjali » de Sri Swami Satchidananda et « Shantaram » de Gregory David Roberts

Anreise	An der Südküste von Koh Samui am Laem Sor Beach gelegen, 45 min Fahrt vom Flughafen
Yoga	Ashtanga, Pranayama, Prenatal, Restorative, Yin Yoga, Yoga Anatomie, Teacher Training
Lehrer	Paul Dallaghan, Richard Freeman, Sri O.P. Tiwari, Simon Low, Claudia Jones, Elonne Stockton, Stephen Thomas, Kino MacGregor
Zimmer	28 Zimmer
Küche	Asiatisch-europäisch, frisch zubereitet mit Produkten der Region, gelegentlich Fisch und Eier, Saftbar, Rohkost
Anwendungen	Ayurveda-Detox, Wellness, Gewichtsreduktion, Bodywork, Massagen, Infrarotsauna, Dampfbad, Darmspülung durch Colon-Hydro-Therapie
Aktivitäten	Salzwasserpool, Strandspaziergänge, Kochkurse

Accès	Situé sur la côte sud de Koh Samui sur la Laem Sor Beach, à 45 min de l'aéroport
Yoga	Ashtânga, Pranayama, Prénatal, Réparateur, Yin, Yoga Anatomie, Teacher Training
Professeurs	Paul Dallaghan, Richard Freeman, Sri O.P. Tiwari, Simon Low, Claudia Jones, Elonne Stockton, Stephen Thomas, Kino MacGregor
Chambres	28 chambres
Restauration	Asiatique et européenne à base de produits bio de la région, occasionnellement poisson et œufs, jus de fruits et de légumes
Traitements	Détox ayurvédique, bien-être et perte de poids, bodywork, massages, sauna infrarouge, bains de vapeur, hydrothérapie du côlon
Activités	Piscine d'eau salée, promenades sur la plage, cours de cuisine saine

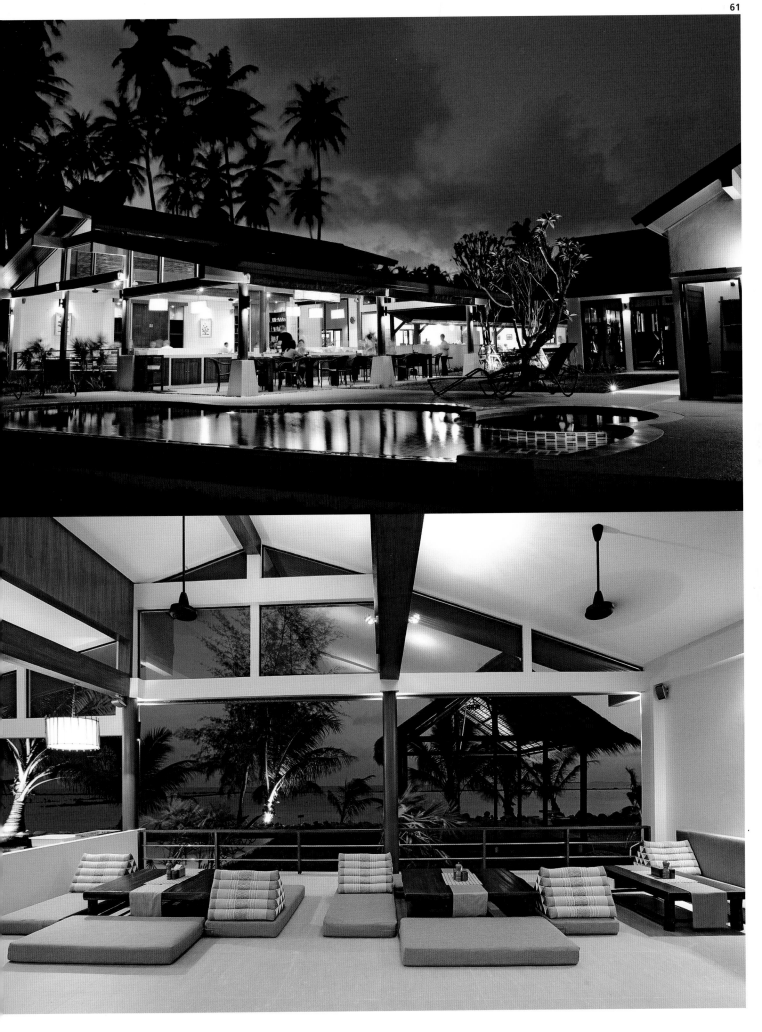

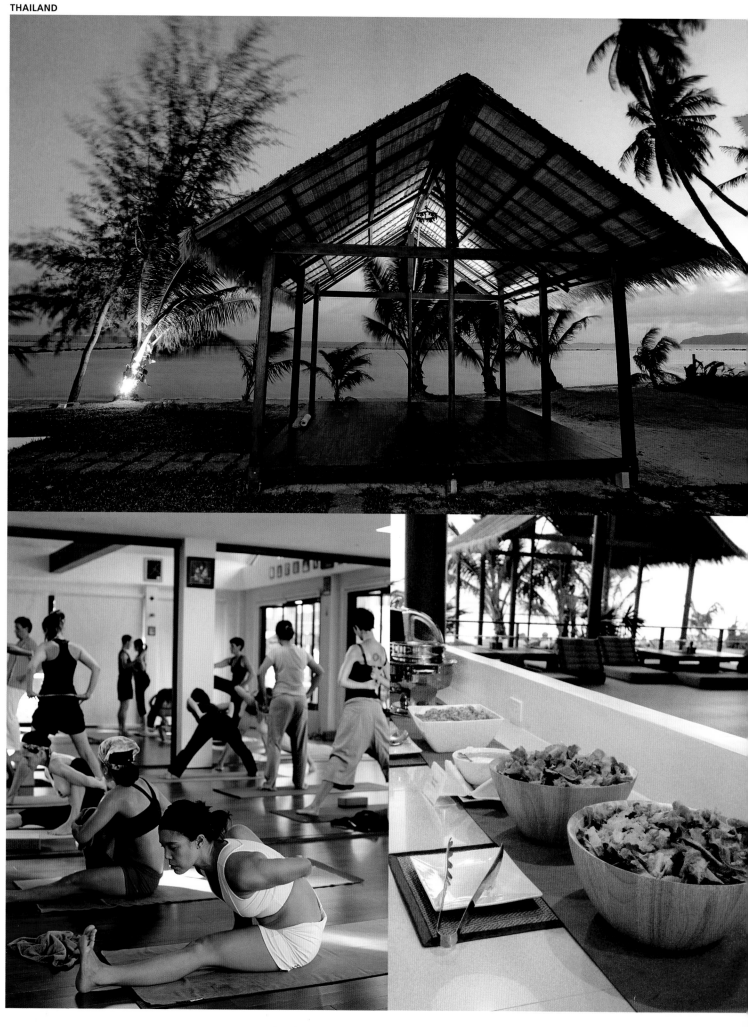

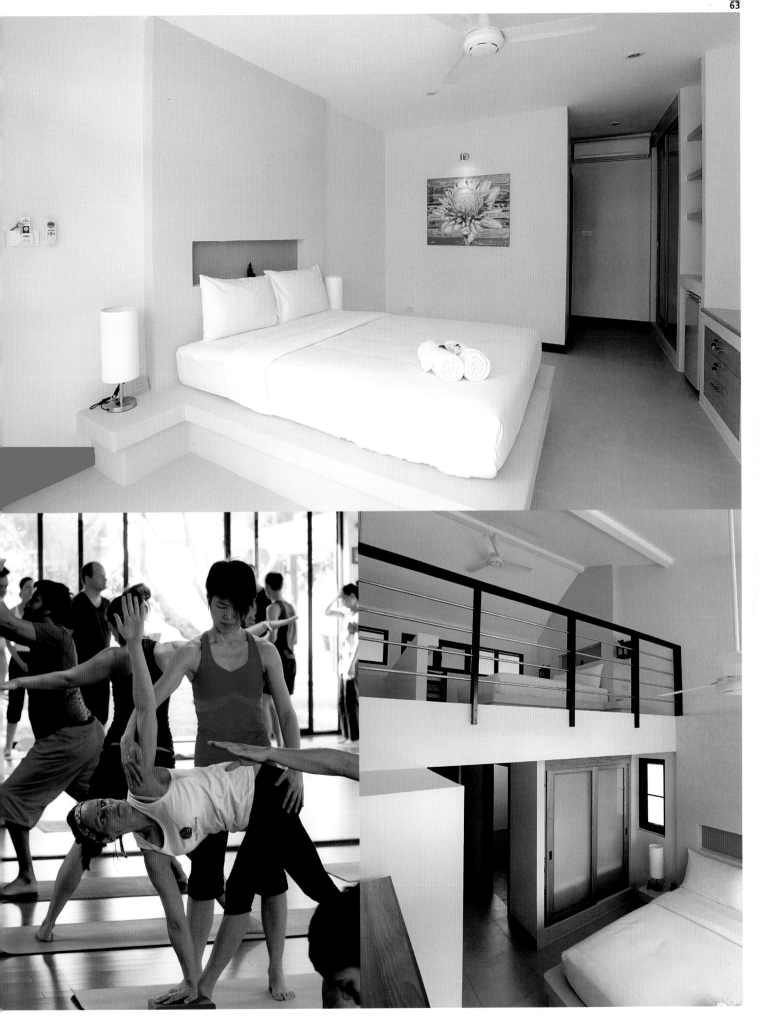

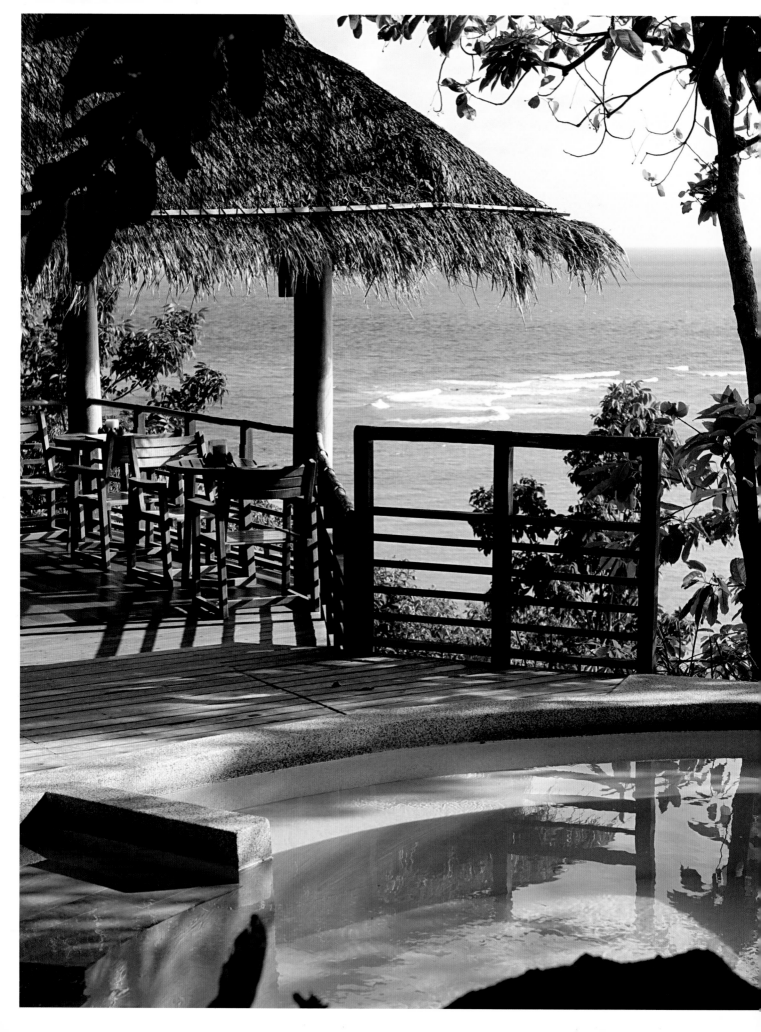

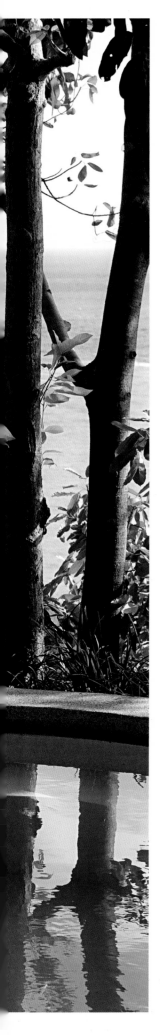

Lotus flowers grow best in a muddy subsoil; their beauty is first revealed at the surface. Translated, Kamalaya means "lotus realm", and this is no exaggeration: they bloom here everywhere in bright pink, well known to the Yogis as a symbol for change. In contrast to other spa resorts the quality of the multiple prize-winning Kamalaya doesn't come from bathrobes that you are allowed to take home along with a light holiday tan. In the middle of the resort between honeysuckle bushes and plunge pools under coconut palms lies the cave in which Buddhist monks have meditated for several hundred years. Located on a steep slope, the site compels you to walk everywhere on shady paths, an activity that leads to its own form of meditation and keeps you from descending into apathy. On the way the quite breathtaking view changes constantly: the Thai coastal landscape, the turquoise-coloured small bay of the resort's own private beach and, in the end, even your perspective on your own significance. And that, finally, is what the yoga taught in a beautiful pavilion up on a cliff is all about. Here, you can create space on all levels, and that includes making room for the outstanding breakfast.

Books to pack: "Autobiography of a Yogi" by Paramahansa Yogananda and "The Beach" by Alex Garland

Kamalaya
Wellness Sanctuary & Holistic Spa

102/9 Moo 3, Laem Set Road
Na-Muang, Koh Samui
Suratthani 84140
Thailand
Tel. +66 77 429 800
Fax +66 77 429 899
info@kamalaya.com
www.kamalaya.com

Directions	Located on the southeastern side of Koh Samui. About 45 min from Koh Samui Airport
Yoga	Hatha, Vinyasa, Kundalini, Ashtanga
Teachers	Lara Baumann, Danny Paradise, Julien Balmer, Simon Low
Rooms	59 hillside rooms and suites for max. 120 guests
Food	Vegetarian dishes, fish, poultry, lamb
Treatments	Chi Nei Tsang (Taoist belly massage), lymph drainage, Reiki, colon hydrotherapy, infra-red sauna, Traditional Chinese medicine, detox, Ayurveda, naturopathy
Leisure	Wellness sanctuary, holistic activity schedule including Yoga, pilates, tai chi, lap pool, painting, kayaking, fitness center, healthy cooking classes

Lotosblüten wachsen am besten in schlammigem Untergrund und entfalten ihre Schönheit erst an der Oberfläche. »Reich des Lotos« heißt Kamalaya übersetzt, was nicht übertrieben ist, denn er blüht hier überall in leuchtendem Rosa, den Yogis wohl-bekannt als Symbol für Veränderung. Anders als gewöhnliche Spa-Resorts bezieht das mehrfach preisgekrönte Kamalaya seine Qualität nicht aus Bademänteln, die man mit nach Hause nehmen darf, und einer leichten Urlaubsbräune. In der Mitte des Resorts zwischen Geißblattbüschen und Badekuhlen unter Kokospalmen liegt die Höhle, in der jahrhundertelang buddhistische Mönche meditierten. An einem steilen Hang gelegen, zwingt einen die Anlage dazu, auf schattigen Wegen überallhin zu Fuß zu gehen, was zu einer eigenen Art von Meditation führt und davor bewahrt, in Apathie zu verfallen. Ständig wechselt dabei die atemberaubende Aussicht auf die thailändische Küstenlandschaft, die türkisfarbene kleine Bucht des eigenen Privatstrands und am Ende sogar die Perspektive auf die eigenen Belange. Darum geht es schließlich im Yoga, das in einem wunderschönen Pavillon oben auf einem Fels unterrichtet wird: Platz schaffen auf allen Ebenen. Nicht zuletzt auch für das hervorragende Frühstück.

Reisebegleiter: »Autobiographie eines Yogi« von Paramahansa Yogananda und »Der Strand« von Alex Garland

Les fleurs de lotus poussent de préférence dans la vase et ne dévoilent toute leur beauté qu'à la surface. Kamalaya signifie littéralement empire du lotus ; de fait, des lotu rose intense fleurissent partout, symbole de la métamorphose, bien connu des yogis. A l'inverse des spas habituels, la qualité du Kamalaya, qui a été plusieurs fois récompensé, ne lui vient pas des manteaux de bain que l'on peut emporter chez soi, ni d'un léger bronzage de vacances. Au centre du domaine, entre les buissons de chèvrefeuille et les cuves de bains sous les cocotiers, se trouve la caverne où, tout au long des siècles, des moines bouddhistes vinrent méditer. Situé sur une pente escarpée, ce lieu appelle à sillonner tous les chemins ombragés, ce qui génère une forme particulière de méditation et empêche de céder à la léthargie. Ce faisant, la vue époustouflante sur les côtes thaïlandaises évolue en permanence, la petite crique couleur turquoise de la plage privée et, enfin, même le regard que l'on porte sur soi. Car c'est bien de cela qu'il s'agit dans le yoga enseigné dans un magnifique pavillon ou tout en haut d'un rocher. Créer de l'espace à tous les niveaux, entre autres pour le succulent petit-déjeuner.

Livres à emporter : « Autobiographie d'un yogi » de Paramahansa Yogananda et « La Plage » d'Alex Garland

Anreise	Auf der südöstlichen Seite von Koh Samui gelegen, etwa 45 min vom Koh-Samui-Flughafen entfernt
Yoga	Hatha, Vinyasa, Kundalini, Ashtanga
Lehrer	Lara Baumann, Danny Paradise, Julien Balmer, Simon Low
Zimmer	59 Zimmer, Suiten und Villen für max. 120 Gäste
Küche	Rohkost, vegetarisch, Fisch, Geflügel und Lamm
Anwendungen	Chi Nei Tsang (taoistische Bauchmassage), Lymphdrainage, Reiki, Colon-Hydro-Therapie, Infrarotsauna, Traditionelle Chinesische Medizin, Detox, Ayurveda, Naturheilkunde
Aktivitäten	Wellnessbereich, ganzheitliches Sportangebot mit Yoga, Pilates und Tai-Chi, Lap Pool, Malen, Ausflüge, Kajak, Fitnesscenter, Kochkurse

Accès	Situé sur la partie sud-est de Koh Samui, à environ 45 min de l'aéroport de Koh Samui
Yoga	Hatha, Vinyasa, Kundalini, Ashtânga
Professeurs	Lara Baumann, Danny Paradise, Julien Balmer, Simon Low
Chambres	59 chambres suites et villas pour 120 personnes max.
Restauration	Cuisine végétarienne, poisson, volaille, agneau
Traitements	Chi Nei Tsang (massage du ventre), drainage lymphatique, reiki, hydrothérapie du côlon, sauna infrarouge, médecine chinoise traditionnelle, détox, Ayurveda
Activités	Sanctuaire de bien-être, programme holistique incluant yoga , pilates et thai chi, lap pool, peinture, excursions kayak, centre de mise en forme, cours de cuisine

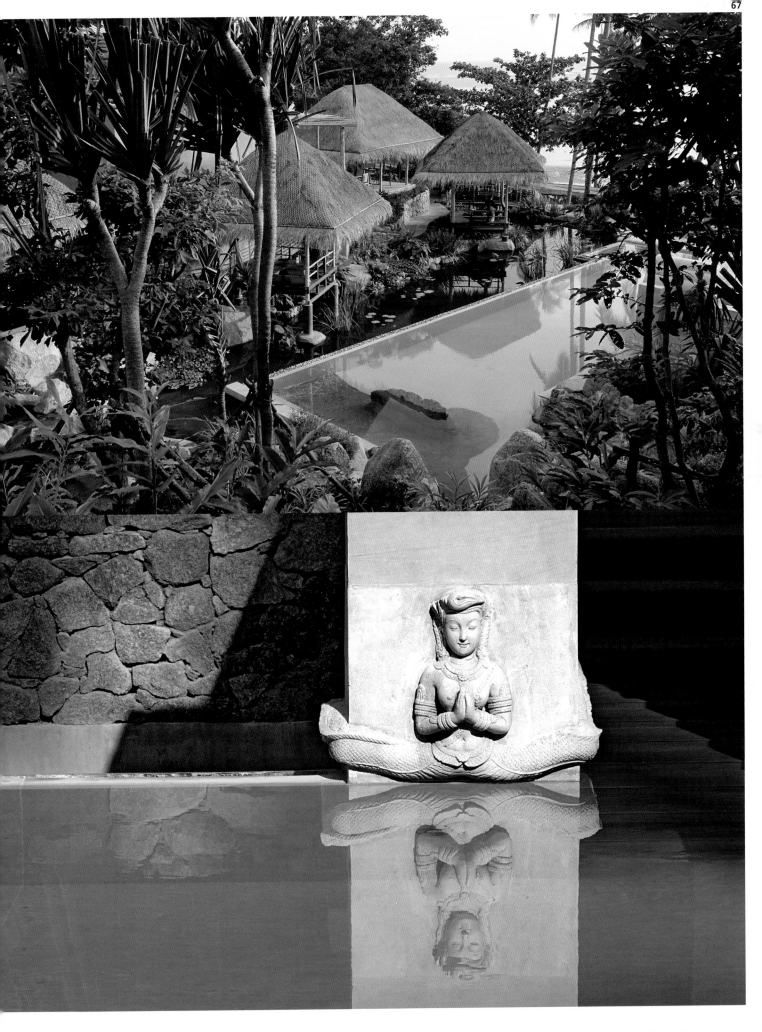

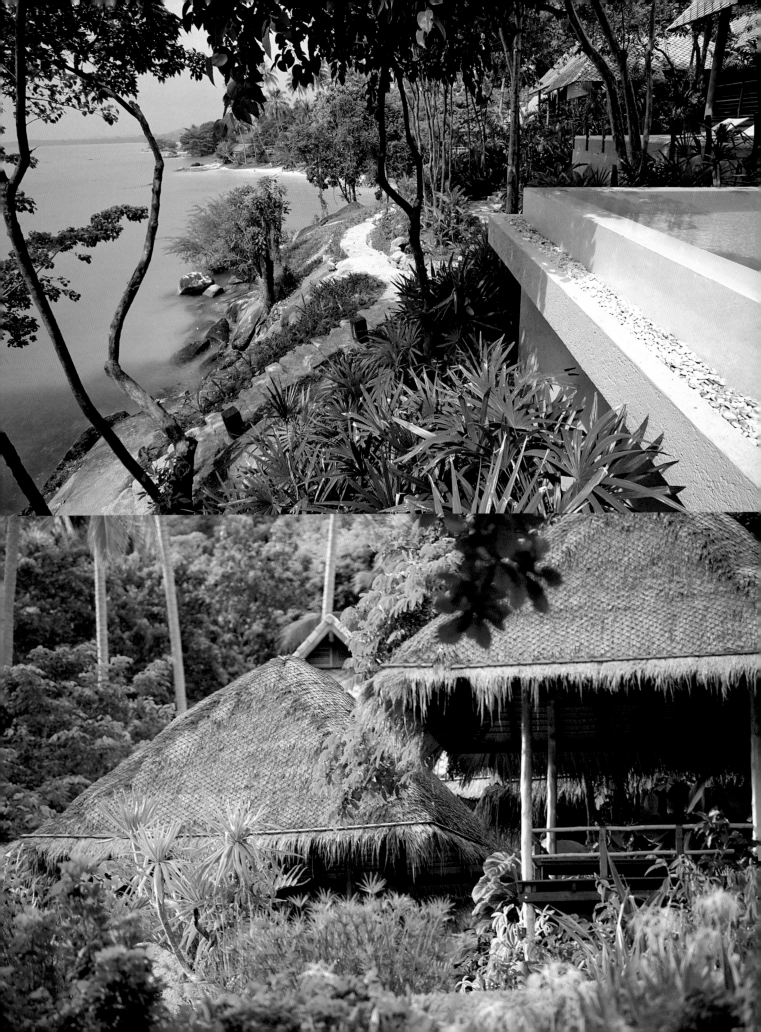

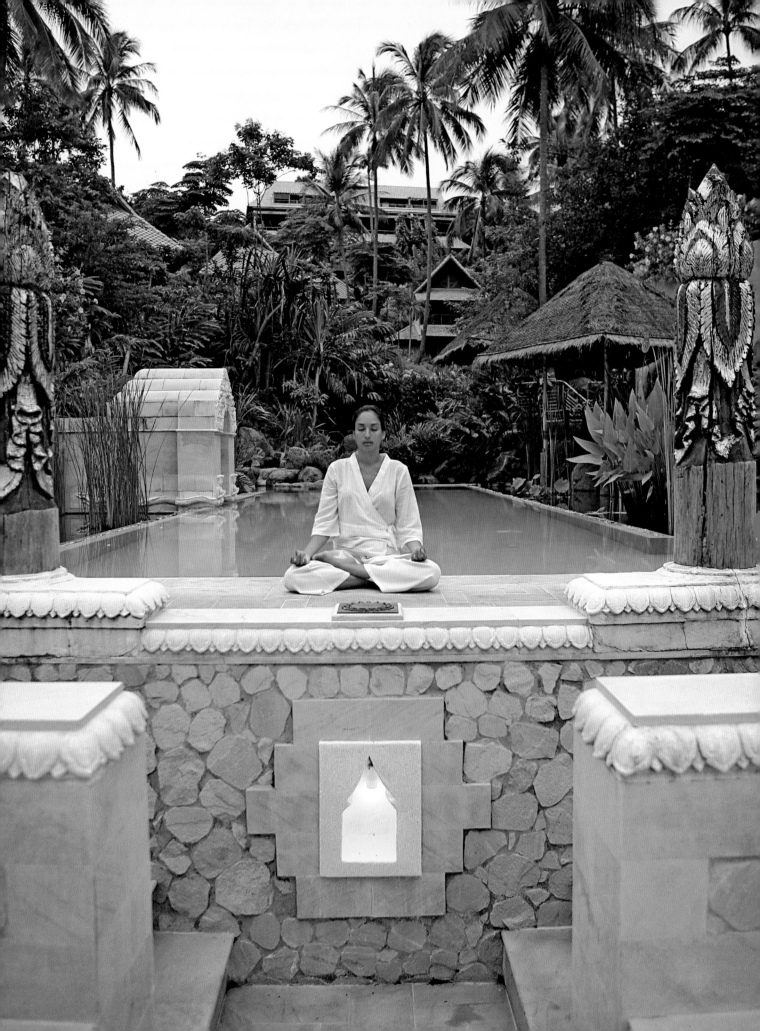

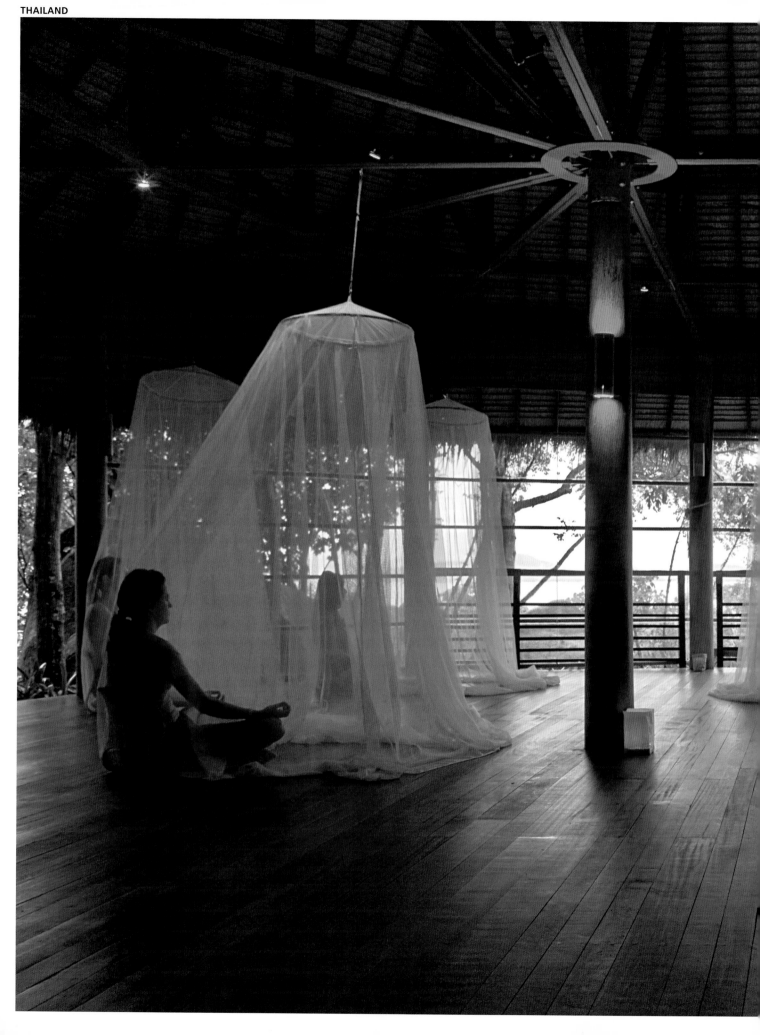

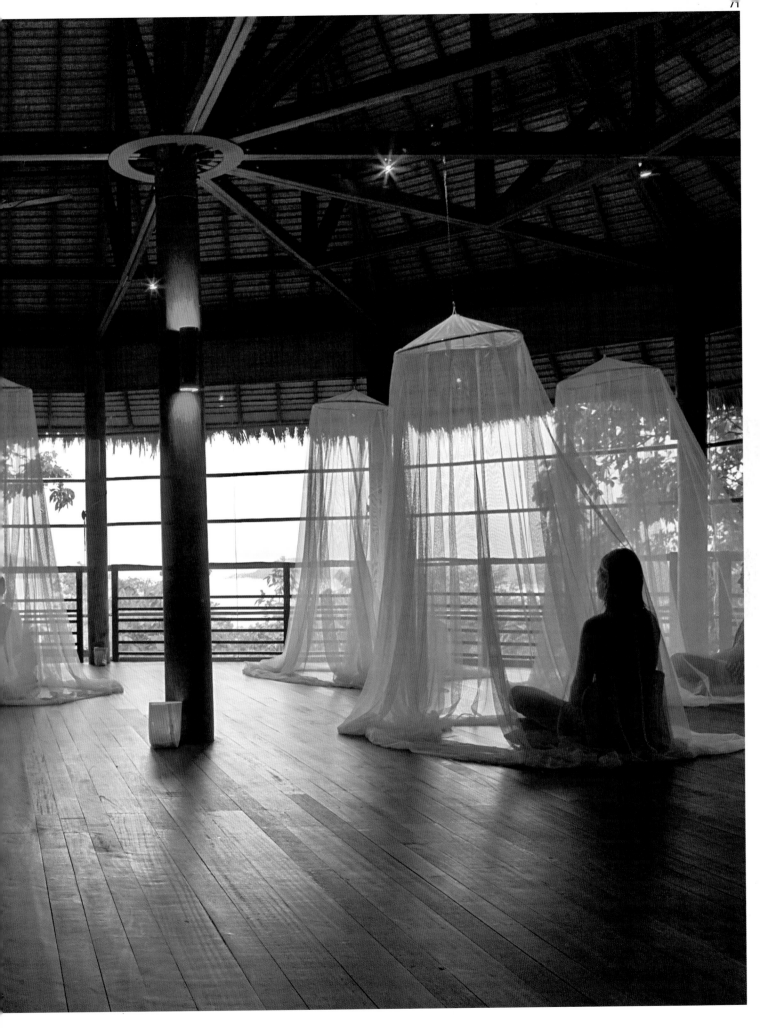

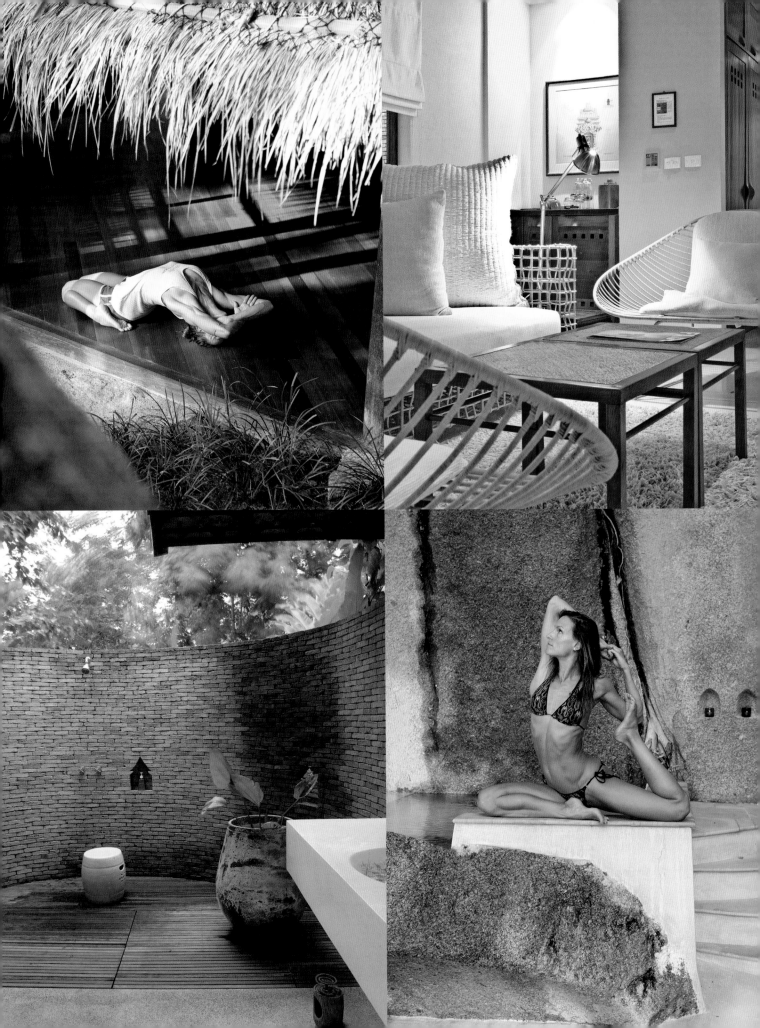

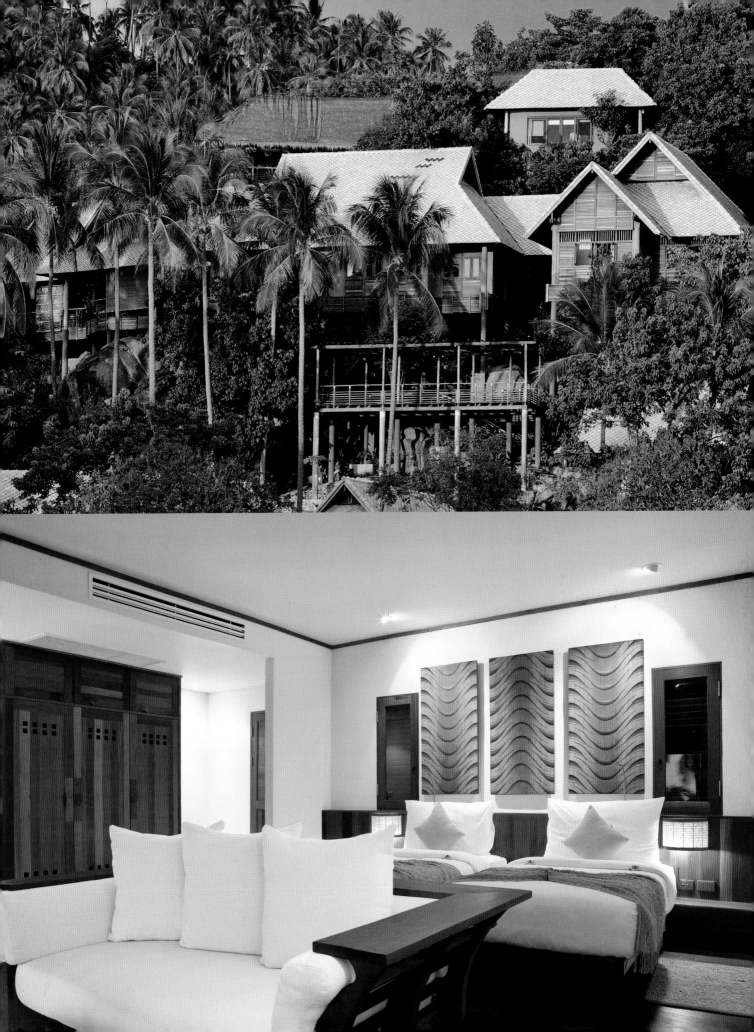

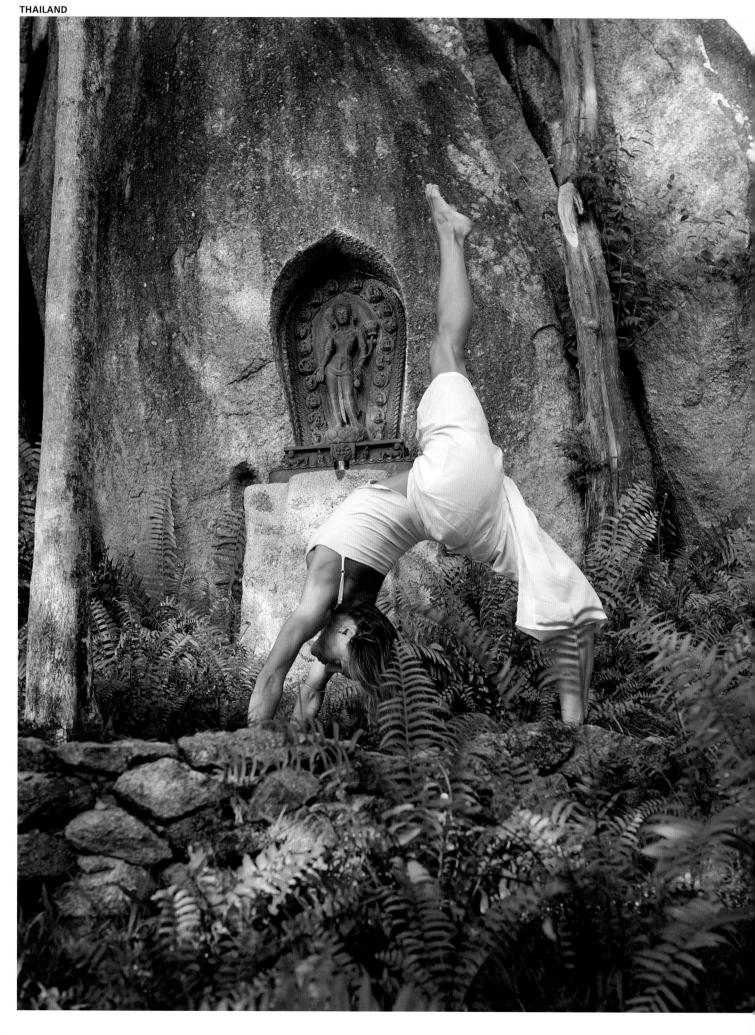

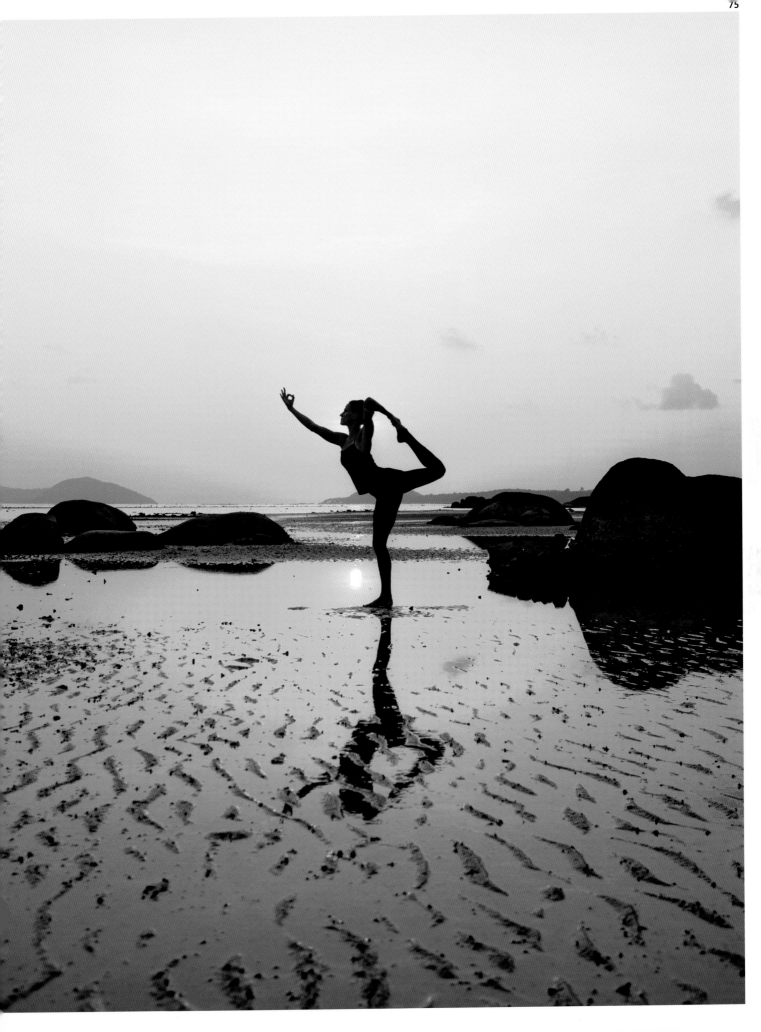

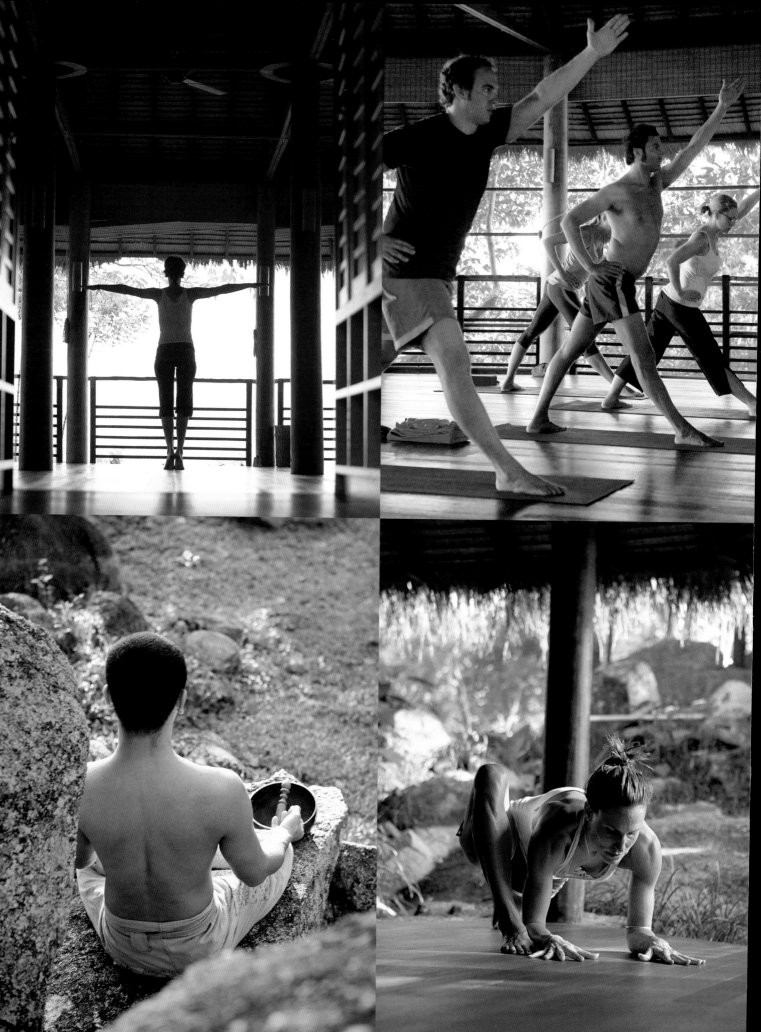

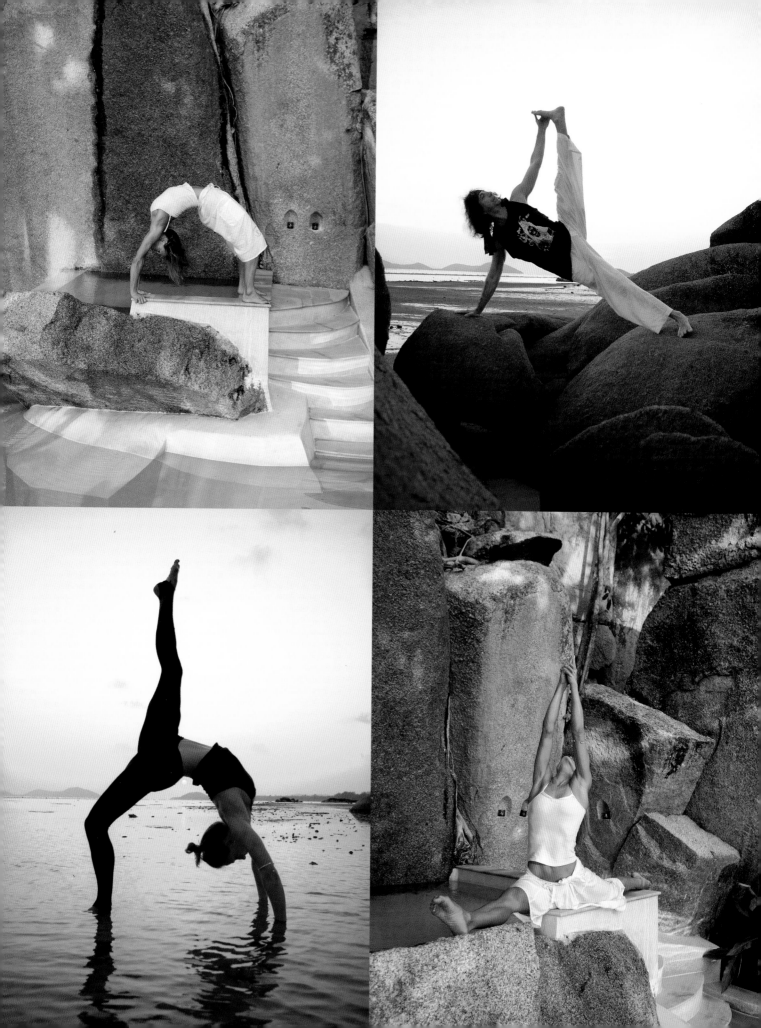

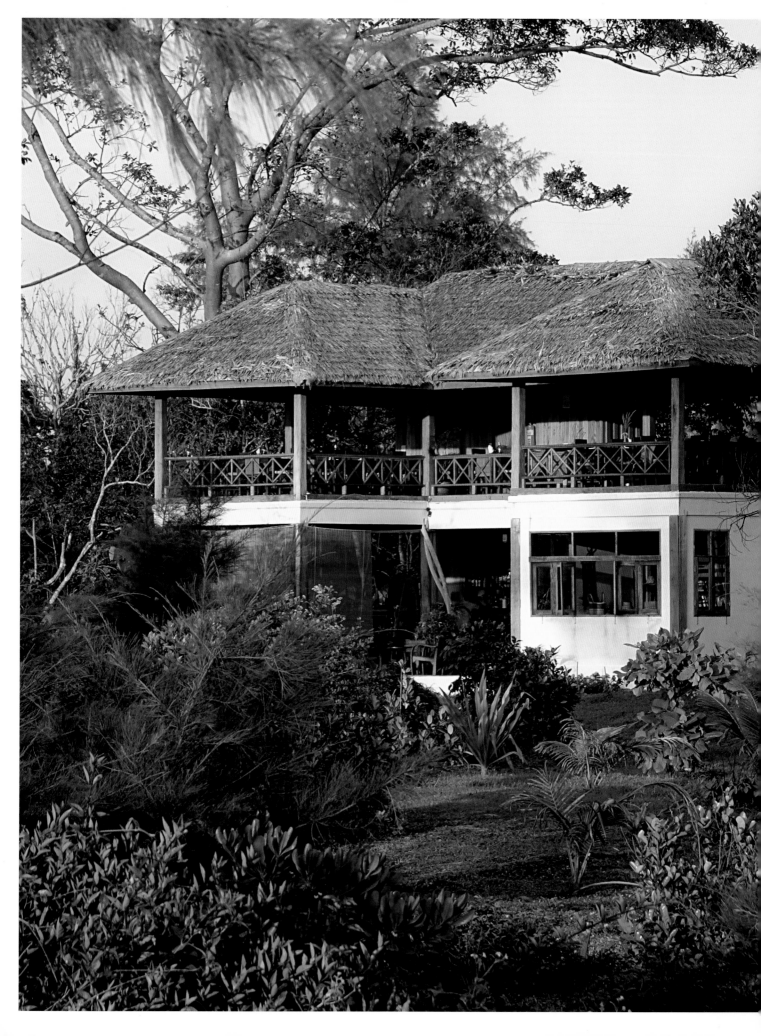

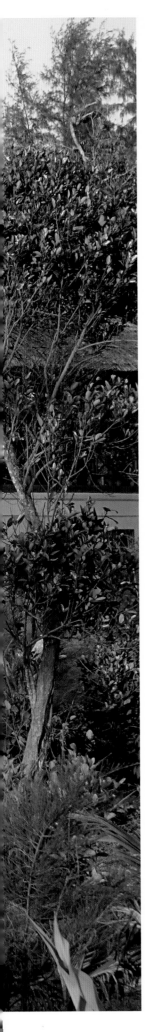

What a wise decision the pirates made in hiding a golden Buddha statue precisely here, on the lonely island of Koh Phra Thong. It lies a couple of hours north of Phuket; enough of a distance away, indeed, to have the feeling of touching down on another planet. Monkeys inhabit their own cliffs here, and white bellied sea eagles soar overhead. The Golden Buddha Beach Resort, an eco lodge that seems as if it was made for dynamic yoga on the beach, lies between green rice fields and dense forest. From the spacious veranda of the wooden stilt houses you look either onto the steep limestone cliffs in the turquoise Andaman Sea or into a small shady wood, where the monkeys romp in the trees. Siddhartha Gautama, the young man from a wealthy background who left his family to seek enlightenment, could well have stopped off here. Or Roger Moore maybe, "the man with the golden gun". One reason to get shipwrecked on the island is without doubt the turtles, elsewhere threatened with extinction, that bury their eggs in the white sand of the ten-mile-long beach in absolute peace and quiet.

Books to pack: "Buddha" by Karen Armstrong and "The Glass Palace" by Amitav Ghosh

Golden Buddha Beach Resort

131 Moo 2, T. Koh Phra Thong
A. Kuraburi, Phang-nga 82150
Thailand
Tel. +66 818 922 208 and +66 818 925 228
info@goldenbuddharesort.com
www.goldenbuddharesort.com

Directions	Some 93 miles away from Phuket Airport, transfer on request
Yoga	Hatha, Vinyasa, Anusara
Teachers	Danny Paradise, Carolina Smilas, Susan Desmarais
Rooms	25 small houses for 2–6 people each
Food	Thai, green papaya salad, pancakes with hibiscus jam, sea bass with coriander and chili
Treatments	Thai Ayurveda massage, aromatherapy massage, Swedish massage, Chakra head massage, foot reflexology massage
Leisure	Hiking, safaris, bird-watching, diving, snorkelling, kayaking

Was für eine weise Entscheidung die Piraten getroffen haben, genau auf dieser einsamen Insel eine goldene Buddha-Statue zu verstecken. Koh Phra Thong liegt ein paar Stunden nördlich von Phuket, weit genug, um das Gefühl zu haben, einen anderen Planeten zu betreten: Affen bewohnen hier ihren eigenen Felsen, Wasserbüffel dösen in der Sonne, weißbauchige Seeadler segeln über ihnen. Und zwischen grünen Reisfeldern und dichten Wäldern liegt das Golden Buddha Beach Resort, eine Öko-Lodge wie geschaffen für dynamisches Yoga am Strand. Von der großzügigen Veranda der auf Stelzen gebauten Holzhäuser sieht man auf die Kalksteinfelsen in der türkisfarbenen Andamanensee oder in ein schattiges Wäldchen, wo die Affen auf den Bäumen turnen. Siddhartha Gautama, der junge Mann aus gutem Haus, der seine Familie verließ, um Erleuchtung zu suchen, könnte hier gut Station gemacht haben. Oder war es Roger Moore, »der Mann mit dem goldenen Colt«? Ein Grund, an diesem Ort vor Anker zu gehen, sind in jedem Fall die vom Aussterben bedrohten Meeresschildkröten, die in aller Ruhe ihre Eier im weißen Sand des 16 Kilometer langen Strandes vergraben.

Reisebegleiter: »Buddha« von Karen Armstrong und »Der Glaspalast« von Amitav Ghosh

Quelle sage décision prirent les pirates qui cachèrent une statue dorée de Bouddha précisément sur cette île déserte. Koh Phra Thong se trouve à quelques heures au nord de Phuket, assez loin pour qu'on ait l'impression d'accéder à une autre planète. Ici, les singes sont chez eux dans les rochers, et des aigles de mer aux ventres blancs survolent les rizières vertes et les forêts touffues. C'est ici que s'étend le Golden Buddha Beach Resort, la station écologique idéale pour l'exercice dynamique du yoga sur la plage. Depuis la vaste véranda des maisons de bois construites sur pilotis, le regard se pose sur les falaises de calcaire surplombant une mer d'Andaman aux reflets turquoise ou sur un bosquet ombragé où les singes virevoltent dans les arbres. Siddhartha Gautama, le jeune homme de bonne famille qui quitta sa famille pour trouver l'Eveil, pourrait bien avoir fait halte ici. Ou était-ce Roger Moore, « l'homme au pistolet d'or » ? En tout cas, les tortues marines menacées d'extinction, qui viennent, en toute quiétude sur la plage longue de 16 kilomètres enfouir leurs œufs dans le sable blanc vous donneraient bien envie de faire naufrage ici.

Livres à emporter : « Bouddha » de Karen Armstrong et « Le Palais des miroirs » d'Amitav Ghosh

Anreise	150 km südlich vom Phuket Airport entfernt, Transfer auf Wunsch
Yoga	Hatha, Vinyasa, Anusara
Lehrer	Danny Paradise, Carolina Smilas, Susan Desmarais
Zimmer	25 Häuschen für je 2–6 Personen
Küche	Thai, grüner Papayasalat, Pfannkuchen mit Hibiskusmarmelade, Loup de mer mit Koriander und Chili
Anwendungen	Thai-Ayurveda-Massage, Aromatherapie-Massage, Schwedische Massage, Kopf-Chakra-Massage, Fußreflexzonen-Massage
Aktivitäten	Wandern, Safari, Vogelbeobachtung, Tauchen, Schnorcheln, Kajak

Accès	À 150 km de l'aéroport de Phuket, transport sur demande
Yoga	Hatha, Vinyasa, Anusara
Professeurs	Danny Paradise, Carolina Smilas, Susan Desmarais
Chambres	25 maisonnettes pour 2 à 6 personnes l'une
Restauration	Thaïlandaise, salade verte de papayes, crêpes à la confiture d'hibiscus, loup de mer au coriandre et au chili
Traitements	Massage ayurvédique thaïlandais, aromathérapie, massage suédois, massage crânien et des chakras, massage réflexe des pieds
Activités	Promenades, safaris, observations des oiseaux, plongée sous-marine, plongée libre, kayak

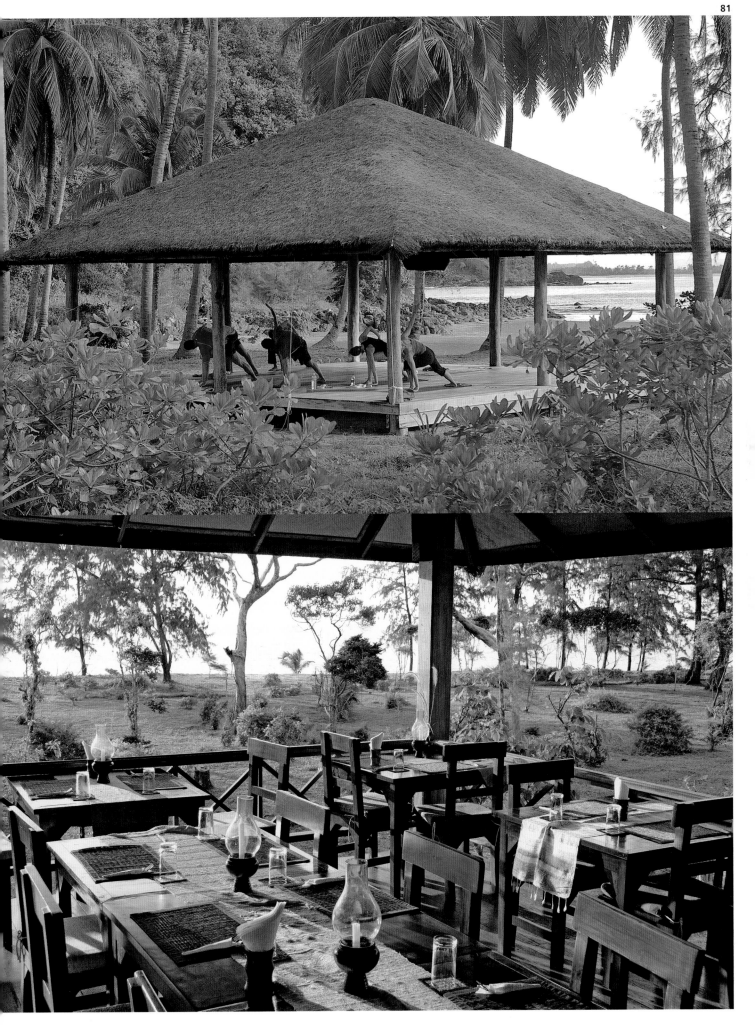

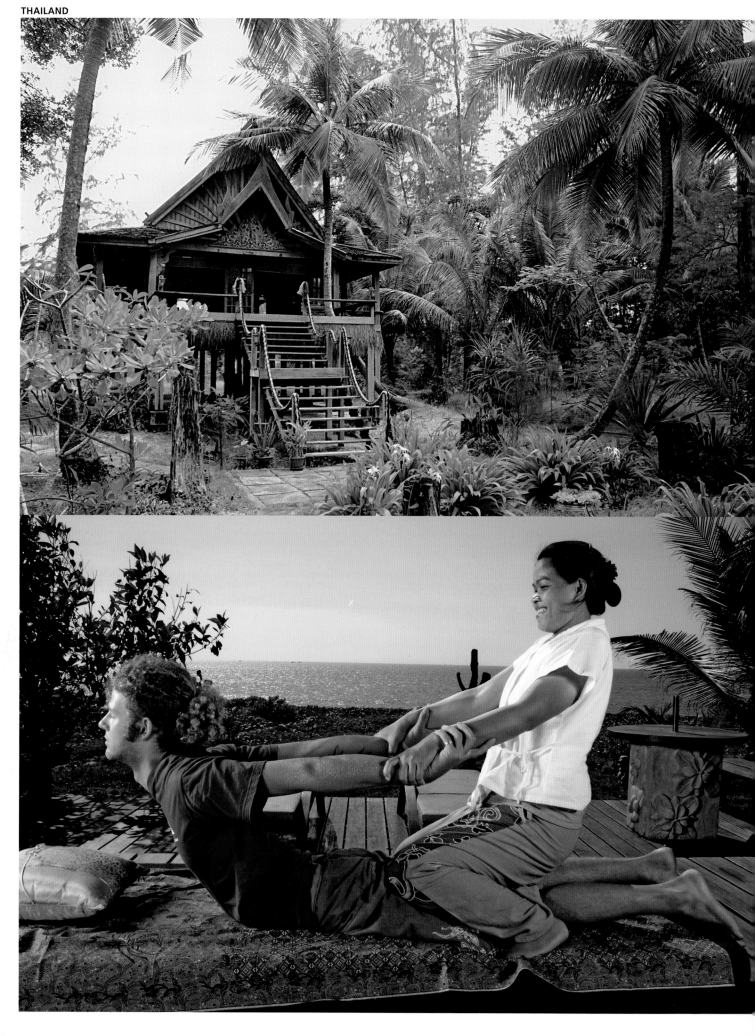

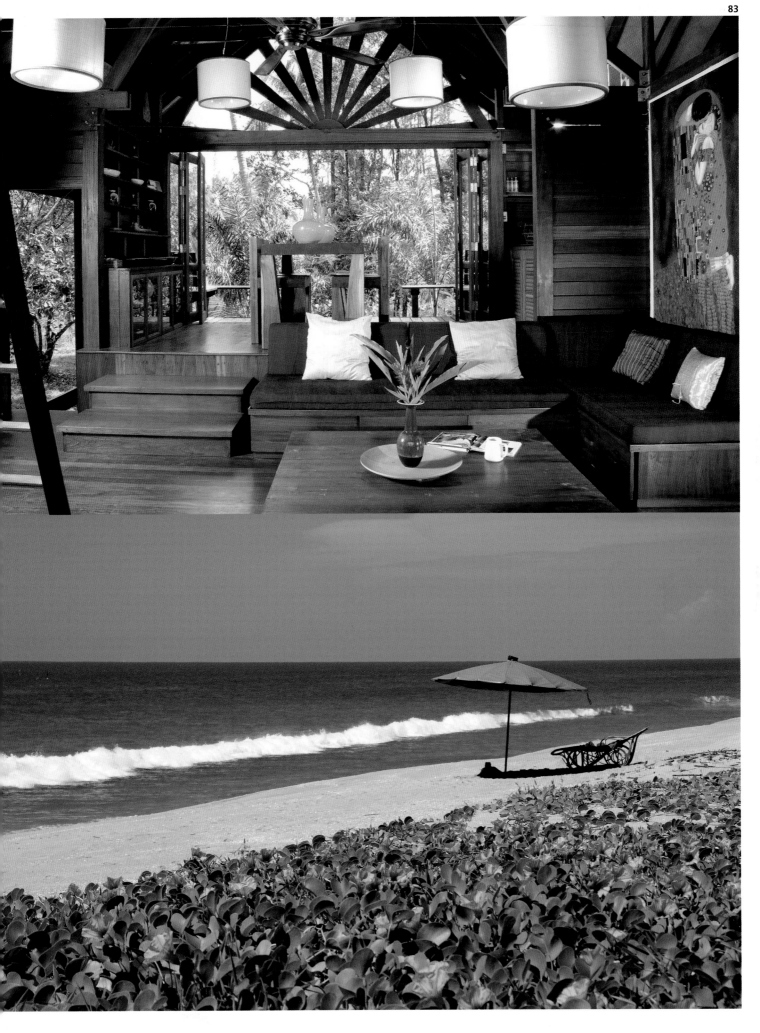

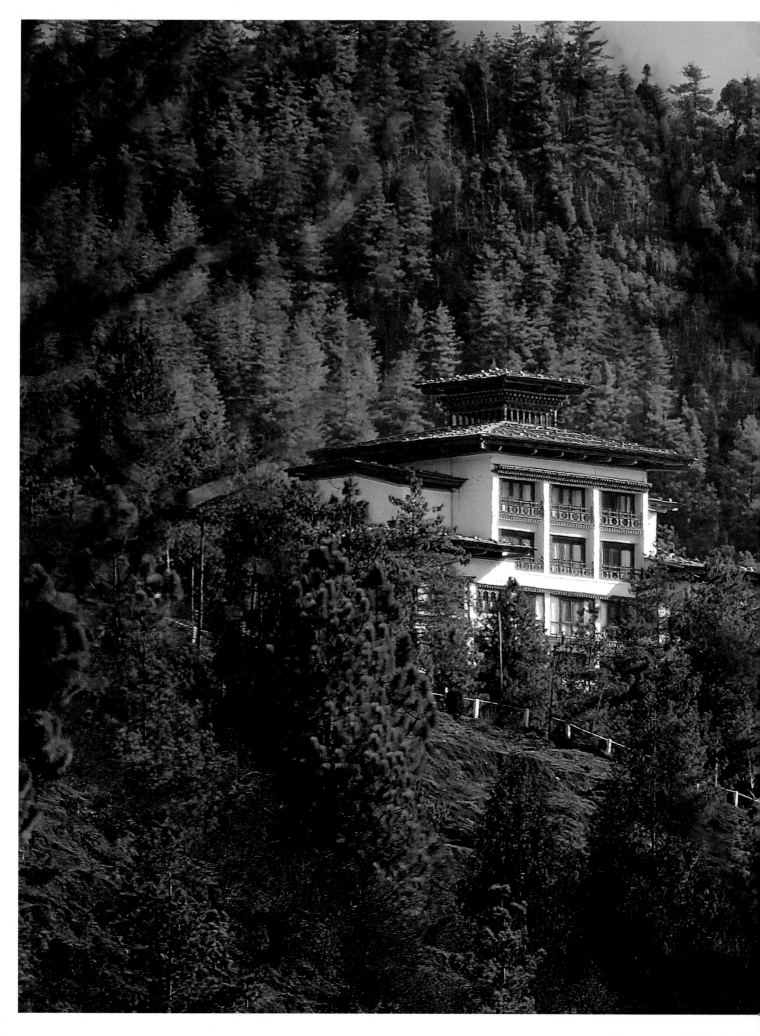

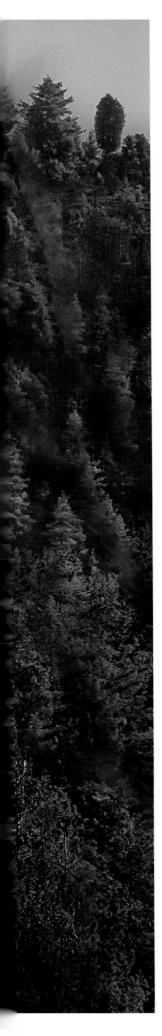

The heart violently pumps oxygen into all the body's cells. Slowly the pulse steadies, and the muscles breathe a sigh of relief. Enjoy hours of yoga a day here on the polished sprung parquet of the open-air pavilion, from which the eyes are gently drawn towards nature. The white magnolia flowers sparkle like stars between Bhutan pines and Himalayan cypresses in the garden, brightly coloured flags flutter in the wind and the sky over the Paro valley is a cobalt blue. The ringing of the prayer wheel, turned by the monks to cleanse their Karma, is audible from far off. Is there a better place than this to meditate? In the 8th century the religion's founder, Guru Rinpoche, after his flight over the Himalayas on the back of a tigress, is said to have landed here in order to free the people from the curse of the outraged spirits of nature and to convert them to Buddhism. Today, the white walls of the Taktsang monastery cling to the steep rock face at this spot. After a day trip to one of the many monasteries, drinking a green tea martini or a chai-spiced hot chocolate, the saffron and burgundy coloured robes of the monks still in your mind's eye, or being treated in the spa on hot stones with herbs from Bhutan, it is easy to live in the here and now.

Books to pack: "Tibetan Book of the Dead" by Sogyal Rinpoche and "Seven Years in Tibet" by Heinrich Harrer

Uma by COMO

P.O. Box 222
Paro
Bhutan
Tel. +975 827 1597
Fax +975 827 1513
info.paro@uma.como.bz
www.uma.paro.como.bz

Directions	Via Bangkok to Paro; 10 min away from the airport there
Yoga	Hatha
Teachers	Eileen Hall, Ming Lee
Rooms	29 guest rooms and suites
Food	Holistic Bhutanese-Indian and Western cuisine
Treatments	Holistic therapies, Ayurveda. Bhutanese hot-stone bath with hot boulders and massage
Recreation	Hot-stone bath house, indoor pool, camping and trekking tours, mountain biking, temple visits

Heftig pumpt das Herz Sauerstoff in alle Körperzellen, langsam beruhigt sich der Puls, und die Muskeln entspannen sich. Mehrere Stunden Yoga täglich werden hier auf dem federnden, polierten Parkett des Open-Air-Pavillons unterrichtet, von dem der Blick sanft in die Natur schweift. Wie weiße Sterne blitzen die Blüten der Magnolien im Garten zwischen Tränenkiefern und Himalaja-Zypressen, knallbunt wehen kleine Fahnen im Wind, und kobaltblau strahlt der Himmel über dem Paro-Tal. Von Weitem ist das helle Klingeln der Gebetsmühlen zu hören, die die Mönche drehen, um ihr Karma zu reinigen. Gibt es einen besseren Platz, um zu meditieren? Im 8. Jahrhundert soll der Religionsstifter Guru Rinpoche – nach einem Flug über den Himalaja auf dem Rücken einer Tigerin – hier gelandet sein, um die Menschen vom Fluch der aufgebrachten Naturgeister zu befreien und sie zum Buddhismus zu bekehren. Heute kleben an dieser Stelle die weißen Mauern des Taktsang-Klosters in der steilen Felswand. Nach einem Ausflug zu einem der vielen Klöster am Kaminfeuer im Salon einen Green Tea Martini oder eine Chai-gewürzte heiße Schokolade zu trinken, die safran- und burgunderfarbenen Roben der Mönche noch vor Augen, oder im Spa auf heißen Steinen mit Kräutern aus Bhutan behandelt zu werden, macht es einem leicht, im Hier und Jetzt zu leben.

Reisebegleiter: »Das tibetische Buch vom Leben und vom Sterben« von Sogyal Rinpoche und »Sieben Jahre in Tibet« von Heinrich Harrer

Avec ardeur le cœur pompe l'oxygène dans toutes les cellules du corps, le pouls ralentit peu à peu et les muscles se détendent. Les cours de yoga sont prodigués cinq heures par jour sur le parquet souple et luisant du pavillon en plein air, d'où le regard s'élève doucement vers la nature environnante. Dans le jardin, entre pins pleureurs et cyprès de l'Himalaya, les fleurs des magnolias brillent comme des étoiles blanches, les petits drapeaux colorés flottent dans le vent et le ciel bleu de cobalt resplendit au-dessus de la vallée de Paro. Au loin retentit le son clair des moulins à prières que les moines font tourner pour purifier leur karma. Existe-t-il un meilleur endroit pour méditer ? Au 8e siècle, dit-on, le fondateur de la religion connu sous le nom de Guru Rinpoché aurait atterri ici, après avoir survolé l'Himalaya sur le dos d'une tigresse, pour libérer les hommes de la malédiction des esprits de la nature alors furieux, et les convertir au bouddhisme. Aujourd'hui, à cet endroit, les murs blancs du monastère de Taktshang s'accrochent à la paroi rocheuse s'élevant à pic. Après une excursion dans l'un des nombreux cloîtres, boire un martini au thé vert ou un chocolat chaud aromatisé au chai devant le feu de cheminée du salon, les robes couleur safran ou bordeaux des moines encore en mémoire, ou dans le spa sur les pierres chaudes s'adonner à un traitement aux herbes de Bhoutan, rien de tel pour vivre l'ici et maintenant.

Livres à emporter : « Le livre tibétain de la vie et de la mort » de Sogyal Rinpoché et « Sept ans d'aventures au Tibet » de Heinrich Harrer

Anreise	Über Bangkok nach Paro, dort 10 min vom Flughafen entfernt
Yoga	Hatha
Lehrer	Eileen Hall, Ming Lee
Zimmer	29 Gästezimmer und Suiten
Küche	Ganzheitlich bhutanisch-indisch und westlich
Anwendungen	Ganzheitliche Therapien, Ayurveda, Bhutanisches Hot-Stone-Bad mit heißen Flusssteinen und Massage
Aktivitäten	Hot-Stone-Badehaus, Indoor-Pool, Camping- und Trekkingtouren, Mountainbiking, Tempelbesuche

Accès	Par Bangkok pour aller à Paro, situé à 10 min de l'aéroport
Yoga	Hatha
Professeurs	Eileen Hall, Ming Lee
Chambres	29 chambres d'hôtes et suites
Restauration	Cuisine intégrale indo-bhoutanaise et occidentale
Traitements	Thérapies intégrales, Ayurveda, bain bhoutanais sur galets chaud et massages
Activités	Pavillon de bains aux pierres chaudes, piscine couverte, camping et trekking, VTT, visites de temples

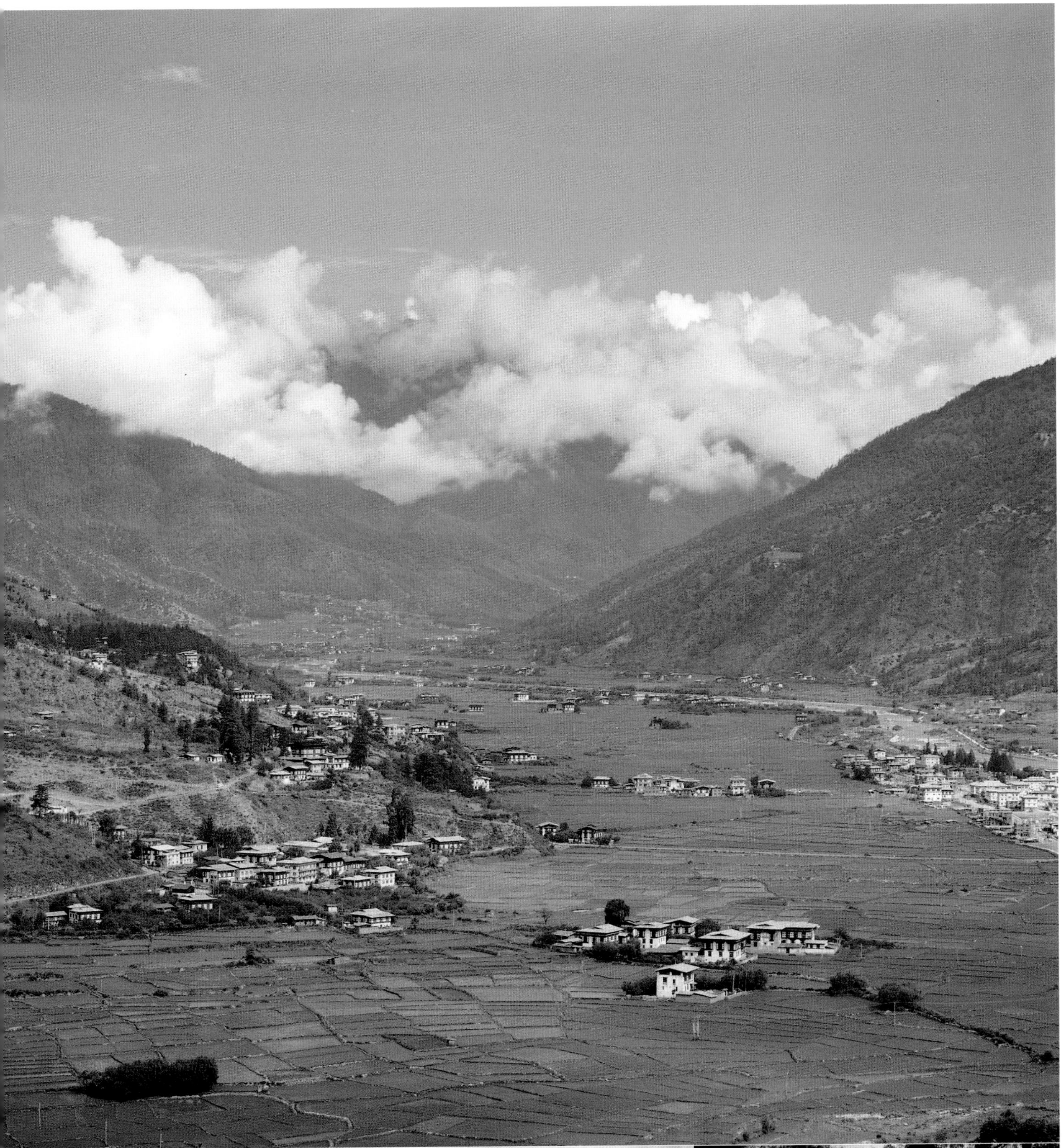

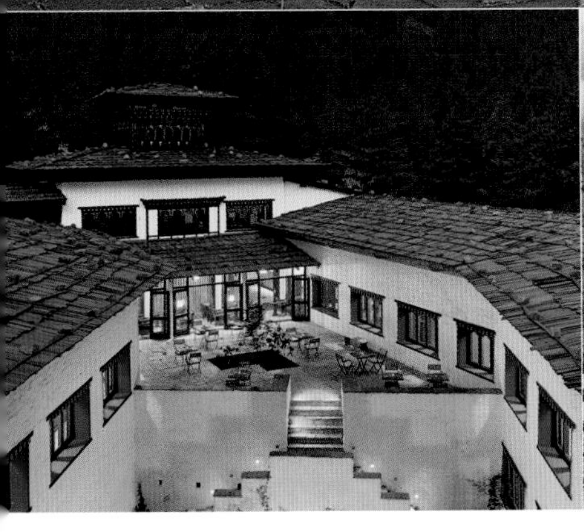

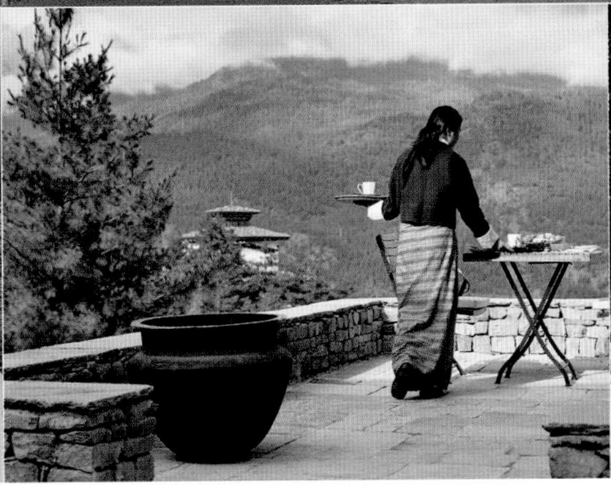

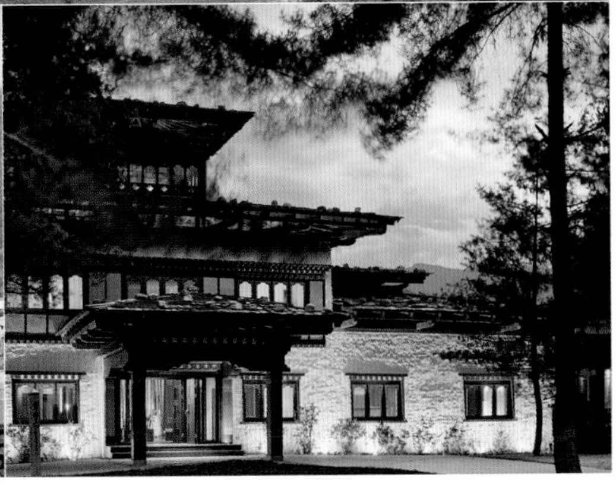

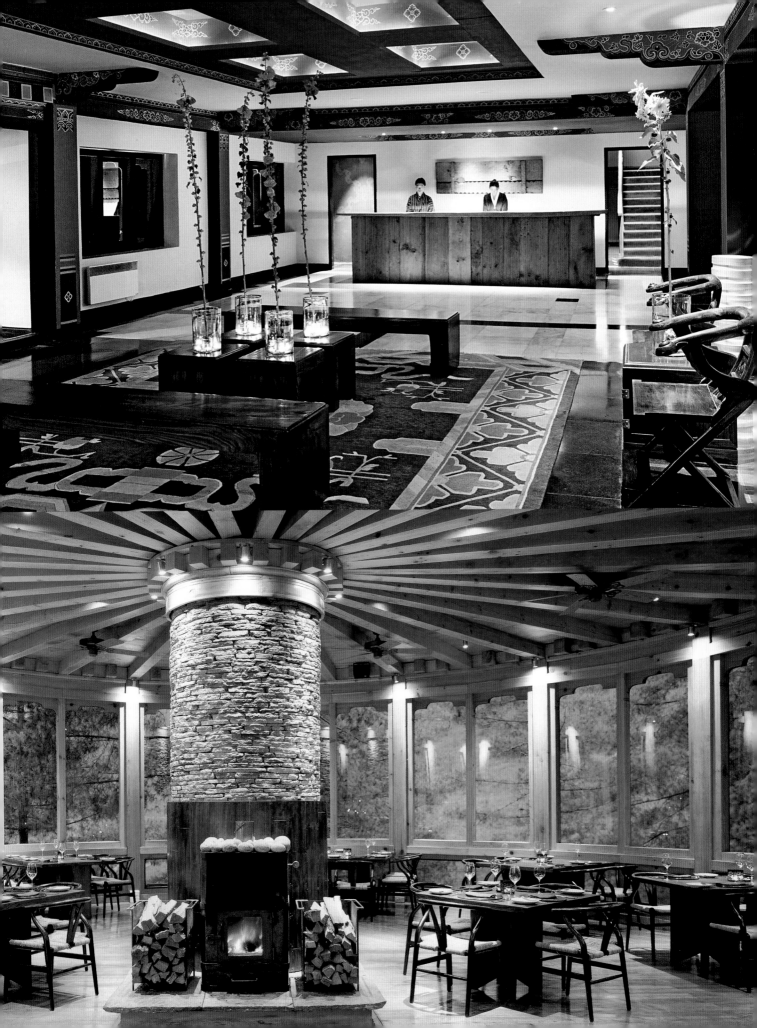

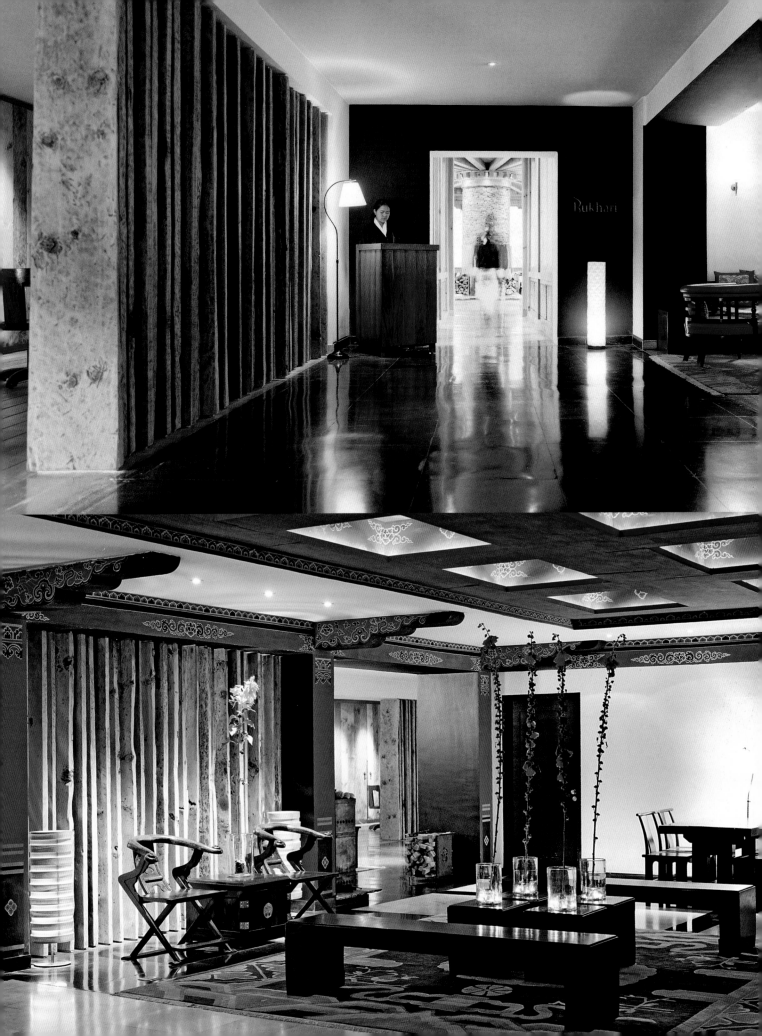

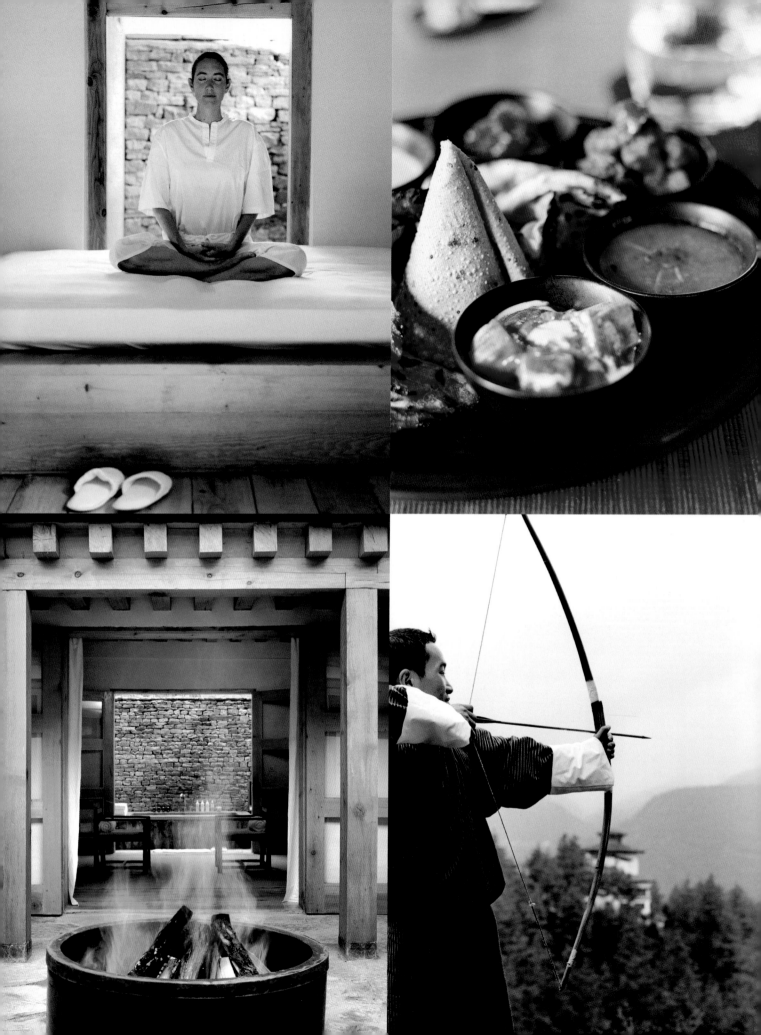

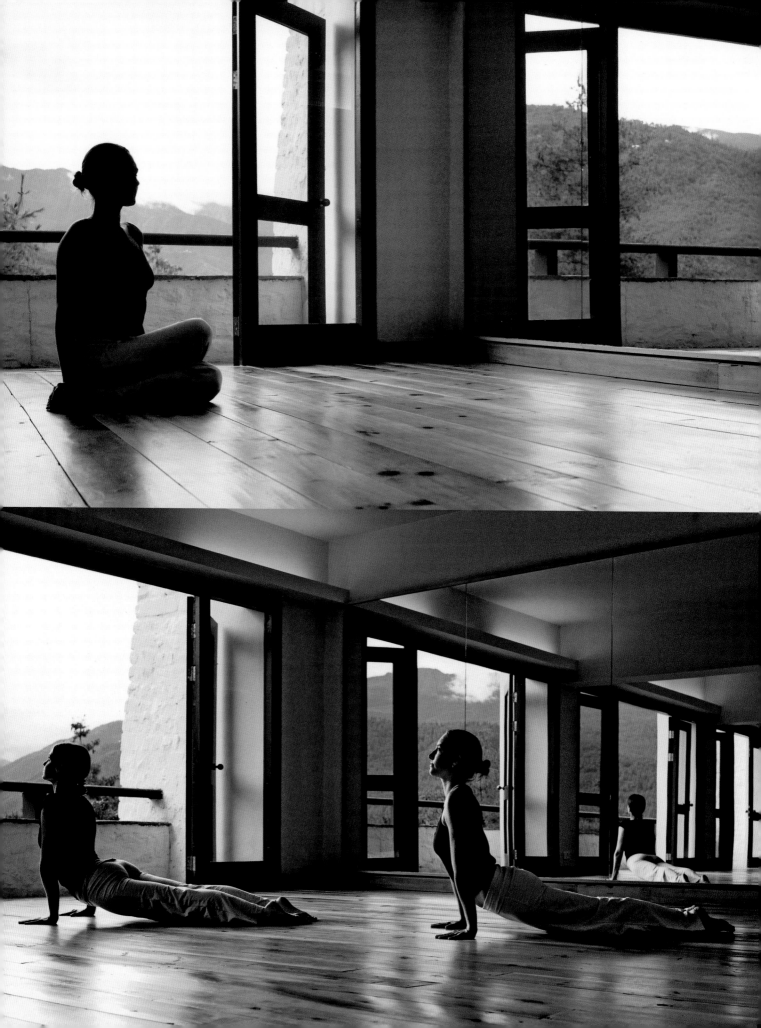

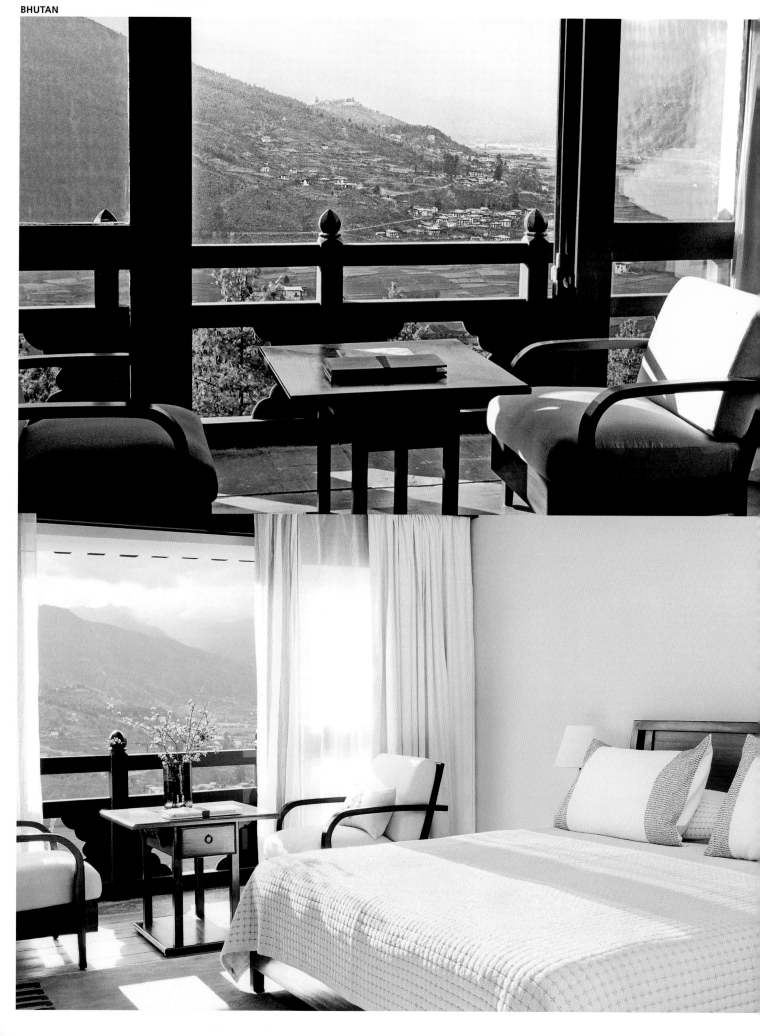

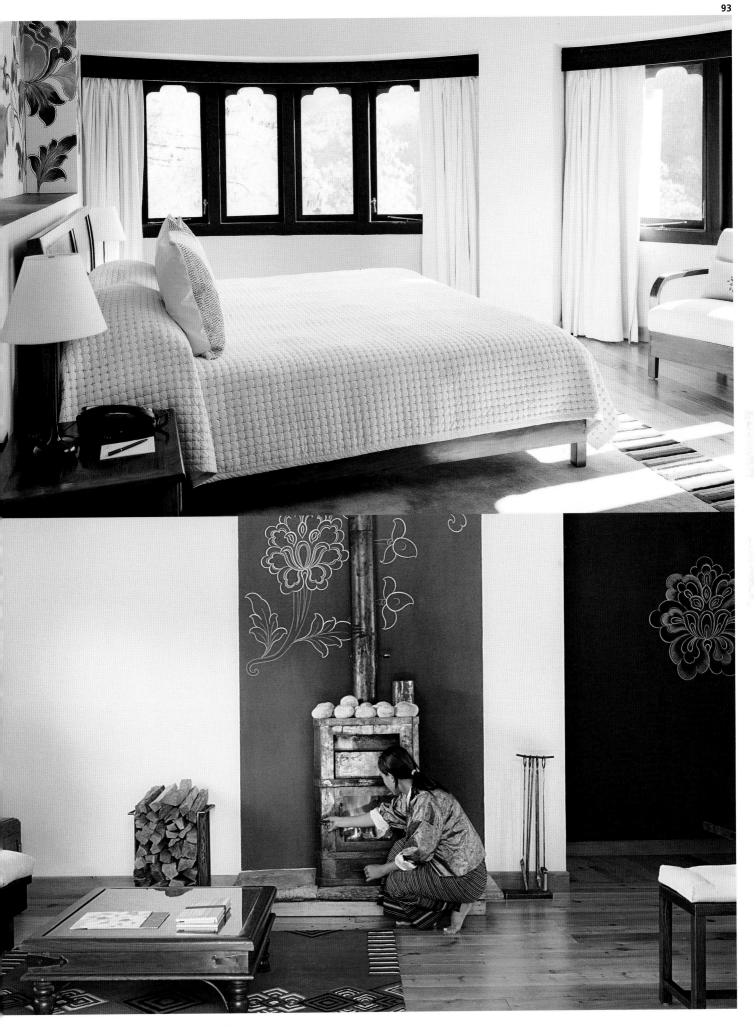

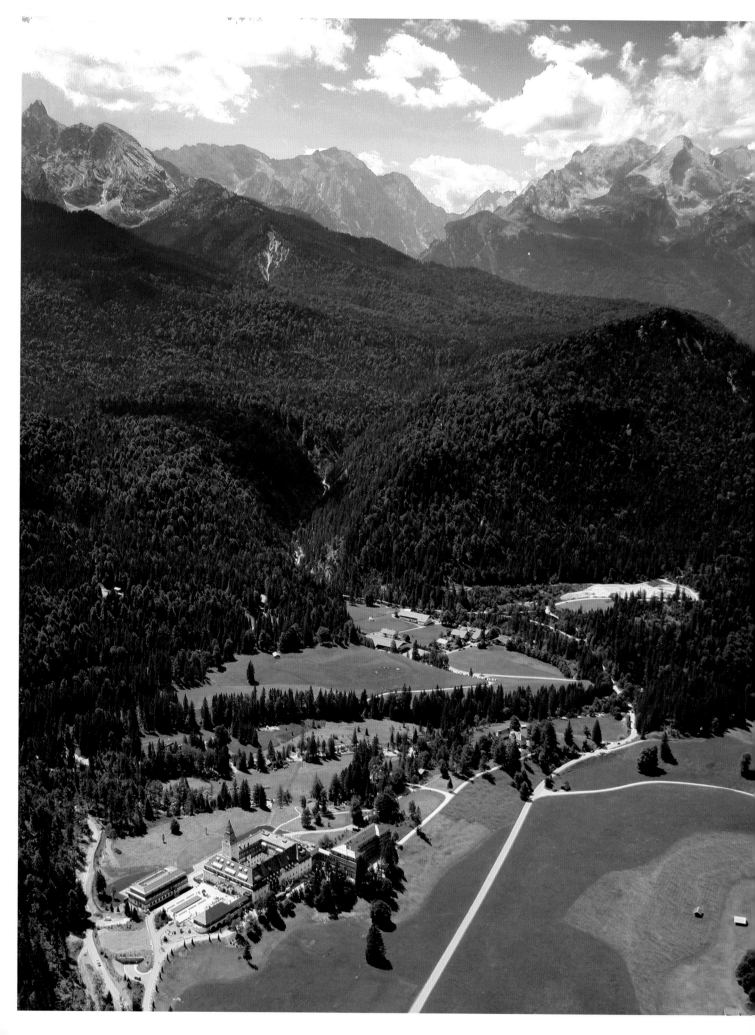

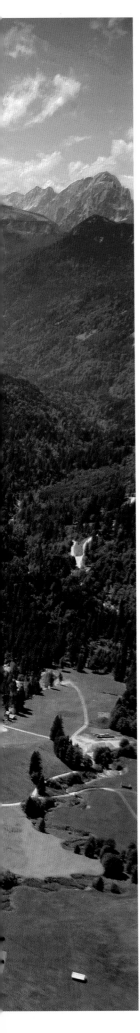

Beyond Garmisch, when the little barrier across the road rises and the Wetterstein massif, at the foot of which Schloss Elmau lies in solitude, seems to get huger with every metre, something strange happens to city dwellers: they take a deep breath. Nestling in gently rising, undulating meadows, whose hollows you can have to yourself in the summer, lies a place that takes you away from the breathlessness of our times. Built between 1914 and 1916 with the support of an aristocratic female admirer by the practical philosopher Johannes Müller and his brother-in-law, the famous architect Carlo Sattler, this place of refuge in Elmau was restored with expert care in 2006–07. Older regular guests still tell of the era of the German economic miracle, when television and radio were frowned upon here and only chamber music by Yehudi Menuhin or Friedrich Gulda was permitted to overlay the concert of nature, when well-brought-up daughters from the surrounding area served tea to north German aristocrats and polka dances were held on two evenings a week. The aristocracy is still here, and now comes from London, the silence has remained, and some of the old floorboards still creak as they used to. When, however, in the heated roof-top pool beneath wide Bavarian skies after a challenging session with yoga aces such as Patrick Broome, Patricia Thielemann or Timo Wahl, your gaze wanders over the snow-covered peaks, nostalgia doesn't take over completely. Enlightenment could hardly be more luxurious.

Books to pack: None—browsing the latest & greatest reading matter in the hotel's spacious book store is just too much fun!

Schloss Elmau

Luxury Spa & Cultural Hideaway
82493 Elmau
Germany
Tel. +49 882 3180
Fax +49 882 318 177
schloss@elmau.de
www.schloss-elmau.de

Directions	Situated 12 miles from the Bavarian town of Garmisch-Partenkirchen, 87 miles south of Munich airport
Yoga	Daily Jivamukti lessons; courses and retreats in Anusara, Hatha, Iyengar, Vinyasa, Spirit Yoga and Aerial Yoga
Teachers	Johannes Mikenda, Gabriela Bozic, Patrick Broome, Michael Forbes, Barbra Noh, Patricia Thielemann, Timo Wahl and others
Rooms	110 rooms and 20 suites
Food	Four restaurants offering a wide range from gourmet with a Michelin star to rustic, from Mediterranean to Asian cuisine
Leisure	Tai Chi, Pilates, swimming, hiking, golf, tennis, cross-country skiing, spa with hammam and sauna, classical and jazz concerts, readings by renowned authors.

Sobald sich weit hinter Garmisch die kleine Straßenschranke hebt, und mit jedem Meter das Wettersteinmassiv noch mächtiger wirkt, an dessen Fuße einsam Schloss Elmau liegt, passiert Großstädtern etwas Eigenartiges: Sie atmen durch. Eingebettet in sanft ansteigende Buckelwiesen, in deren Kuhlen man im Sommer ganz für sich sein kann, liegt ein Ort, der einen aus der Atemlosigkeit unserer Zeit entführt. Von 1914 bis 1916 mit Unterstützung einer adligen Verehrerin von dem Lebensphilosophen Johannes Müller und seinem Schwager, dem berühmten Architekten Carlo Sattler, erbaut, wurde das Elmauer Refugium 2006/07 mit versierter Behutsamkeit renoviert. Ältere Stammgäste erzählen noch von der Wirtschaftswunder-Ära, als hier Fernsehen und Radio verpönt waren und nur Kammermusik von Yehudi Menuhin oder Friedrich Gulda das Konzert der Natur übertönen durfte, als wohlerzogene Töchter aus der Umgebung dem norddeutschen Adel den Tee servierten und zweimal wöchentlich Tanzabende mit Polka stattfanden. Der Adel ist geblieben und kommt jetzt auch aus London, die Stille ist geblieben, und manche alte Diele knarrt sogar noch wie damals. Doch wenn man nach einer herausfordernden Stunde bei Yoga-Cracks wie Patrick Broome, Patricia Thielemann oder Timo Wahl im geheizten Dachpool unter weitem, bayrischem Himmel treibt, den Blick auf schneebedeckte Gipfel gerichtet, hält sich die Wehmut in Grenzen. Luxuriöser lässt sich Erleuchtung nicht denken.

Reisebegleiter: »Das Frühstücksei« von Loriot, der Stammgast war. Falls zuhause keine Zeit blieb: Im unfassbar geräumigen und wohlsortierten Buchladen des Hotels danach fragen!

Après avoir franchi la petite barrière routière loin derrière Garmisch et en allant à la rencontre du massif Wetterstein qui, à chaque pas, devient de plus en plus imposant et aux pieds duquel se trouve isolé le château d'Elmau, les habitants des grandes villes font une expérience bizarre : ils respirent à pleins poumons. Encastré au milieu de prairies pommelées aux pentes douces, où l'on peut goûter la solitude en été, ce lieu nous arrache à la trépidation de notre époque. Construit de 1914 à 1916 avec le soutien d'une aristocrate admiratrice du philosophe Johannes Müller et du beau-frère de ce dernier, le célèbre Carlo Sattler, le refuge d'Elmau a été rénové en 2006/07 avec précaution et savoir-faire. Les clients les plus âgés parlent encore de l'époque du miracle économique lorsque la télévision et la radio étaient mal vues ici et que seule la musique de chambre de Yehudi Menuhin ou de Friedrich Gulda avait le droit de couvrir le concert de la nature, lorsque les filles bien élevées des environs servaient le thé aux aristocrates du nord de l'Allemagne et qu'il y avait deux fois par semaine des soirées dansantes avec polka. Les aristocrates sont restés et viennent même de Londres, le silence est resté et certains vieux planchers grincent comme avant. Mais après une heure exigeante de yoga auprès de cracks comme Patrick Broome, Patricia Thielemann ou Timo Wahl, quand on se prélasse sur la piscine chauffée sur le toit, sous le vaste ciel bavarois, le regard dirigé vers les monts enneigés, la mélancolie est nuancée. Difficile d'imaginer un éveil plus luxueux.

Livres à emporter : Aucun – la spacieuse librairire de l'hôtel vous propose un choix incomparable de livres.

Anreise	20 km von Garmisch-Partenkirchen gelegen, 140 km südlich des Münchner Flughafens
Yoga	Tägliche Jivamukti-Klassen, Kurse und Retreats in Anusara, Hatha, Iyengar, Vinyasa, Air Floating Yoga, Spirit Yoga
Lehrer	Johannes Mikenda, Gabriela Bozic, Patrick Broome, Michael Forbes, Barbra Noh, Patricia Thielemann, Timo Wahl u. a.
Zimmer	110 Zimmer und 20 Suiten
Küche	Vier Restaurants, die ein breites Spektrum bieten – von Michelin-besternt bis herzhaft regional, von italienischer bis zu asiatischer Spa-Küche
Aktivitäten	Tai Chi, Pilates, Schwimmen, Wandern, Golf, Tennis, Skilanglauf, Spa mit Hammam und Sauna, Klassik- und Jazzkonzerte, Lesungen prominenter Autoren

Accès	Situé à 20 km de Garmisch-Parten-kirchen et à 140 km au sud de l'aéroport de Munich
Yoga	Jivamukti quotidien, en plus des cours de Anusara, Hatha, Iyengar, Vinyasa, Yoga aérien, Spirit Yoga
Professeurs	Johannes Mikenda, Gabriela Bozic, Patrick Broome, Michael Forbes, Barbra Noh, Patricia Thielemann, Timo Wahl et al.
Chambres	110 chambres et 20 suites
Restauration	Quatre restaurants proposant des cuisines diversifiées : restaurant étoilé, régional, italien et asiatique
Activités	Tai Chi, Pilates, natation, randonnées, golf, tennis, ski de fond, spa avec hammam et sauna, concerts classiques et de jazz, séances de lecture par des auteurs connus

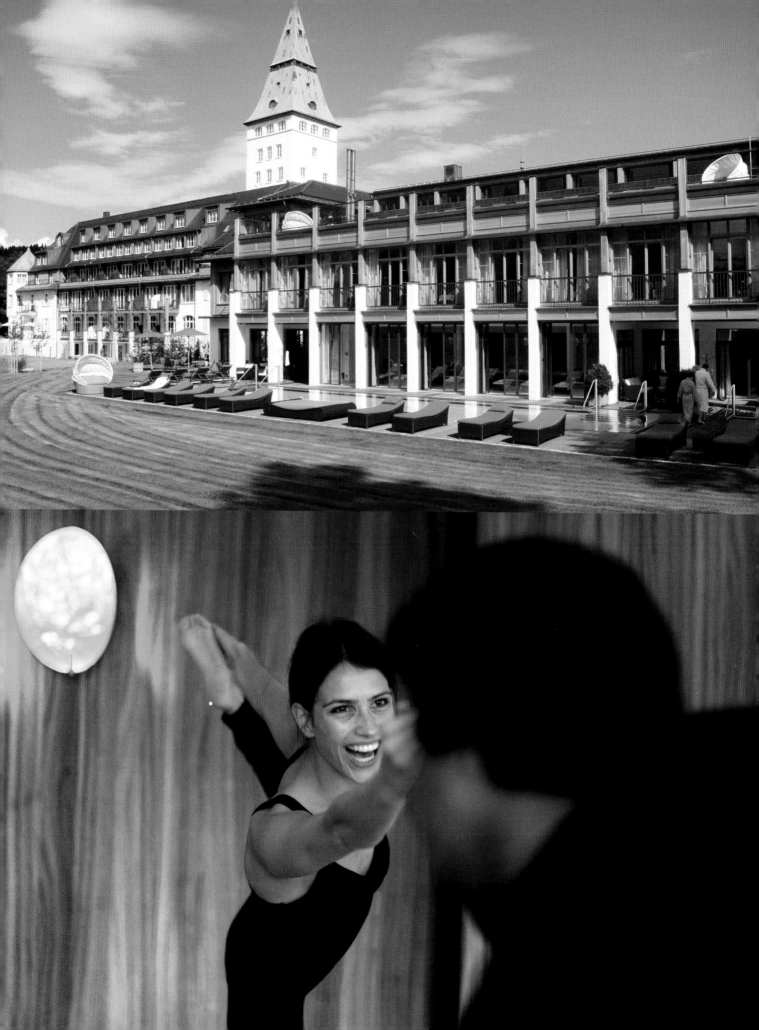

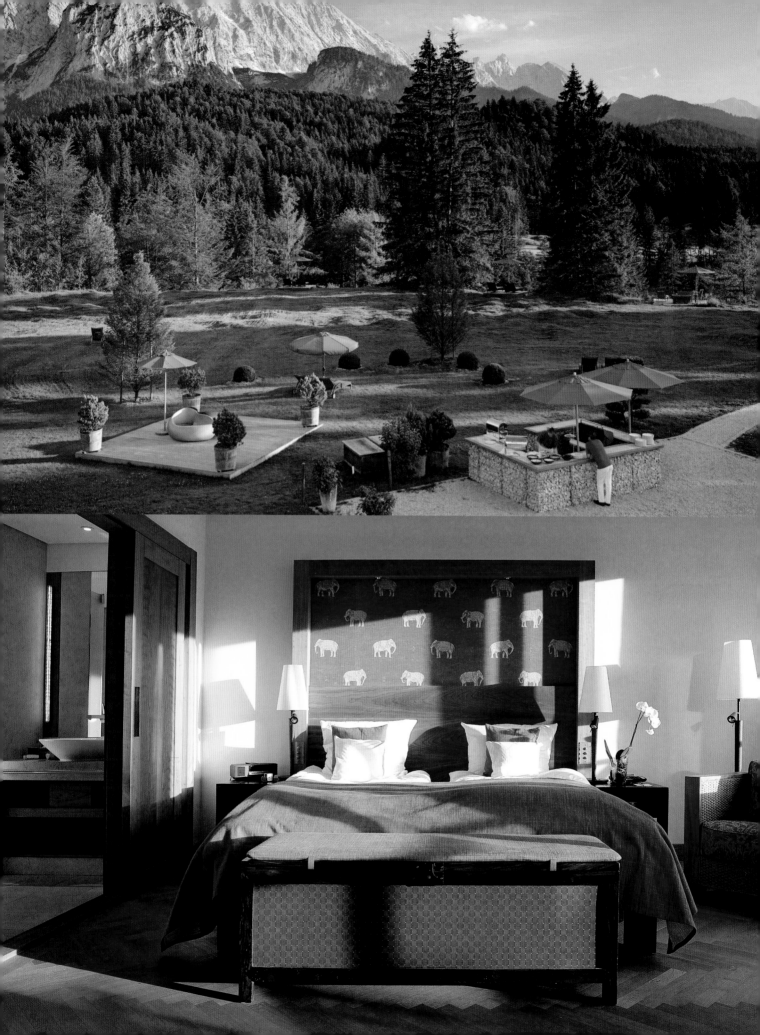

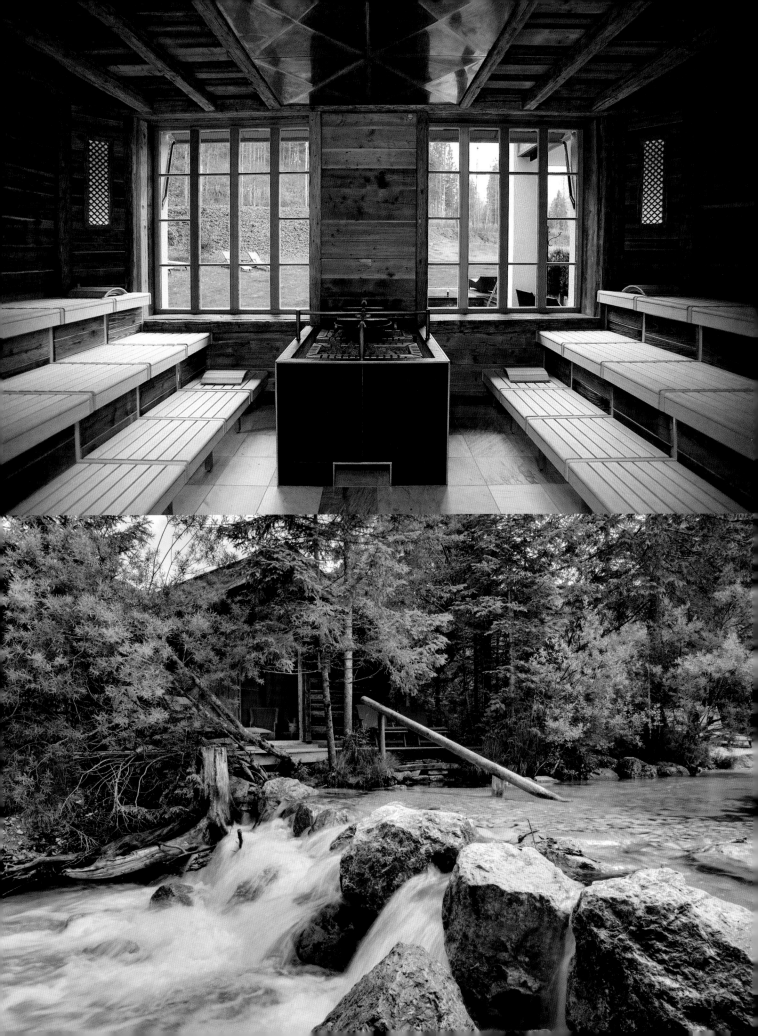

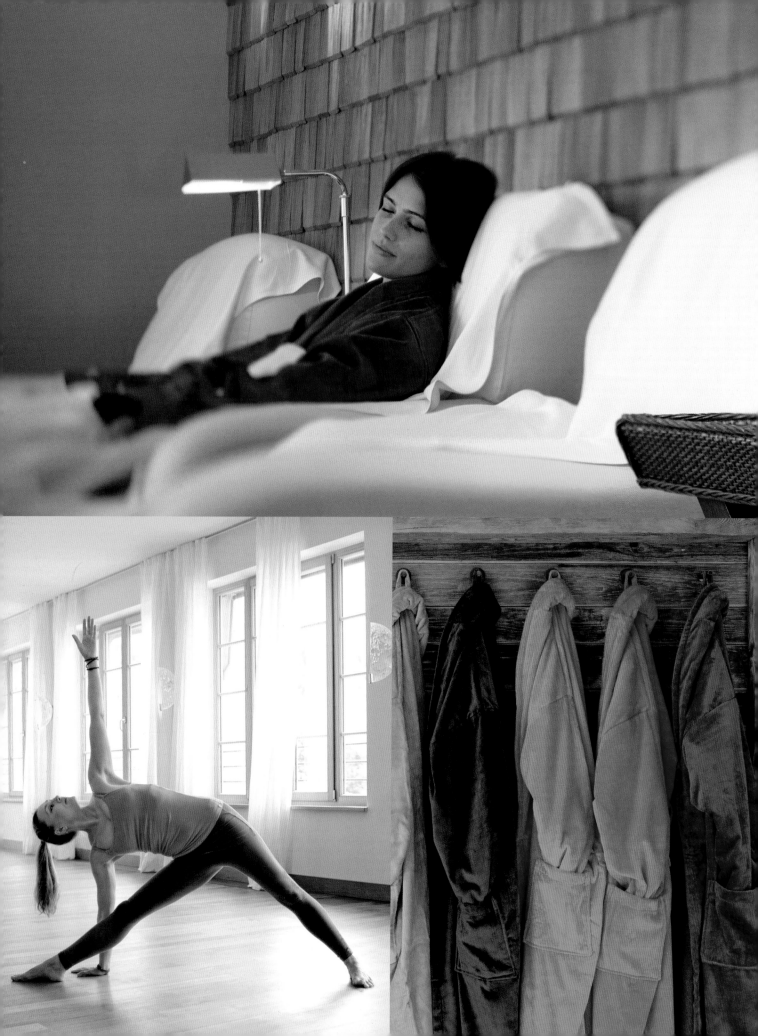

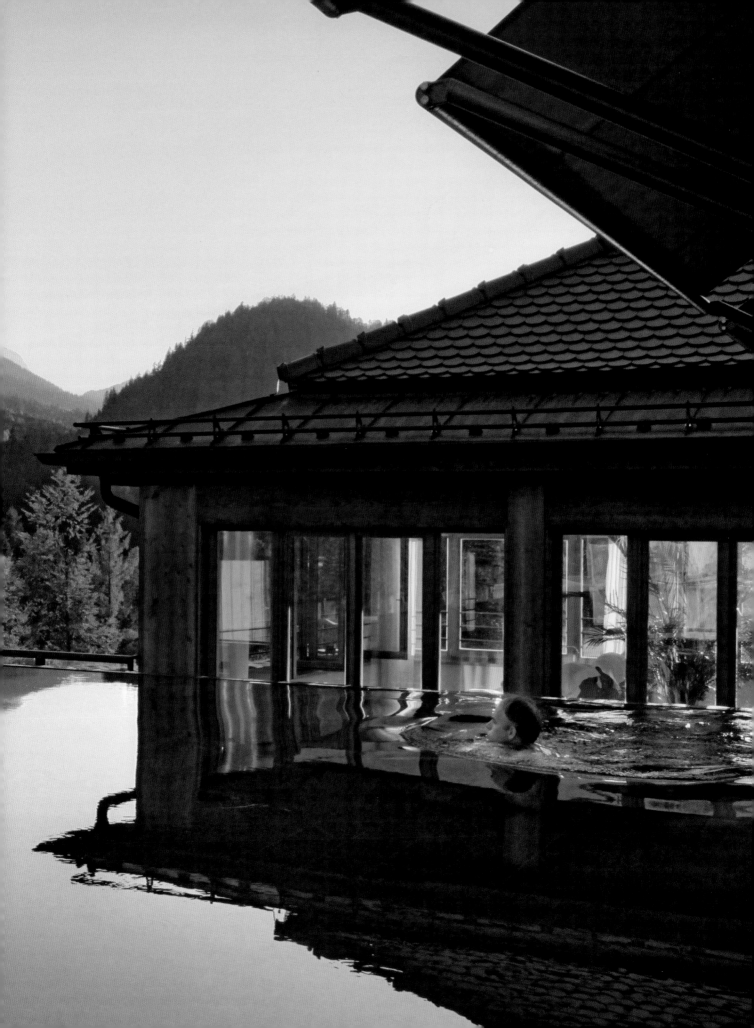

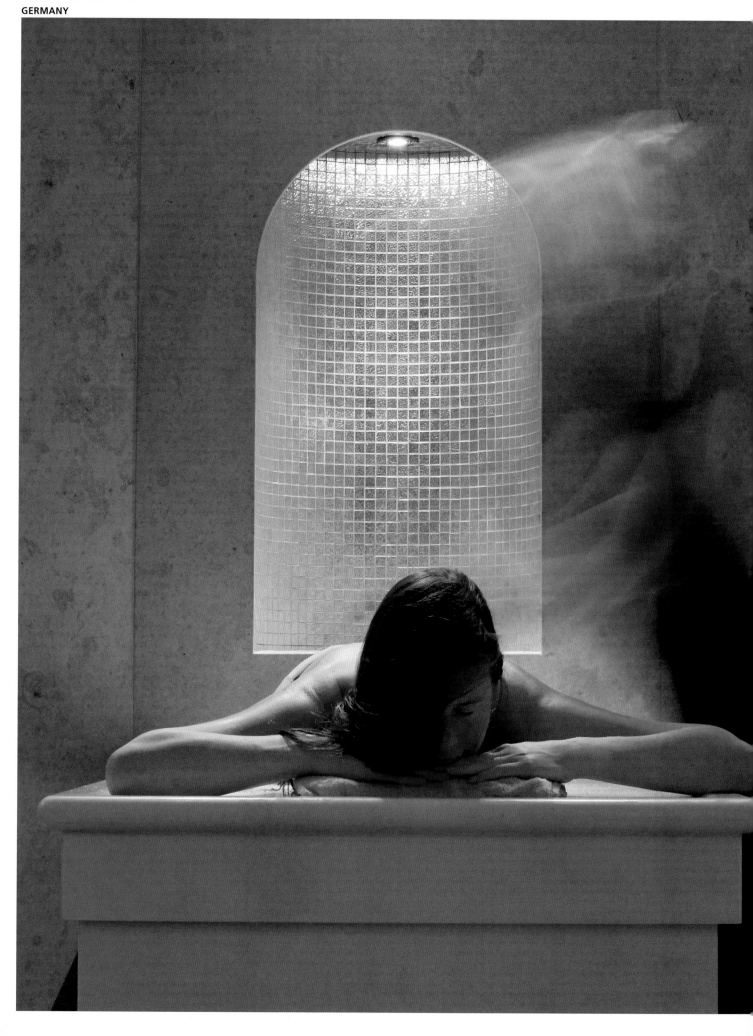

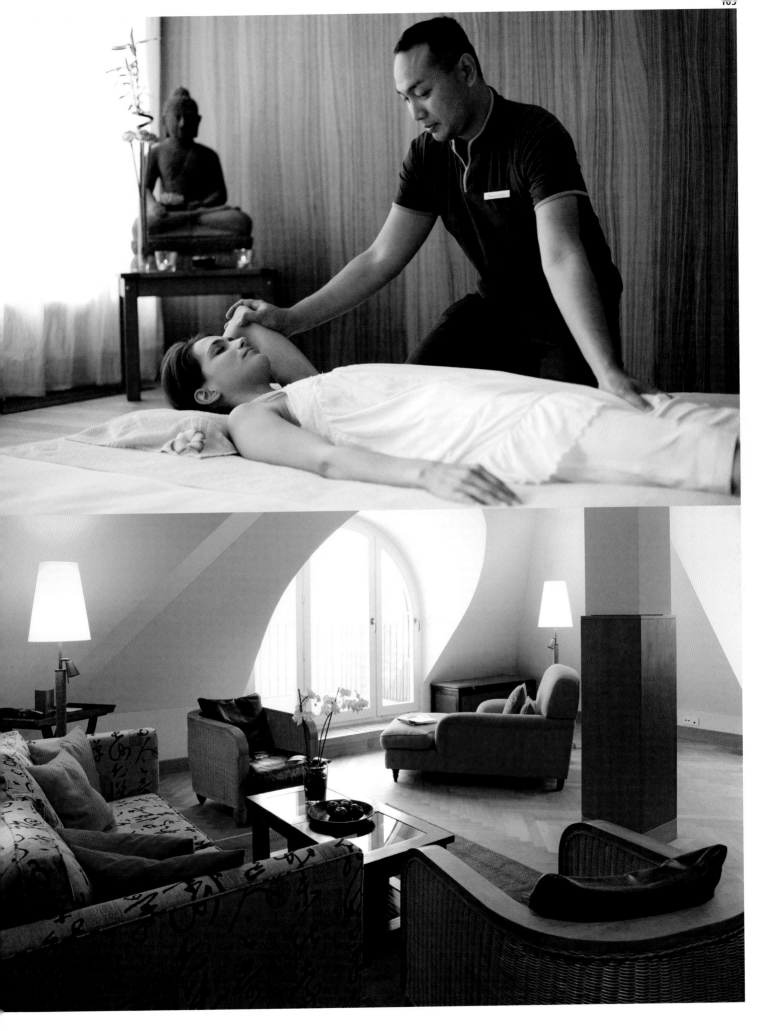

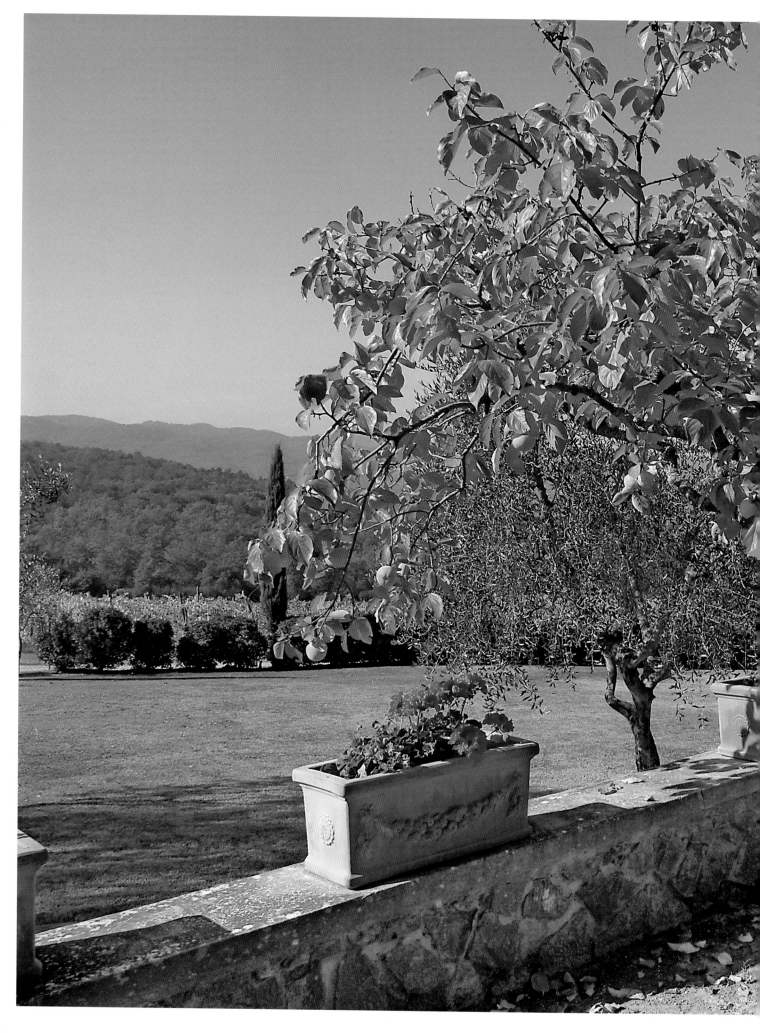

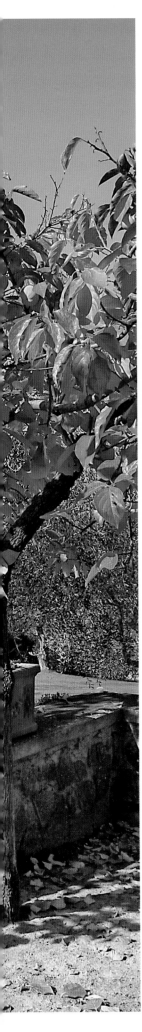

A last look across the vineyards, gently sloping down into the valley in the first light of dawn, and then the eyes are closed for meditation, until the aromas of toast and fresh orange juice announce the end of the extended yoga session. A brisk march lasting several hours, undertaken in silence, through dried-out river beds and hip-high grasses, gorse, myrtle and rose hip bushes, past gnarled shrubs and shady pine forests, in the hills between Arezzo, Siena and Florence further clears the thoughts and sharpens the senses. How intense suddenly is the scent of the rosemary and the wild thyme, the oleander and the lemon trees. Frogs, butterflies, geckos and deer cross the path. At lunch the rescinded vow of silence and a delicious zucchini quiche provide for a lively cheerfulness. Contrary to the example set by "The Ashram" in Malibu, the organiser of Yogahikes, British film producer and yoga fan Ian Flooks, sets great store by good food. A lazy afternoon by the pool, with the silvery olive trees around you and the wide azure sky above, is also tolerated. We are in Italy after all, *Madonna*!

Books to pack: "An Enigma by the Sea" by Carlo Fruttero and Franco Lucentini and "The English Patient" by Michael Ondaatje

Borgo Iesolana

Località Iesolana
52021 Bucine, Tuscany
Italy
Tel. +44 7768 117 413
mail@yogahikes.com
www.yogahikes.com and www.iesolana.it

Directions	From Florence, Pisa or Milan, exit Valdarno on the A1 Florence-Rome in the direction of Montevarchi, at the next intersection continue in the direction of Levane, Bucine and Borgo Iesolana
Yoga	Workshops only through www.yogahikes.com
Teachers	Alexa Harris
Rooms	3 one-bedroom apartments and 16 single-occupancy rooms with bath
Food	Vegetarian; specialities: sautéed mushrooms, aubergine parmigiana, fennel bake
Treatments	Massages
Leisure	2 swimming pools, hill walking, Prada outlet

Noch ein letzter Blick über die im Morgengrauen sanft abfallenden Weinberge hinunter ins Tal – und schon schließen sich die Augen zur Meditation, bis der Geruch nach Toast und frischem Orangensaft das Ende der ausgedehnten Yogastunde ankündigt. Ein mehrstündiger strammer Marsch, schweigend unternommen, durch ausgetrocknete Flussbetten und hüfthohe Gräser, Ginster, Myrte und Hagebuttensträucher, vorbei an knorrigen Büschen und schattigen Pinienwäldern in den Hügeln zwischen Arezzo, Siena und Florenz klärt weiter die Gedanken und schärft die Sinne. Wie stark auf einmal Rosmarin und wilder Thymian duften, der Oleander und die Zitronenbäume. Frösche, Schmetterlinge, Geckos, Rehe kreuzen den Weg. Beim Mittagessen sorgen das aufgehobene Schweigegebot und eine köstliche Zucchini-Quiche für ausgelassene Fröhlichkeit. Anders als beim Vorbild »The Ashram« in Malibu legt der Veranstalter von Yogahikes, der britische Filmproduzent und Yogafan Ian Flooks, größten Wert auf gute Küche. Ein fauler Nachmittag am Pool, die silbrigen Olivenbäume vor sich und darüber der weite azurfarbene Himmel, ist ebenfalls geduldet. Wir sind schließlich in Italien, *Madonna*!

Reisebegleiter: »Das Geheimnis der Pineta« von Carlo Fruttero und Franco Lucentini und »Der englische Patient« von Michael Ondaatje

Un dernier regard, à l'aube naissante, sur les vignobles glissant en pente douce vers la vallée, et déjà les yeux se ferment pour la méditation jusqu'à ce que l'odeur de toast et de jus d'orange frais annonce la fin de la longue séance de yoga. Une marche soutenue de plusieurs heures, effectuée en silence à travers lits de fleuve desséchés et hautes herbes, genêts, myrtes et buissons de cynorhodon, devant les arbustes noueux et les forêts de pins ombragées des collines ondulant entre Arezzo, Sienne et Florence finit d'éclaircir l'esprit en aiguisant les sens. Avec quelle intensité soudaine le romarin et le thym sauvage, les lauriers roses et les citronniers n'embaument-ils pas ! Grenouilles, papillons, geckos et biches croisent le chemin. Pendant le déjeuner, la consigne de silence levée et une délicieuse quiche aux courgettes permettent à une joyeuse convivialité de s'installer. Se démarquant du modèle « The Ashram » à Malibu, l'organisateur de Yogahikes Ian Flooks, producteur de films britannique et adepte du yoga, attache la plus grande importance à une cuisine raffinée. De même, un après-midi à se prélasser au bord de la piscine, les oliviers argentés devant soi et l'immense ciel bleu azur au-dessus, peut être envisagé. Après tout, nous sommes dans la « bella Italia » !

Livres à emporter : « Place de Sienne, coté ombre » de Carlo Fruttero et Franco Lucentini et « Le Patient anglais » de Michael Ondaatje

Anreise	Von Florenz, Pisa oder Mailand, Ausfahrt Valdarno auf der A1 Florenz–Rom, Richtung Montevarchi, an der nächsten Kreuzung Richtung Levane, Bucine und Borgo Iesolana
Yoga	Nur Workshops über www.yogahikes.com
Lehrer	Alexa Harris
Zimmer	3 Einzimmerapartments und 16 Einzelzimmer mit Bad
Küche	Vegetarisch, Spezialitäten: sautierte Pilze, Auberginen parmigiana, Fenchelauflauf
Anwendungen	Massagen
Aktivitäten	Bergwandern, 2 Pools, Prada-Outlet

Accès	Venant de Florence, Pise ou Milan, sortie Valdarno sur l'A1 Florence-Rome, direction Montevarchi, au prochain carrefour, direction Levane, Bucine und Borgo Iesolana
Yoga	Stages uniquement via www.yogahikes.com
Professeurs	Alexa Harris
Chambres	3 suites d'une chambre et 16 chambres individuelles avec salle de bain
Restauration	Végétarienne, spécialités : champignons sautés à la poêle, aubergines au parmesan, gratin de fenouil
Traitements	Massages
Activités	Randonnées en montagne, 2 piscines, espace Prada

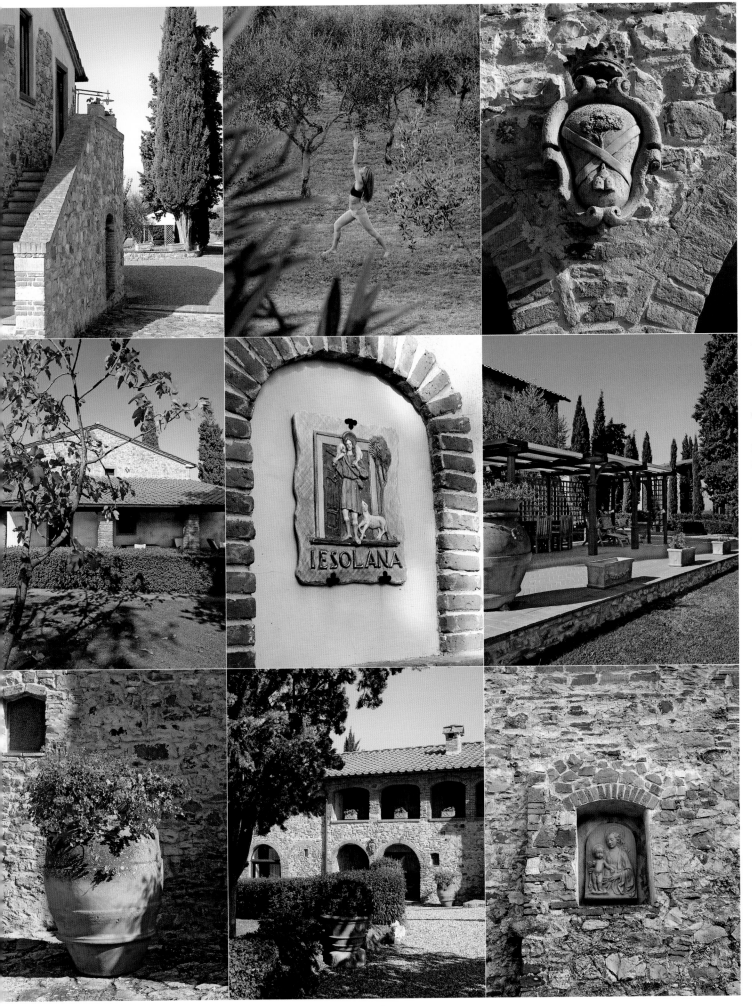

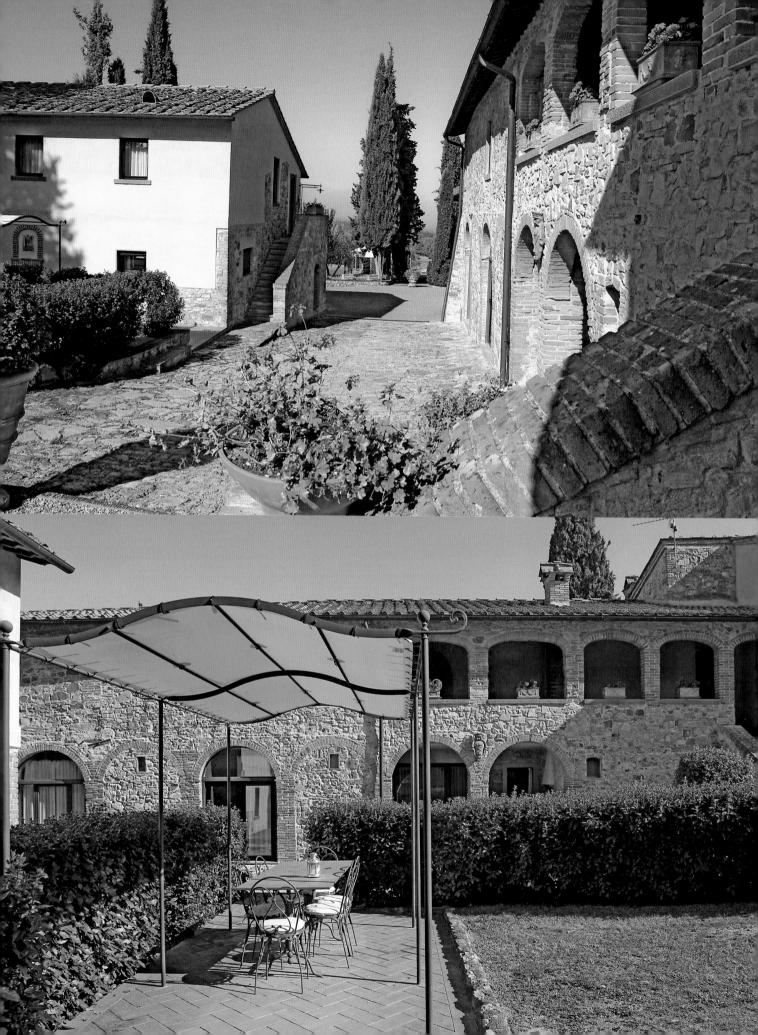

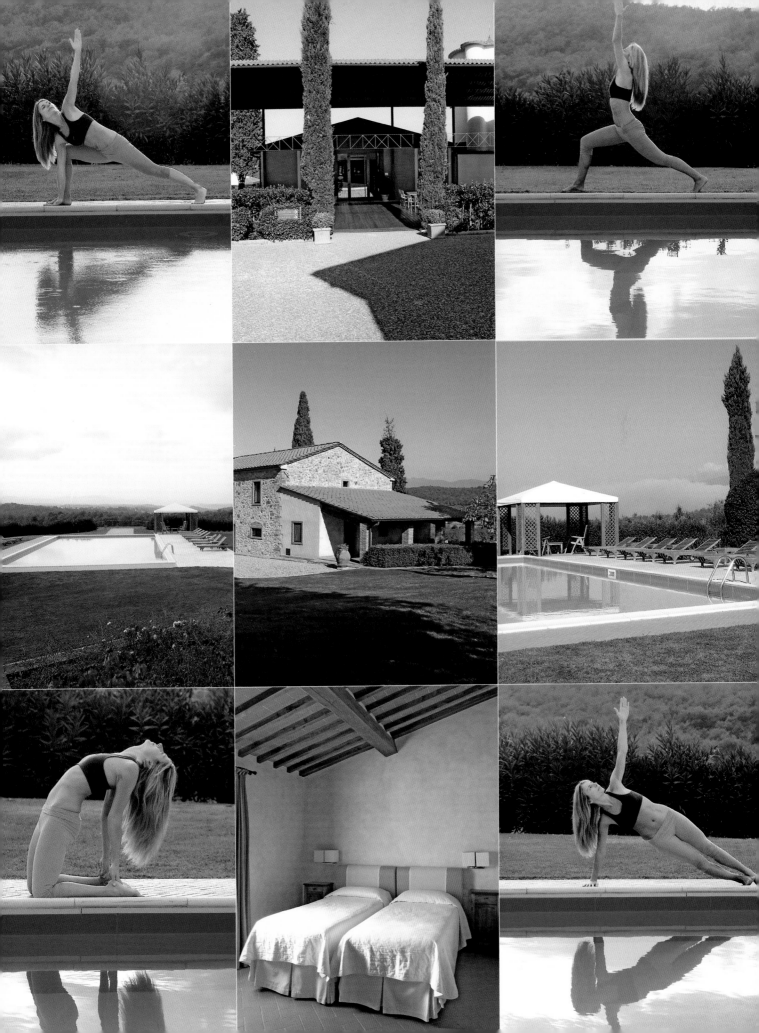

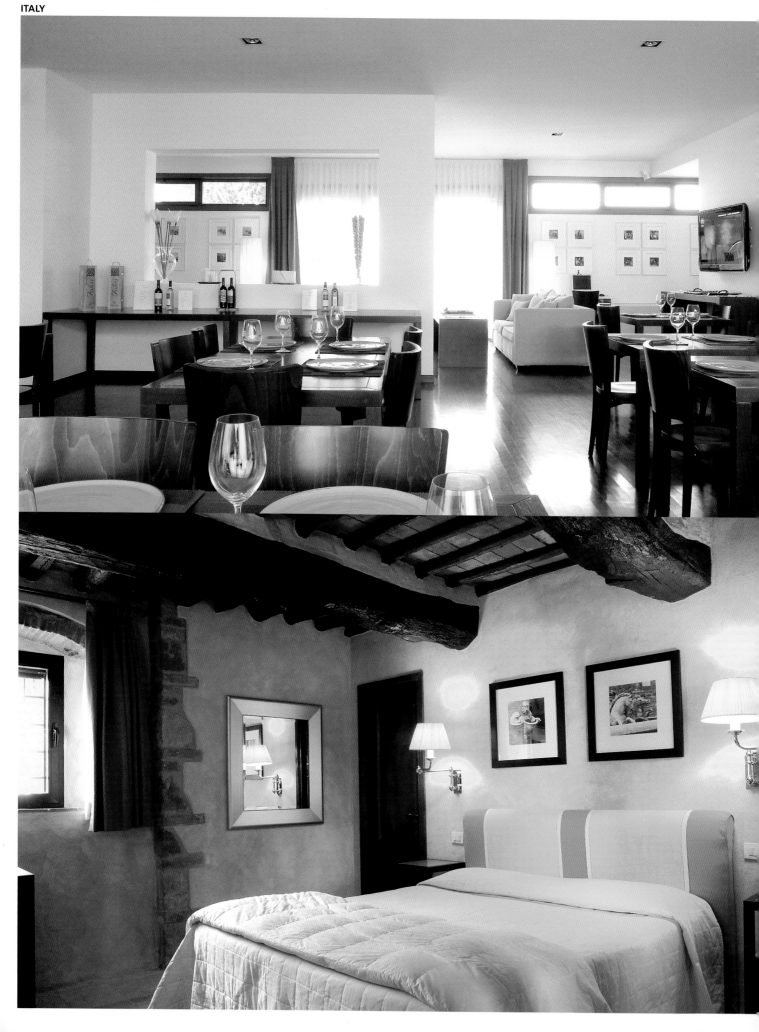

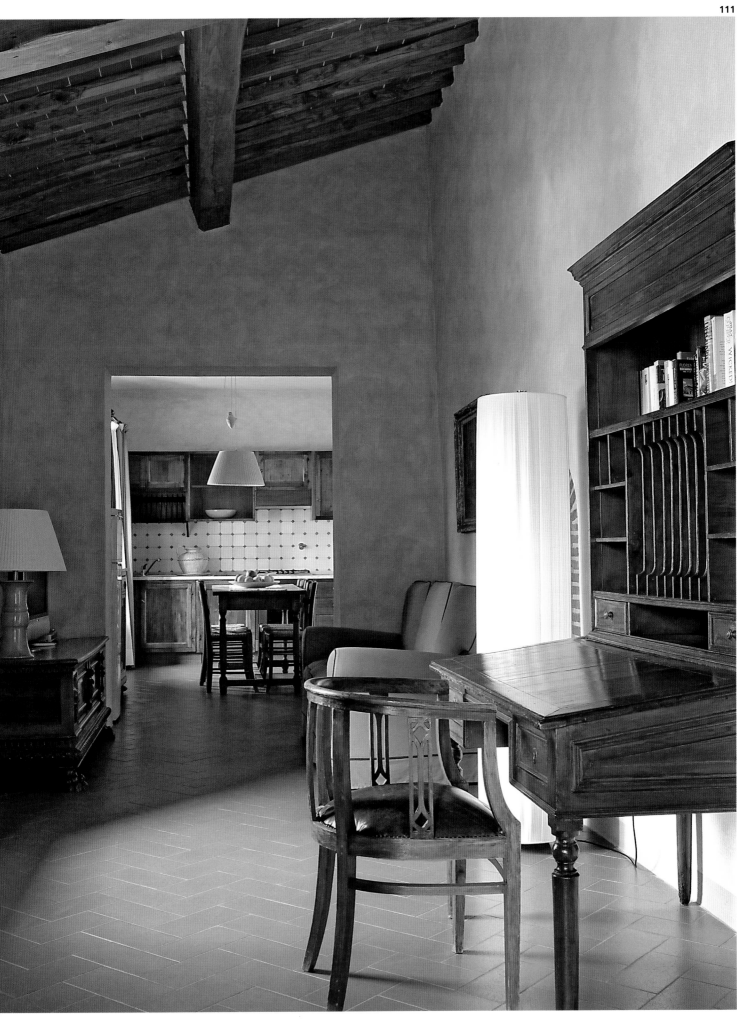

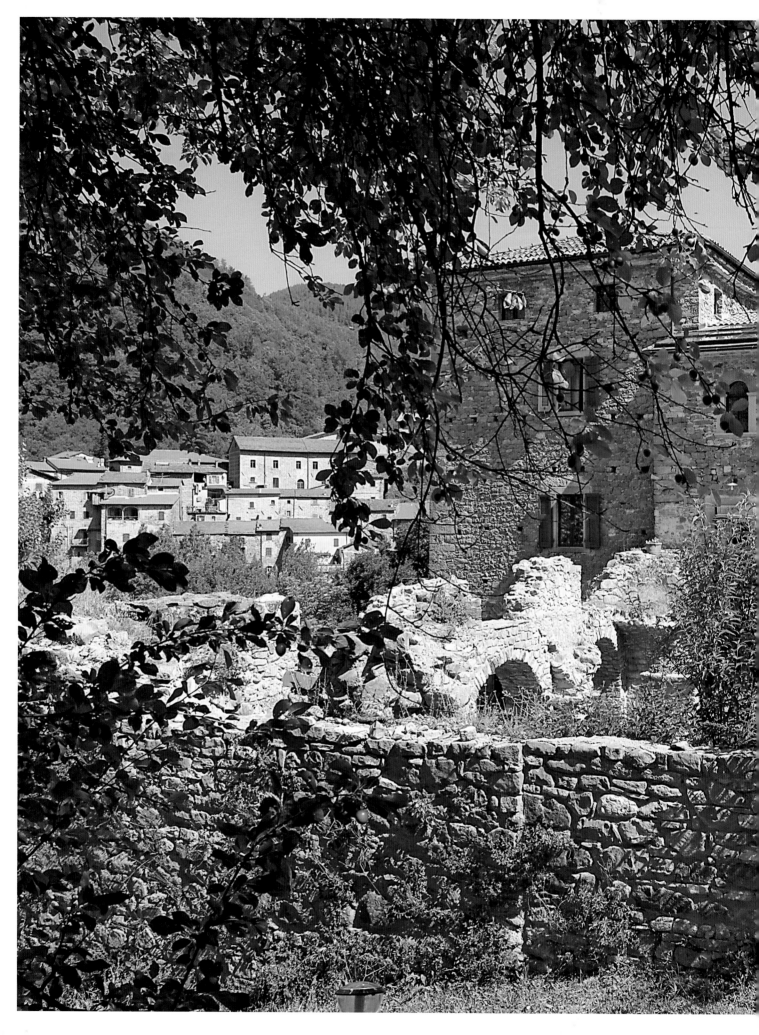

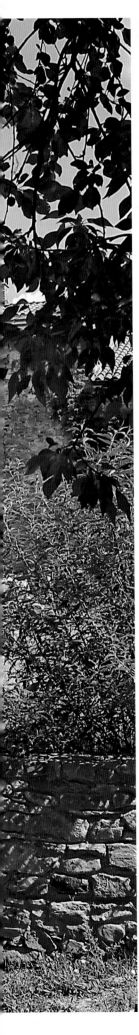

When a dancer and a meditating Marxist look for a place to stay together, a former convent is really the only thing that fits the bill. Il Convento, built in 1549, accommodated the nuns of Santa Marta for over three centuries. St Martha is the patron saint of housekeeping and often depicted with cooking utensils and a bunch of keys, but she is also responsible for painters and sculptors. Lunigiana, an area of countryside between Parma and Florence as yet little developed for tourism, captivates through its green hills, vineyards, endless chestnut forests, olive groves and river sources, the mountain pasture of the Apennines and the peaks of the Apuan Alps on the horizon. Time and time again, friends and relations lent money to the couple, who brought up their children here, until from the half-dilapidated masonry a charming place of retreat emerged. In the vault of the former wine cellar, yoga is now practised; guests sleep in simple whitewashed rooms and read by the fireplace. The overall impression is still somewhat monastic, but in compensation the view into the valley is anything but restrained, and the cuisine is sensually Italian. You can, by the way, also find accommodation as a working guest and participate intellectually and materially, directly or indirectly in this small family's big project to create a place of peace and contemplation. But don't worry: the sisters of Santa Marta are sure to have giggled on occasion, too.

Books to pack: "The Name of the Rose" by Umberto Eco and "The Palace" by Lisa St. Aubin de Terán

Il Convento

Casola in Lunigiana, 54014
Italy
Tel. +39 585 900 75
Fax +39 585 900 75
convento.seminar@tin.it
www.il-convento.net

Directions	Il Convento in Casola lies 2 hrs north of Florence Airport
Yoga	Vinyasa, Iyengar, Satyananda, Vedanta Philosophy, Meditation, Lord Vishnu's Couch, Sunrise Yoga, Dream Journeys
Rooms	15 rooms for max. 35 guests
Food	The vegetarian menu is inspired by regional Tuscan cuisine, and the use of fresh herbs makes each meal a colorful event; with each meal, wine and fresh spring water are served
Leisure	Meditation, hiking

Wenn eine Tänzerin und ein meditierender Marxist zusammen eine Bleibe suchen, kann eigentlich nichts anderes herauskommen als ein ehemaliges Kloster. Il Convento, 1549 gebaut, beherbergte über drei Jahrhunderte den Frauenorden Santa Marta, der heiligen Martha, die als Patronin der Häuslichkeit gerne mit Kochgerät und Schlüsselbund dargestellt wird, aber auch für Maler und Bildhauer zuständig ist. Die Lunigiana, eine touristisch noch wenig erschlossene Landschaft zwischen Parma und Florenz, besticht durch ihre grünen Hügel, Weinberge, endlosen Kastanienwälder, Olivenhaine und Quellflüsse – am Horizont die Bergwiesen des Appenins und die Gipfel der Apuanischen Alpen. Freunde und Verwandte haben dem Paar, das hier seine Kinder aufzog, immer wieder Geld geliehen, bis aus dem halb verfallenen Gemäuer ein bezaubernder Ort des Rückzugs wurde. Im Gewölbe des ehemaligen Weinkellers wird jetzt Yoga geübt, in weiß gekalkten, schlichten Zimmern wird geschlafen, am Kaminfeuer gelesen. Die gesamte Anmutung ist noch immer etwas klösterlich, dafür ist der Blick ins Tal alles andere als zurückhaltend und die Küche sinnlich italienisch. Man kann übrigens auch als Working Guest unterkommen und sich gedanklich und materiell, direkt oder indirekt beteiligen am großen Lebensprojekt der kleinen Familie, einen Ort der Ruhe und Selbstbesinnung zu schaffen. Aber keine Angst: Die Schwestern von Santa Marta haben sicher auch gelegentlich gekichert.

Reisebegleiter: »Der Name der Rose« von Umberto Eco und »Der Palast« von Lisa St. Aubin de Terán

Quand une danseuse et un marxiste épris de méditation cherchent ensemble un logis, il ne peut s'agir que d'un ancien cloître. Il Convento, construit en 1549, hébergea pendant plus de trois siècles l'ordre religieux féminin Santa Marta, de sainte Marthe patronne des foyers, souvent représentée munie d'ustensiles de cuisine et d'un trousseau de clés, également patronne des peintres et sculpteurs. La Lunigiane, région encore peu ouverte aux touristes entre Parme et Florence, séduit par ses vertes collines, ses vignobles, ses infinies forêts de châtaigniers, ses bosquets d'oliviers, ses sources jaillissantes, et, à l'horizon, les prairies de l'Appenin et les sommets des Alpes apuanes. Des amis et parents ont régulièrement prêté de l'argent au couple, qui a élevé ses enfants ici, jusqu'à ce que ces murs en ruine se transforment en un lieu de retraite envoûtant. Sous la voûte de l'ancien cellier ont lieu désormais des séances de yoga, les austères chambres blanchies à la chaux invitent au sommeil, les feux de cheminée à la lecture. Si l'atmosphère générale est restée quelque peu monastique, le panorama de la vallée est des plus vastes et la cuisine italienne succulente à souhait. De plus, il est possible d'y séjourner en tant que working guest, en participant sur le plan spirituel et matériel, directement ou indirectement, au grand projet d'ensemble de la petite famille : créer un lieu de paix et de recueillement. Mais n'ayez crainte : il est sûrement arrivé aussi aux religieuses de sainte Marthe de rire en douce.

Livres à emporter : « Le Nom de la rose » d'Umberto Eco et « The Palace » de Lisa St. Aubin de Terán

Anreise	Il Convento in Casola liegt 2 Std. nördlich des Flughafens Florenz
Yoga	Vinyasa, Iyengar, Satyananda, Vedanta Philosophy, Meditation, Lord Vishnu's Couch, Sunrise Yoga, Yogatraumreisen
Zimmer	15 Zimmer für max. 35 Gäste
Küche	Vegetarische Mahlzeiten – ein farbenfrohes Ereignis, mit frischen Kräutern, inspiriert von der regionalen toskanischen Küche; zum Essen wird Landwein und frisches Quellwasser serviert
Aktivitäten	Meditation, Wandern

Accès	Il Convento in Casola est à 2h au nord de l'aéroport de Florence
Yoga	Vinyasa, Iyengar, Satyananda, philosophie Vedanta, méditation, méditation du Seigneur Vishnu, Yoga de l'aube, voyage onirique par le yoga
Chambres	15 chambres pour 35 hôtes max.
Restauration	Le menu végétarien s'inspire de la cuisine toscane et l'utilisation d'herbes fraîches fait de chaque plat un évenement coloré ; les repas sont accompagnés de vin et d'eau de source
Activités	Méditation, randonnées

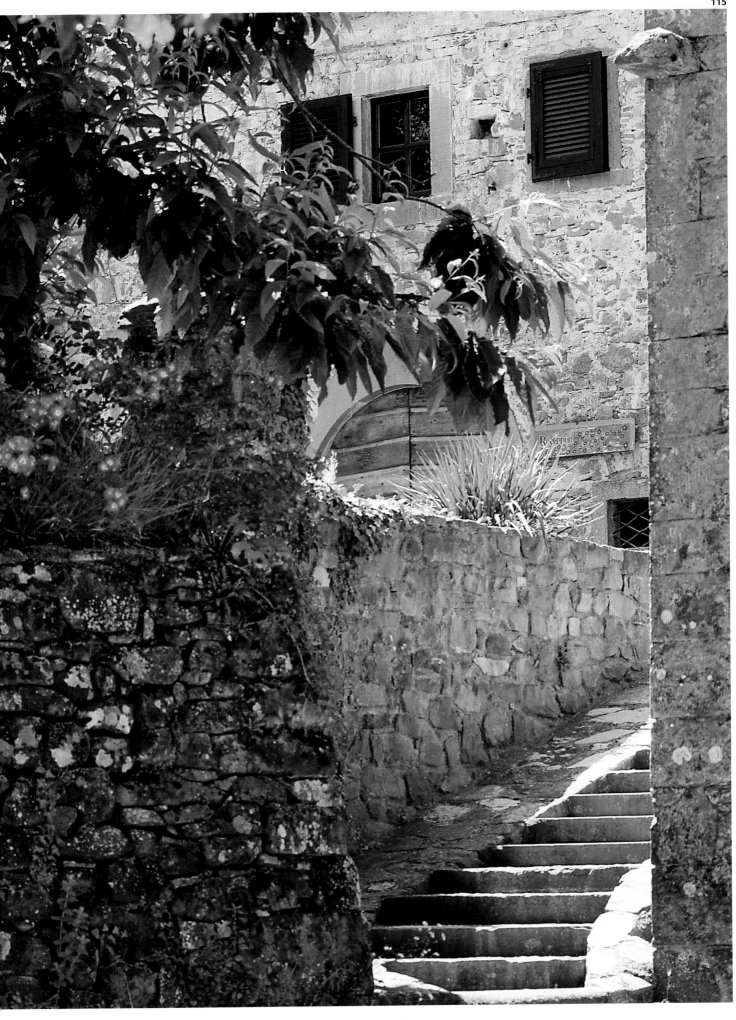

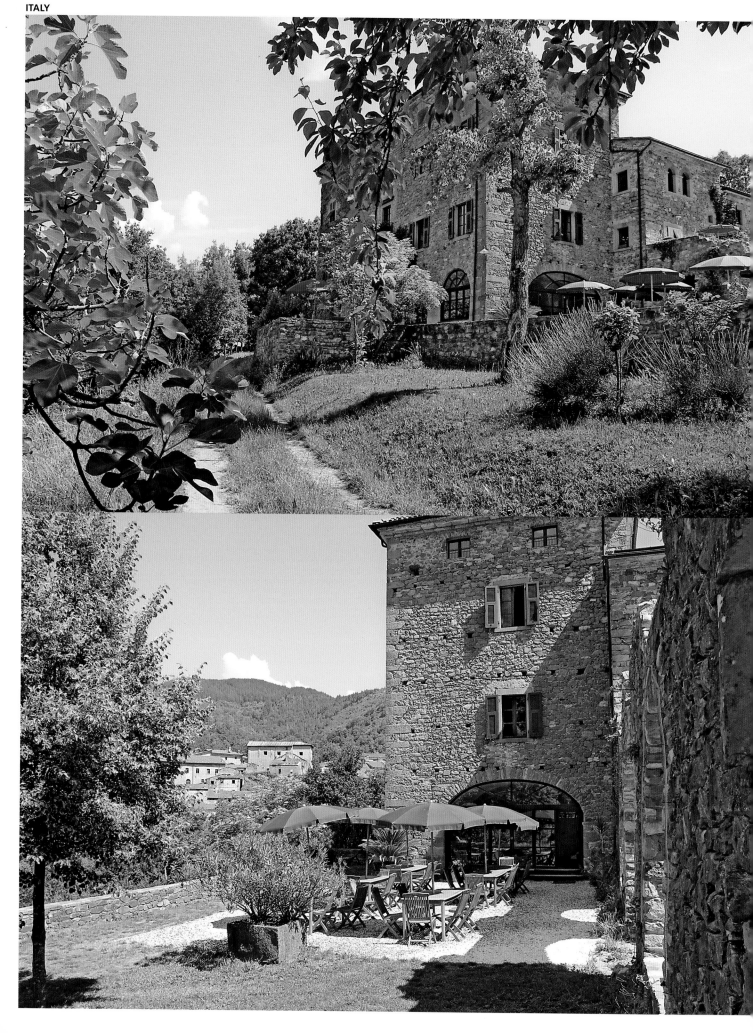

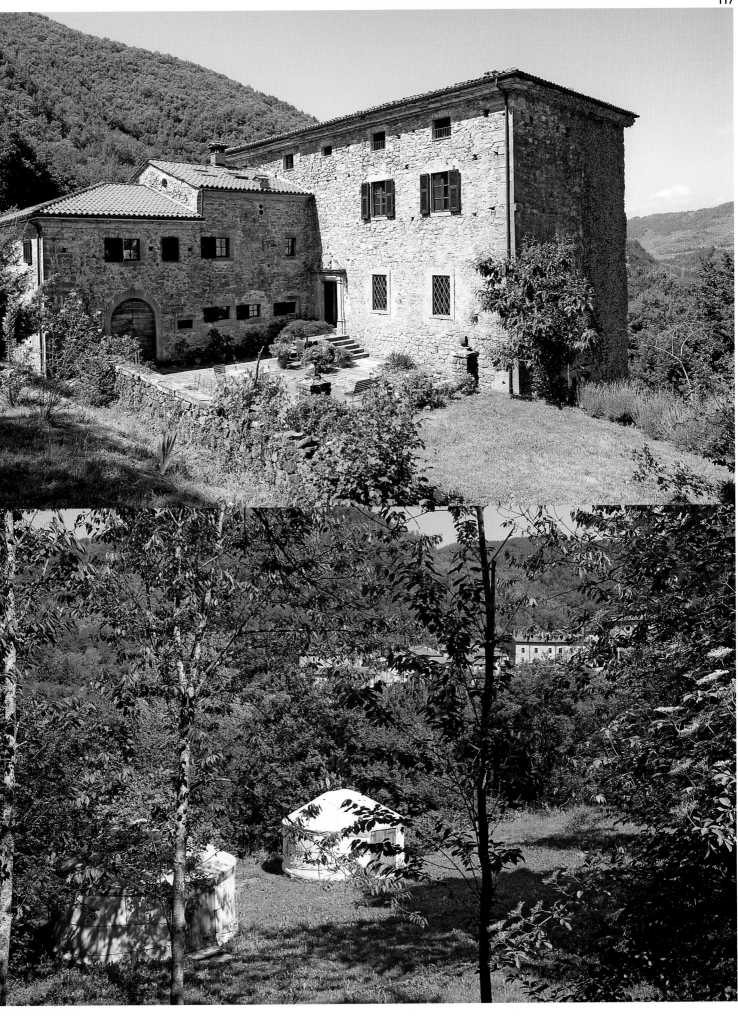

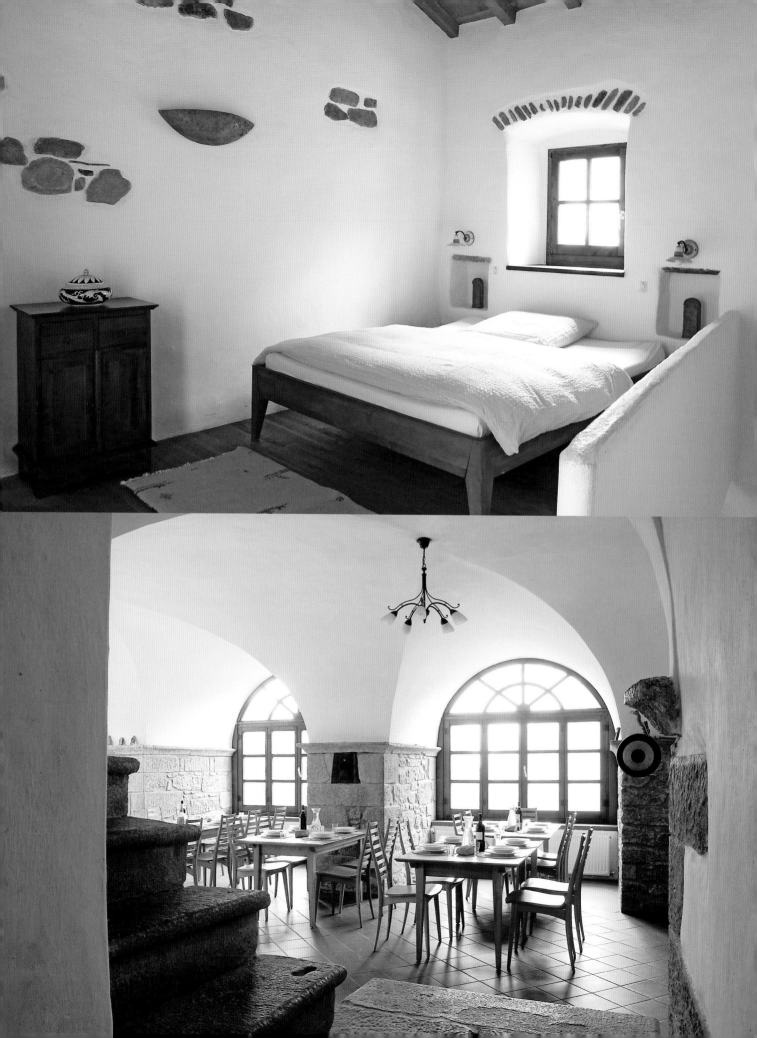

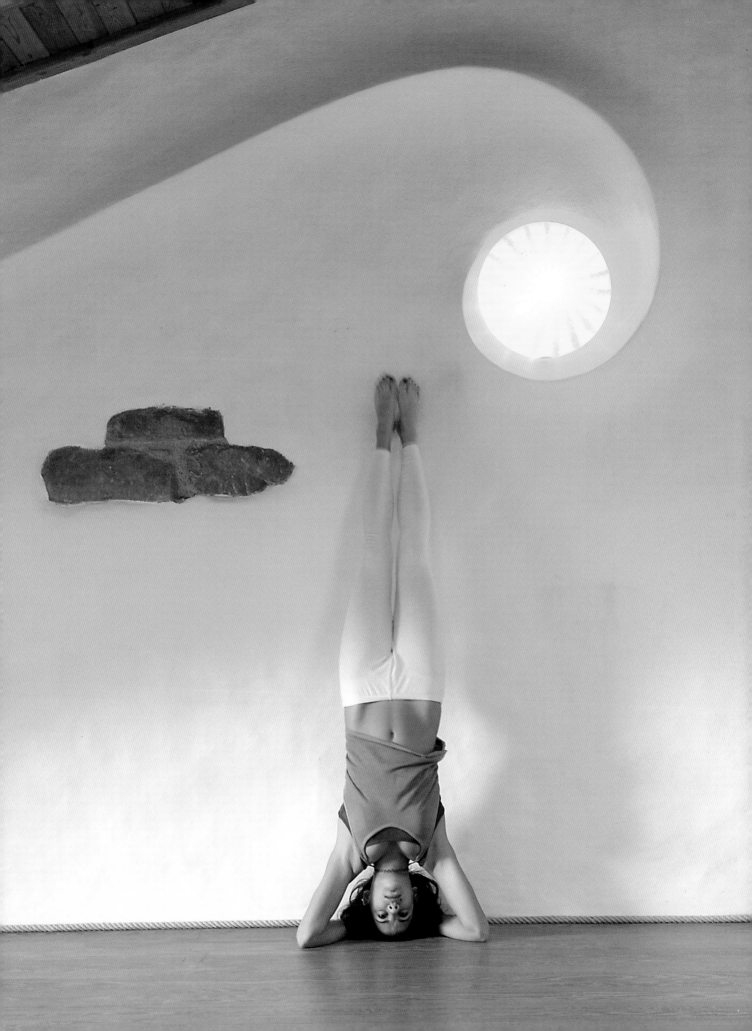

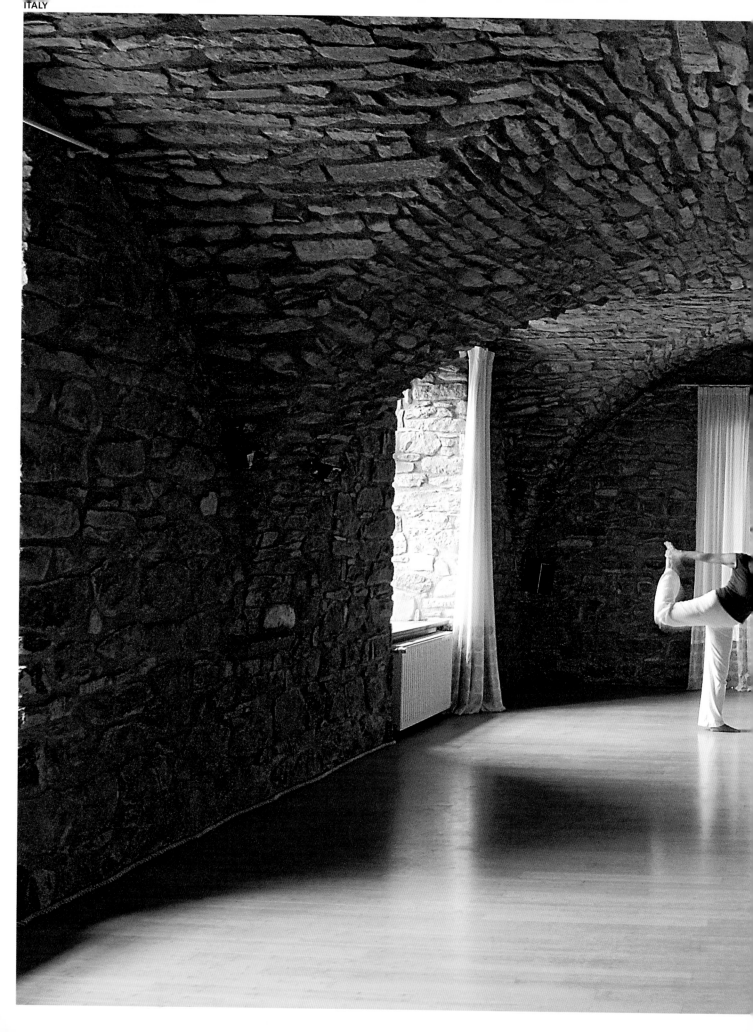

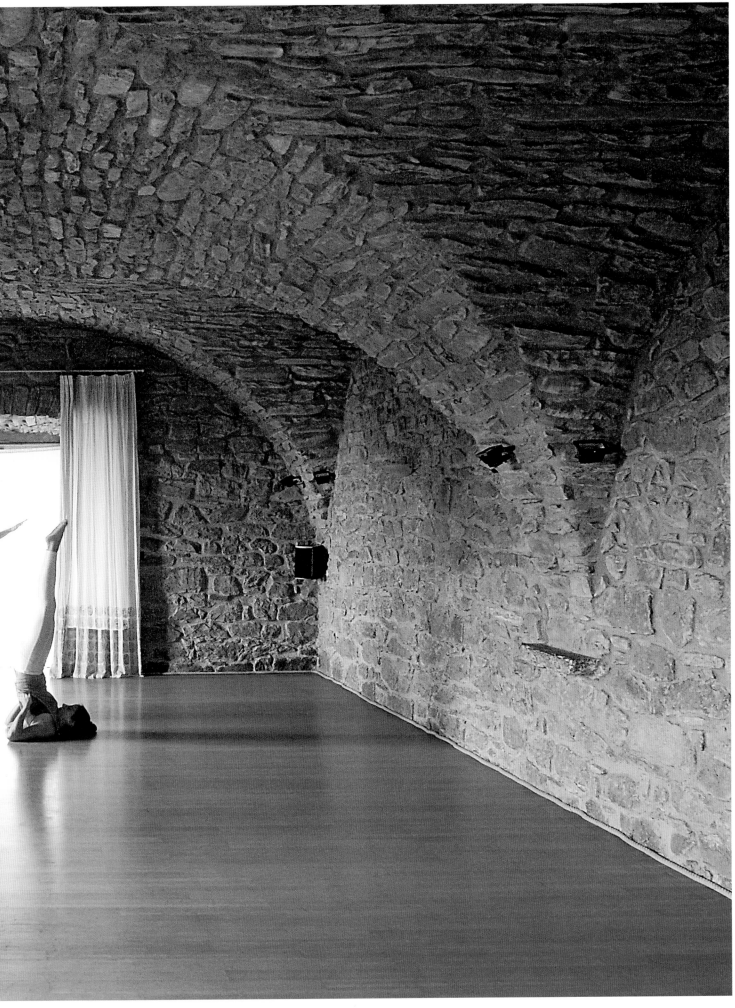

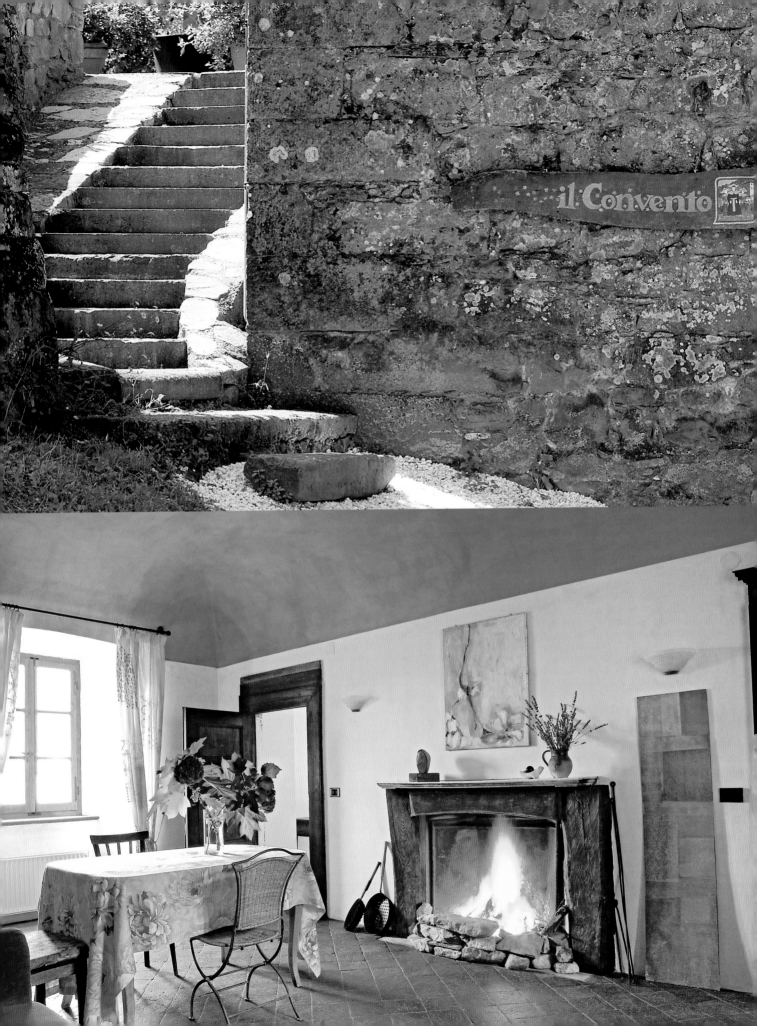

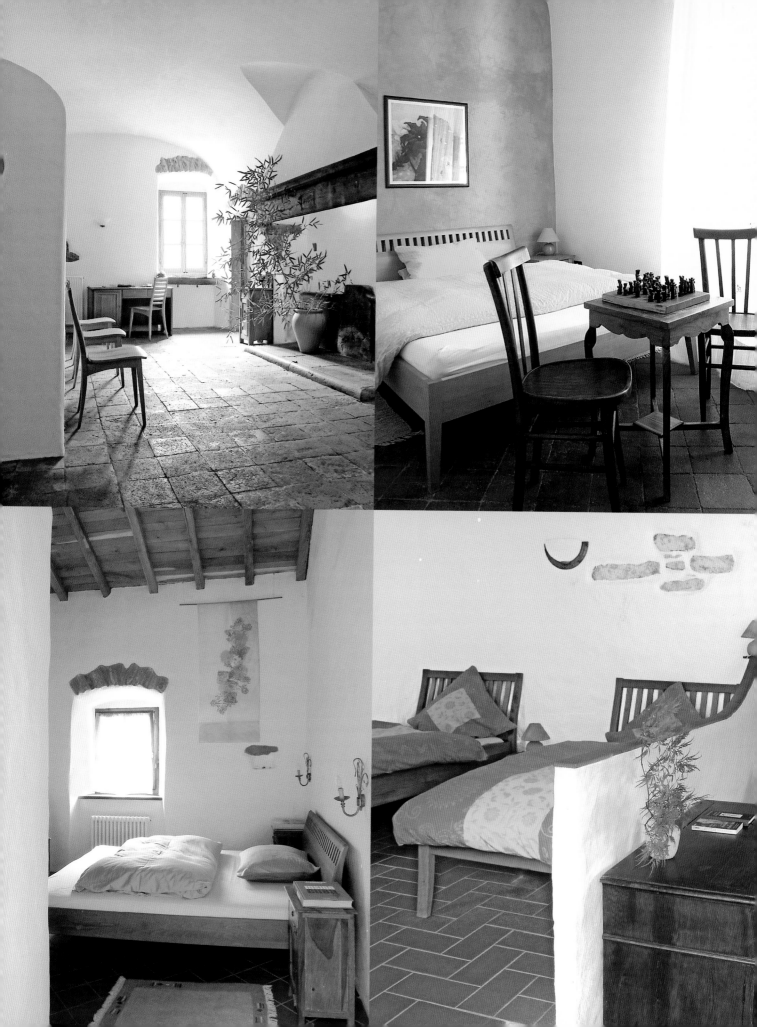

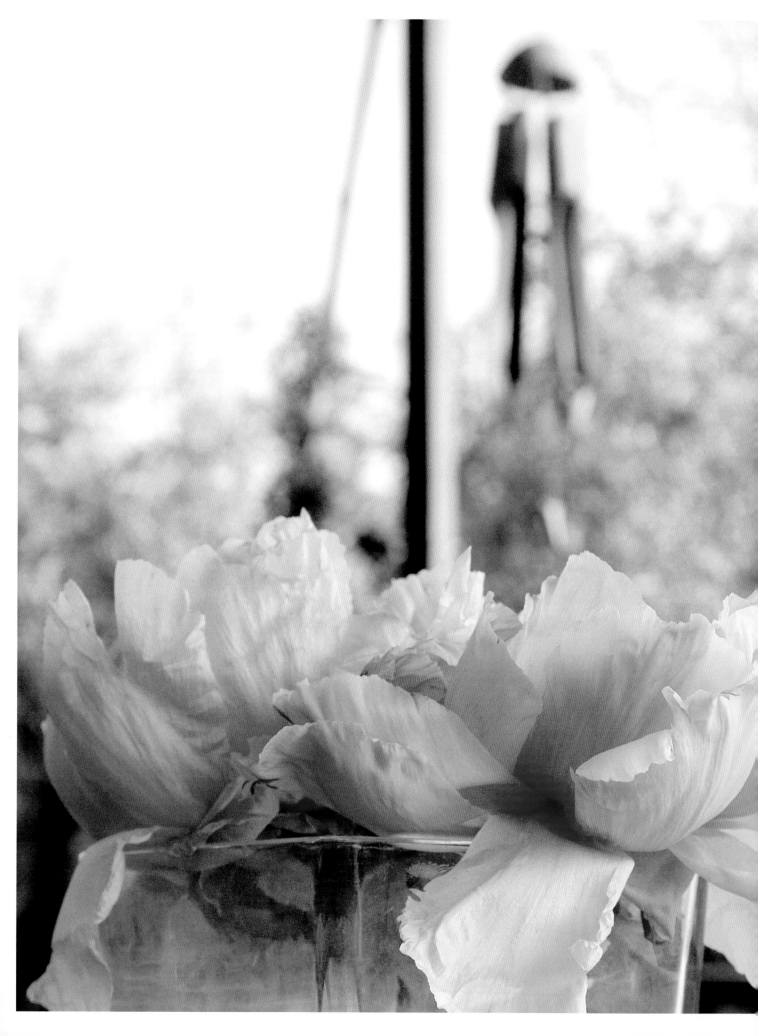

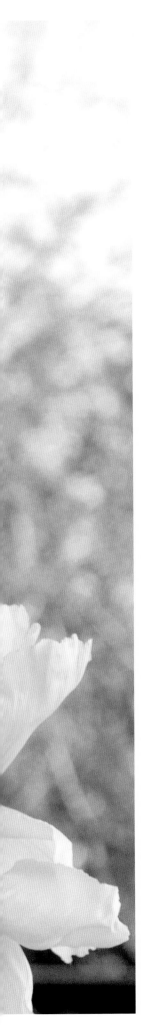

If Rome is the Eternal City, then In Sabina, less than an hour away, has even more of a claim to eternity. Because that's how long you would like to stay within these old 17th-century walls. Located not far from the medieval village of Torri in Sabina between olive groves and fruit trees, from each of the three terraces there is an amazing view of the sunset that stirs even the most unshakable of yogis. Simply and lovingly furnished inside, hammocks and loungers at the pool, a richly laid table in the garden and even a cinema screen in the open air for occasional evening entertainment turn this place into a second home that makes you forget the passing time. The yoga deck, in the midst of the greenery, is protected from the sun by a light, white canvas. yoga arises from the observation of nature, as Patañjali said more than two millennia ago. Another reason to transform yourself into Vrksasana, the tree, and hope that you can stay an eternity.

Books to pack: "One Last Ride on the Merry-Go-Round" by Tiziano Terzani and "Invisible Cities" by Italo Calvino

In Sabina

Via Pizzuti 53
Torri in Sabina Rieti, 02049
Italy
Tel. +39 340 387 6028
www.insabina.com

Directions	47 miles north of Rome, 1 1/2 hrs away from Rome Airport
Yoga	Ashtanga, Sivananda, Iyengar, Scaravelli, Jivamukti, Anusara
Teachers	Glenn Ceresoli, John Stirk, Gingi Lee, Heather Elton
Rooms	1–3-bed rooms for max. 22 people
Food	Organic cuisine with self-grown produce
Treatments	Massages in specially built tree-house
Leisure	Day trips to Orvieto, Assisi, Spoleto and Rome, and to the hot springs of Viterbo; hiking and horseback riding

Wenn Rom die Ewige Stadt ist, dann hat In Sabina, weniger als eine Stunde entfernt, erst Recht Anspruch auf Ewigkeit. So lange möchte man nämlich bleiben in diesen alten Gemäuern aus dem 17. Jahrhundert. Nicht weit von dem mittelalterlichen Dorf Torri in Sabina, zwischen Olivenhainen und Obstbäumen gelegen, hat man von jeder der drei Terrassen einen umwerfenden Blick auf Sonnenuntergänge, die selbst den unerschütterlichsten Yogi rühren. Schlichte, liebevolle Ausstattung im Inneren, Hängematten und Liegestühle am Pool, eine reich gedeckte Tafel im Garten und sogar eine Kinoleinwand im Freien für gelegentliche Abendunterhaltungen machen diesen Platz zu einem Zuhause, das einen die Zeit vergessen lässt. Das mitten ins Grüne gebaute Yoga-Deck wird von einem luftigen weißen Segel gegen die Sonne geschützt. Yoga entsteht aus der Beobachtung der Natur, sagte Patañjali vor über 2000 Jahren. Ein Grund mehr, sich in Vrksasana, den Baum, zu verwandeln und zu hoffen, dass man bleiben darf.

Reisebegleiter: »Noch eine Runde auf dem Karussell: Vom Leben und Sterben« von Tiziano Terzani und »Die unsichtbaren Städte« von Italo Calvino

Si Rome est la Ville éternelle, In Sabina, située à moins d'une heure, peut légitimement prétendre à l'éternité. Car on aimerait rester pour toujours entre ces vieux murs du 17e siècle. A proximité du village médiéval de Torri in Sabina entre les bosquets d'oliviers et les arbres fruitiers, on a, de chacune des trois terrasses, une vue époustouflante sur des couchers de soleil qui émeuvent même le yogi le plus inébranlable. Un intérieur simple, aménagé avec amour, des hamacs et des chaises longues au bord de la piscine, une table copieusement garnie dans le jardin et même un écran de cinéma pour les soirées en plein air donnent à celui qui séjourne ici et oublie le temps, l'impression d'être chez soi. La plate-forme de yoga bâtie dans la verdure est protégée du soleil par une voile blanche aérienne. Le yoga naît de l'observation de la nature, a dit Patañjali il y a plus de 2000 ans. Raison de plus pour se métamorphoser en arbre, en Vrksasana, et espérer qu'on pourra rester.

Livres à emporter : « Un autre tour de manège » de Tiziano Terzani et « Les Villes invisibles » d'Italo Calvino

Anreise	75 km nördlich von Rom, 1,5 Std. vom Flughafen Rom entfernt
Yoga	Ashtanga, Sivananda, Iyengar, Scaravelli, Jivamukti, Anusara
Lehrer	Glenn Ceresoli, John Stirk, Gingi Lee, Heather Elton
Zimmer	Ein- bis Dreibettzimmer für max. 22 Personen
Küche	Biologische Küche mit Produkten aus eigenem Anbau
Anwendungen	Massagen im eigens gebauten Baumhaus
Aktivitäten	Ausflüge nach Orvieto, Assisi, Spoleto und Rom, zu den heißen Quellen von Viterbo; Wandern und Reiten

Accès	Situé à 75 km au nord de Rome, à 1 h 30 de l'aéroport de Rome
Yoga	Ashtânga, Sivananda, Iyengar, Scaravelli, Jivamukti, Anusara
Professeurs	Glenn Ceresoli, John Stirk, Gingi Lee, Heather Elton
Chambres	Chambres de 1 à 3 lits pour 22 personnes max.
Restauration	Cuisine bio à base de produits cultivés sur place
Traitements	Massages dans la maison-arbre spécialement conçue
Activités	Excursions à Orvieto, Assise, Spolète et Rome, aux sources chaudes de Viterbe ; randonnées et équitation

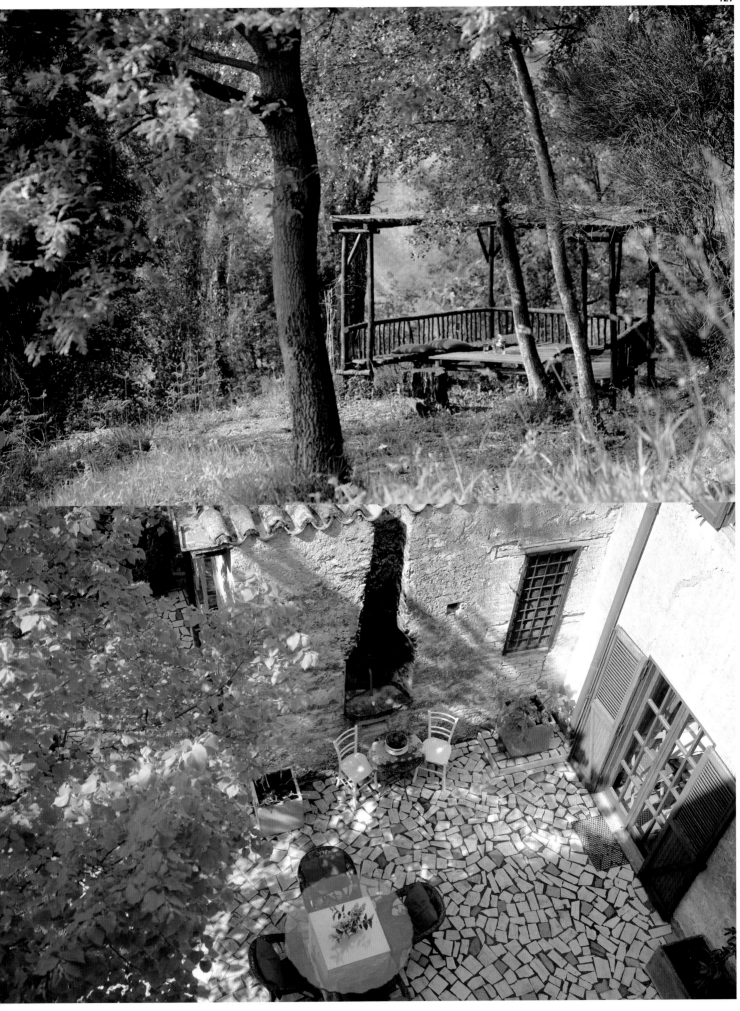

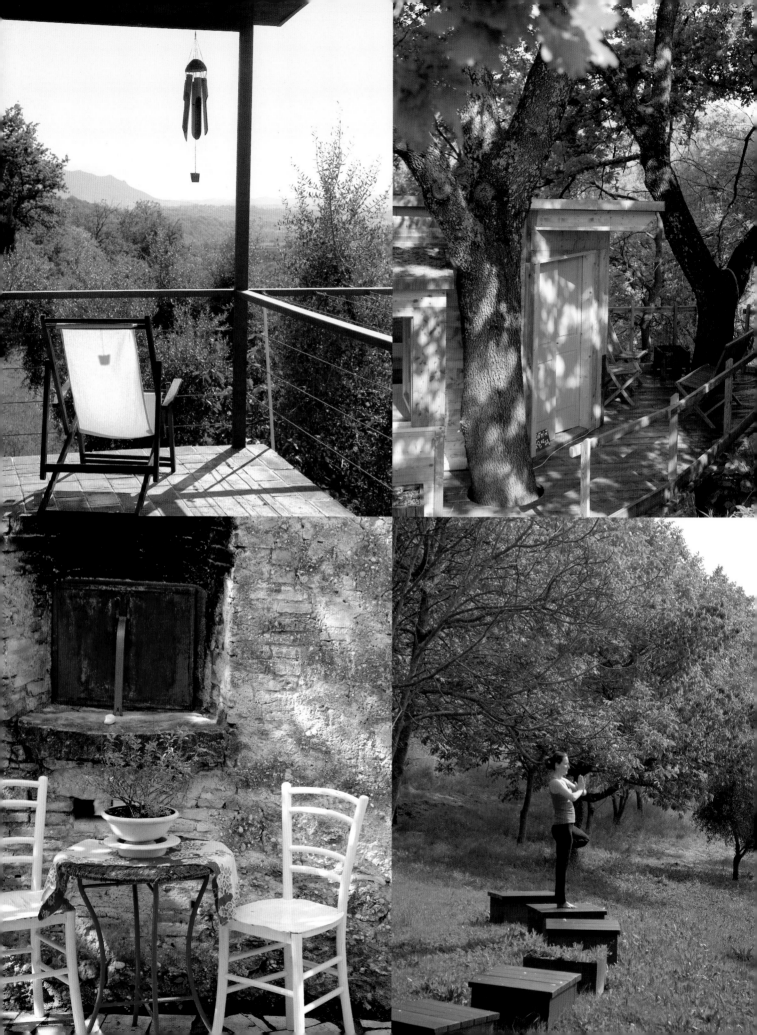

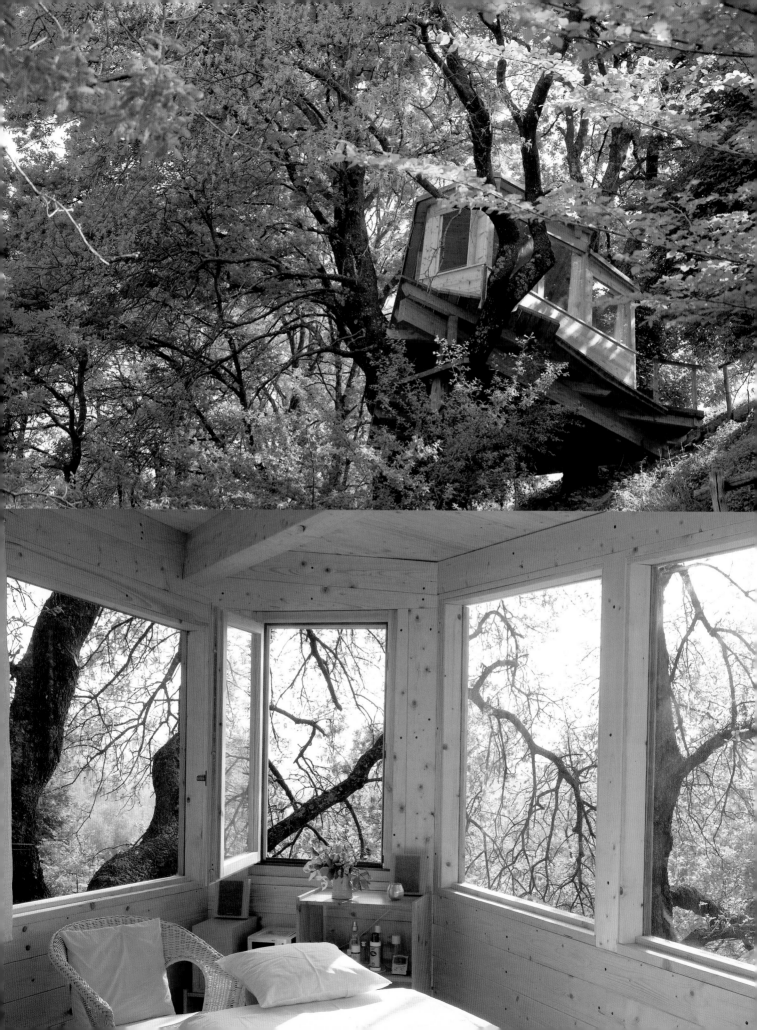

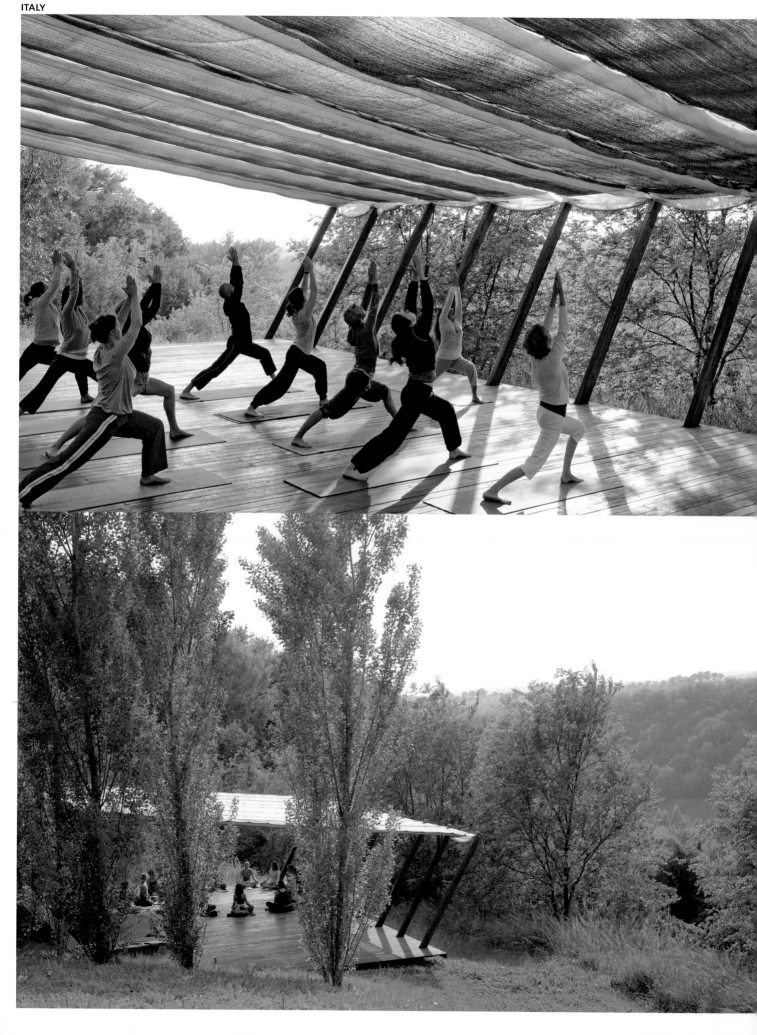

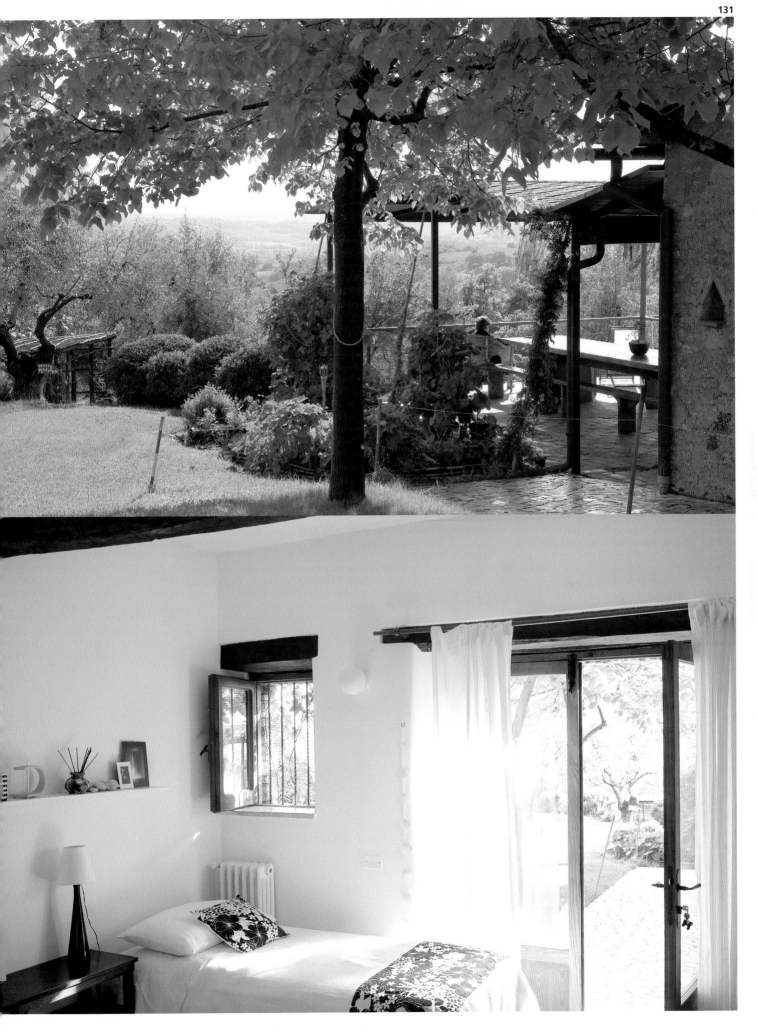

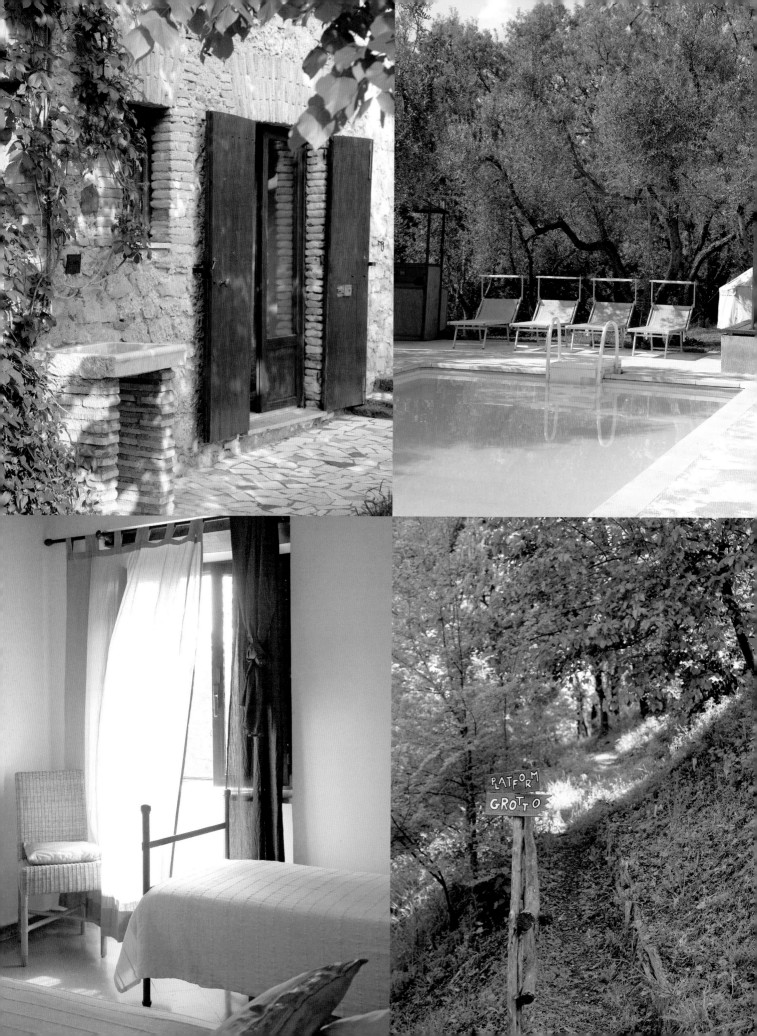

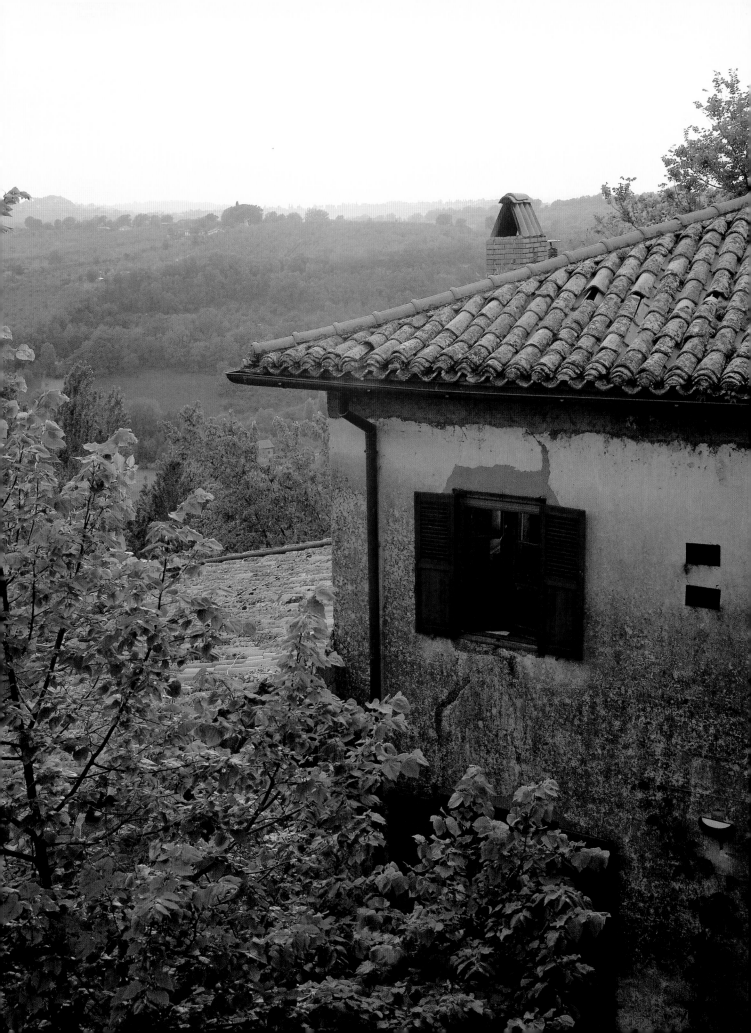

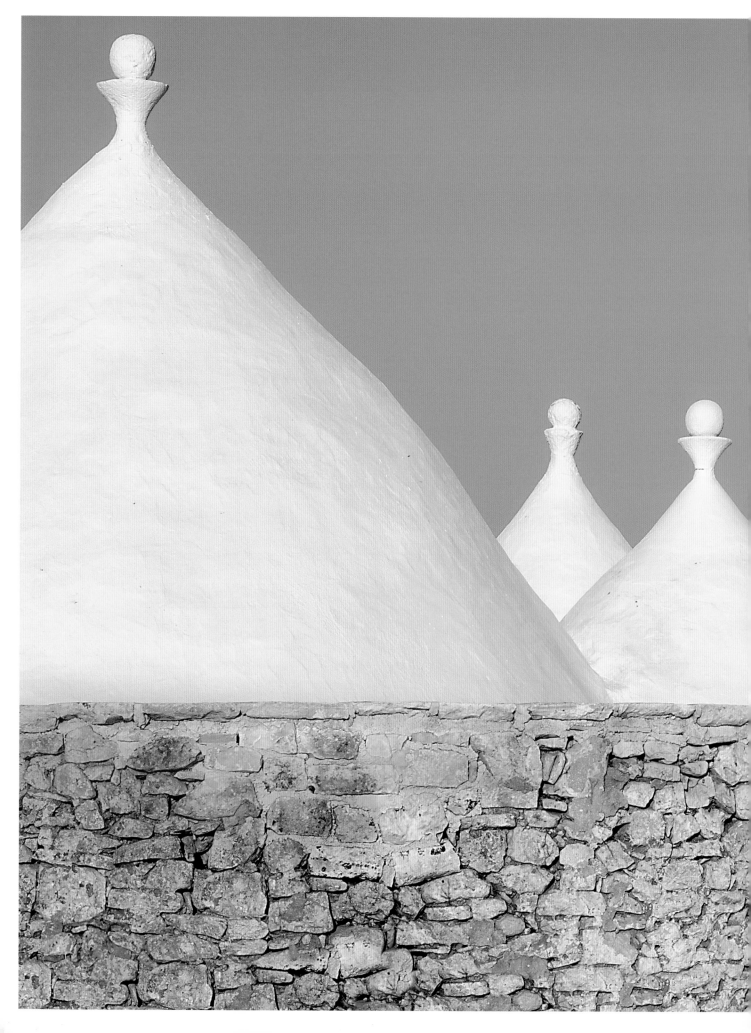

Gleaming white like forgotten pieces of laundry, the little houses of the masseria lie on the plain and defy the Apulian sun. Like a fortress of happiness, the small whitewashed dwellings of the estate, with their conical roofs, pit themselves against the endlessly blue sky. Between the 17th and 19th centuries, farmers lived in these so-called trulli. The walls, up to three feet thick, served as protection from cold and heat and are freshly whitewashed every year as a means of disinfection. Olive trees, grapevines, orange, lemon and almond trees thrive, and dusty blackberry bushes entwine themselves between the low stone walls. The food comes direct from the garden onto the plate and is generously sprinkled with olive oil. Yoga is taught on the hard parquet floor in a fantastically appointed vault, which can also be heated if necessary. Those who are admitted through the sacred walls of the world yoga retreat & healing place La Rosa dei 4 Venti today are a part of a large community sharing the importance of life based on freedom, heart, love, yoga and much more. Women of all ages with open locks and intelligent smiles offer proof that the earth is female—wouldn't you agree?

Books to pack: "Peace Is Every Step" by Thich Nhat Hanh and "A Walk in the Dark" by Gianrico Carofiglio

La Rosa dei 4 Venti

Via Monti del Duca 302
Martina Franca, 74014
Itria Valley
Italy
Tel. +39 080 449 0224
info@larosadei4venti.org
www.larosadei4venti.org

Directions	45 min from Brindisi Airport, 1 h 30 from Bari Airport; the next railway station is Ostuni
Yoga	Hatha, Ashtanga, Iyengar, Bikram, Vinyasa, Jivamukti
Teachers	Bryan Kest, Heather Elton, Anja Kuhnel, Carolina Fischer Waibel, Lina Thurnherr Baggenstos and many others
Rooms	1-, 2- and 3-bed rooms for max. 24 guests
Food	Vegetarian Food Philosophy based on the Alkaline diet
Leisure	Swimming, mountain bike, meditation walks in the forest, day trips to the sea or local ancient villages

Gleißend weiß wie vergessene Wäschestücke liegen die Häuschen der Masseria in der Ebene und trotzen der apulischen Sonne. Wie ein Fort der Fröhlichkeit stemmen sich die kleinen, gekalkten Zipfelmützenhäuser des Landguts dem endlos blauen Himmel entgegen. In diesen sogenannten »trulli« wohnten zwischen dem 17. und 19. Jahrhundert Bauern. Die bis zu einem Meter dicken Mauern dienten zum Schutz vor Kälte oder Hitze und werden jedes Jahr – auch aus Gründen der Desinfektion – frisch gekalkt. Olivenbäume, Weinreben, Orangen-, Zitronen- und Mandelbäume blühen, staubige Brombeerbüsche ranken zwischen den steinernen Mäuerchen hervor. Das Essen kommt direkt aus dem Garten auf den Teller und wird großzügig mit Olivenöl besprenkelt. Die Yoga-Stunden finden auf hartem Parkett in einem fantastisch hergerichteten Gewölbe statt, das bei Bedarf sogar geheizt werden kann. Wer heute Einlass in die heiligen Gemäuer vom World Yoga Retreat & Healing Place La Rosa dei 4 Venti findet, gehört zu einer großen Gemeinde, die den Leitgedanken eines Lebens basierend auf Freiheit, Liebe, Yoga und dergleichen mehr teilt. Frauen jeden Alters mit offenem langem Haar und klugem Lächeln beweisen, dass die Erde weiblich ist – wie könnte es auch anders sein?

Reisebegleiter: »Ich pflanze ein Lächeln« von Thich Nhat Hanh und »In freiem Fall« von Gianrico Carofiglio

D'une blancheur éblouissante, comme des pièces de linge qu'on aurait oubliées, les maisonnettes en pierre à chaux de la Masseria ornent la plaine, bravant le soleil des Pouilles. Telle une citadelle du bonheur, les petites maisons en forme de bonnet de lutin se dressent vers l'azur infini. Entre le 17e et le 19e siècle, des paysans logèrent dans ces « trulli ». Les murs, dont l'épaisseur va jusqu'à un mètre, protégeaient du froid et de la chaleur et sont, chaque année, assainis à la chaux. Oliviers, vignes, orangers, citronniers et amandiers fleurissent, des buissons de mûres grimpent le long des murets en pierre. Les aliments, généreusement aspergés d'huile d'olive, passent directement du jardin à la table. Les cours de yoga ont lieu sur parquet dur dans une salle voûtée magnifiquement restaurée qui peut, au besoin, être chauffée. Ceux qui ont la chance d'être admis entre les murs sacrés du World Yoga Retreat & Healing Place La Rosa dei 4 Venti aujourd'hui font partie d'une vaste communauté ayant en partage l'importance d'une vie basée sur la liberté, le coeur, l'amour, le yoga, et encore tellement plus. Les femmes, tous âges confondus, aux longs cheveux défaits et au sourire subtil sont bien la preuve vivante que la Terre est une femme, non ?

Livres à emporter : « La paix en marche. La paix en soi » de Thich Nhat Hanh et « Les yeux fermés » de Gianrico Carofiglio

Anreise	45 min Fahrt vom Flughafen Brindisi entfernt, 1,5 Std. vom Flughafen Bari, nächster Bahnhof ist Ostuni
Yoga	Hatha, Ashtanga, Iyengar, Bikram, Vinyasa, Jivamukti
Lehrer	Bryan Kest, Heather Elton, Anja Kuhnel, Carolina Fischer Waibel, Lina Thurnherr Baggenstos und viele andere
Zimmer	Ein- bis Dreibettzimmer für max. 24 Gäste
Küche	Vegetarisches Essen, basierend auf der Alkaline-Diät
Aktivitäten	Schwimmen, Mountainbiken, Meditations-Wanderungen, Ausflüge ans Meer oder zu historischen Dörfern

Accès	Situé à 45 min de l'aéroport de Brindisi, à 1 h 30 de l'aéroport de Bari, gare la plus proche : Ostuni
Yoga	Hatha, Ashtanga, Iyengar, Bikram, Vinyasa, Jivamukti
Professeurs	Bryan Kest, Heather Elton, Anja Kuhnel, Carolina Fischer Waibel, Lina Thurnherr Baggenstos et beaucoup d'autres
Chambres	Chambres de un à trois lits pour 24 personnes max.
Restauration	Cuisine végétarienne basée sur le régime alcalin
Activités	Natation, VTT, randonnées méditatives, excursions en bord de mer ou dans des villages historiques

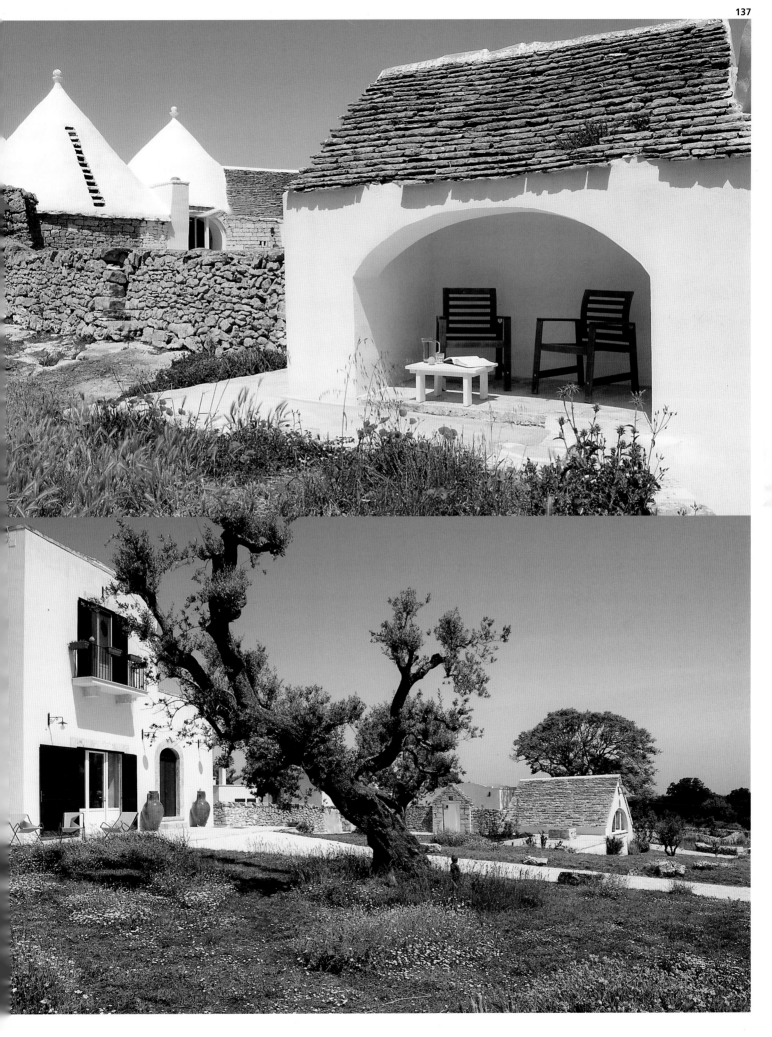

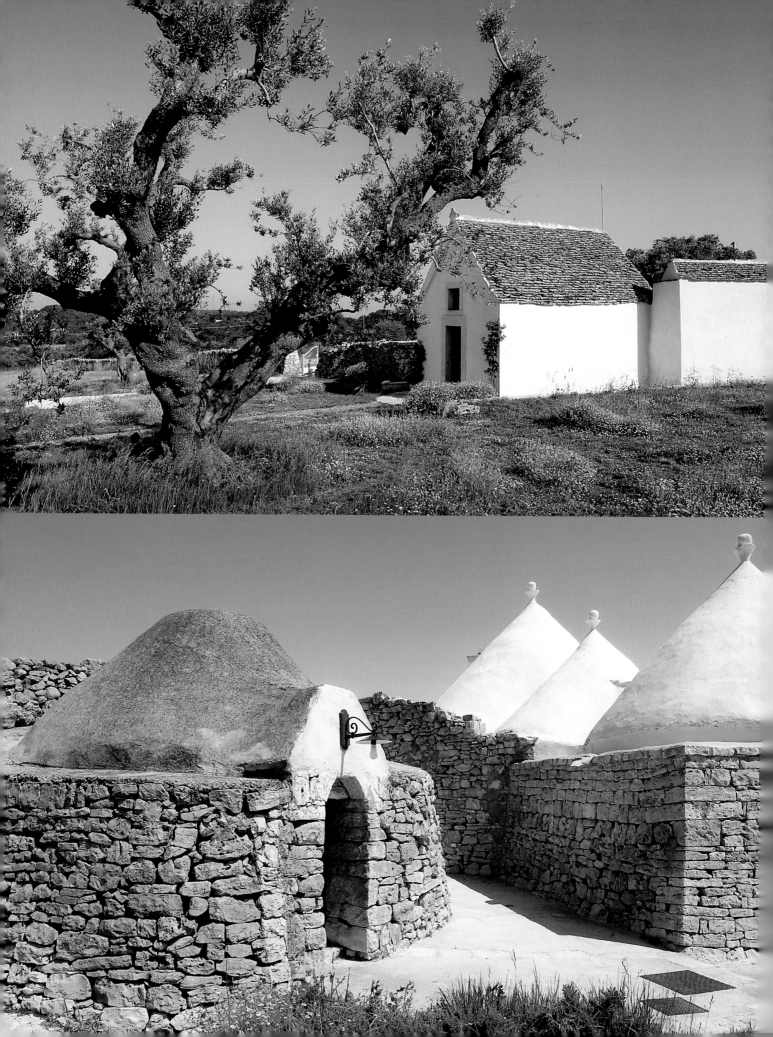

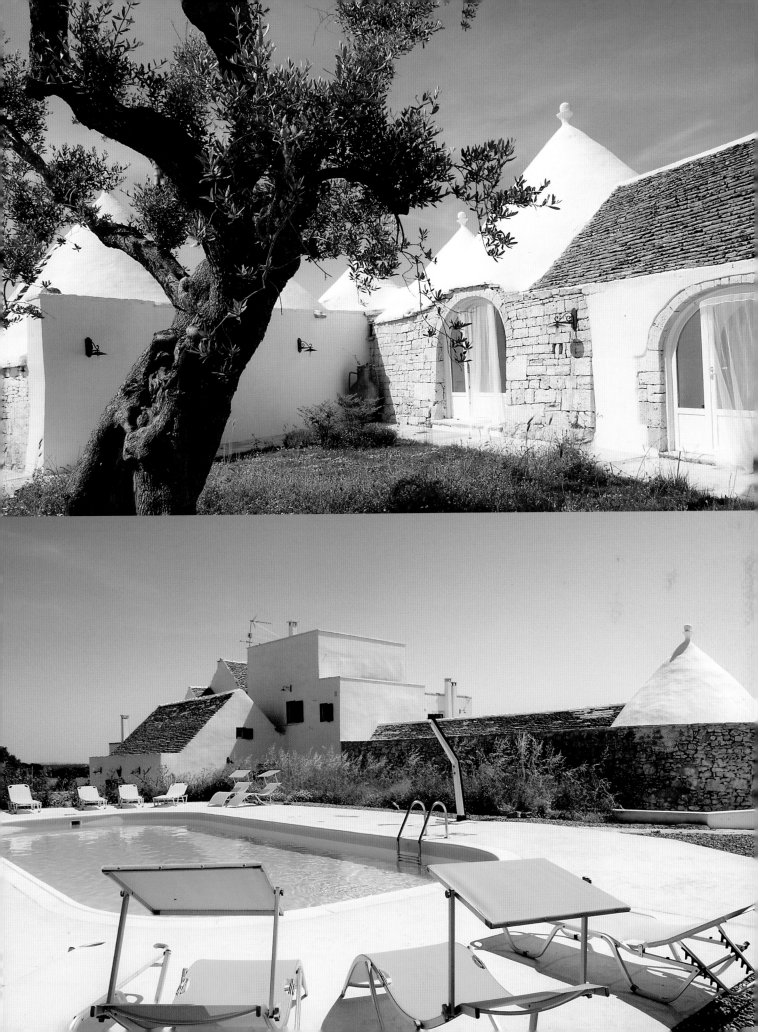

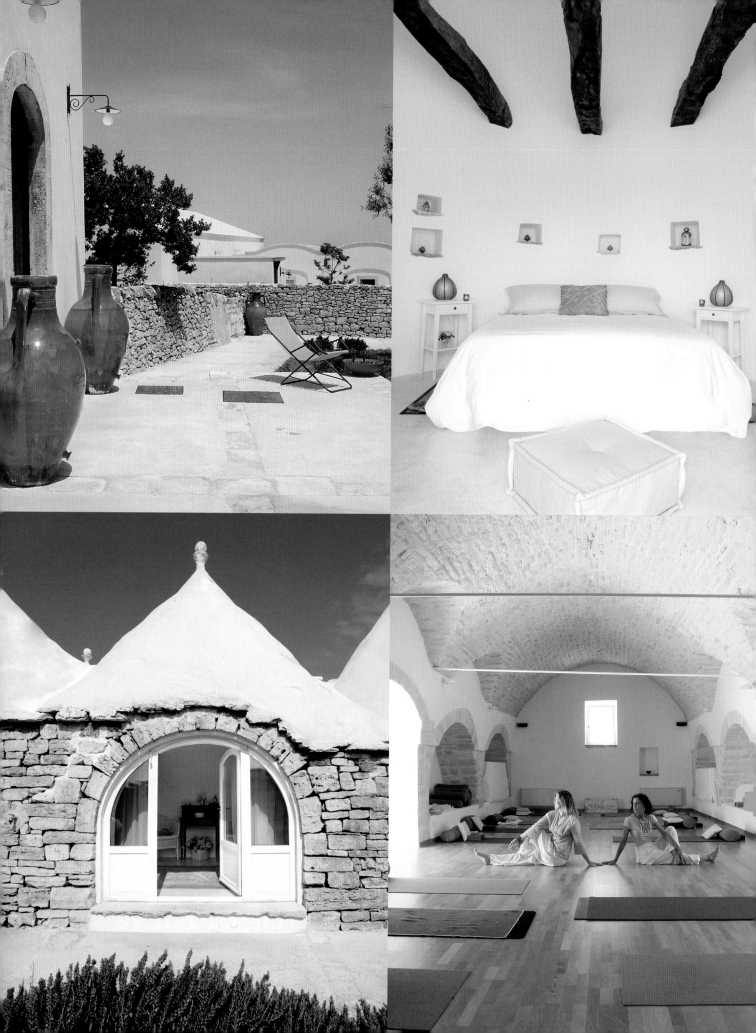

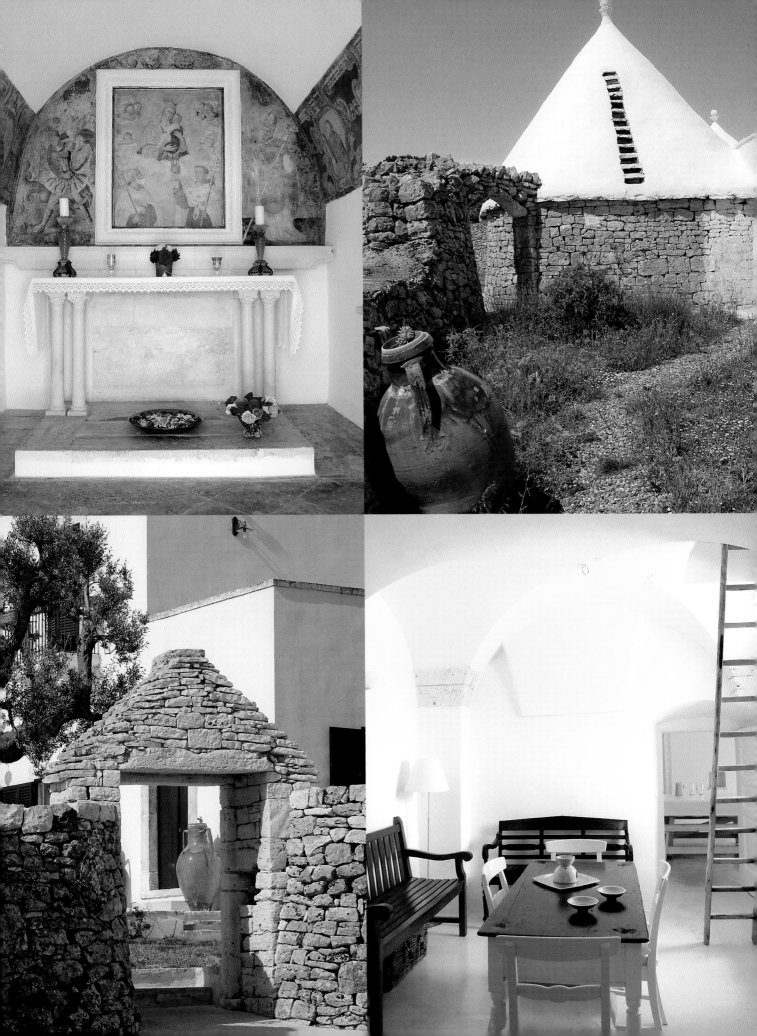

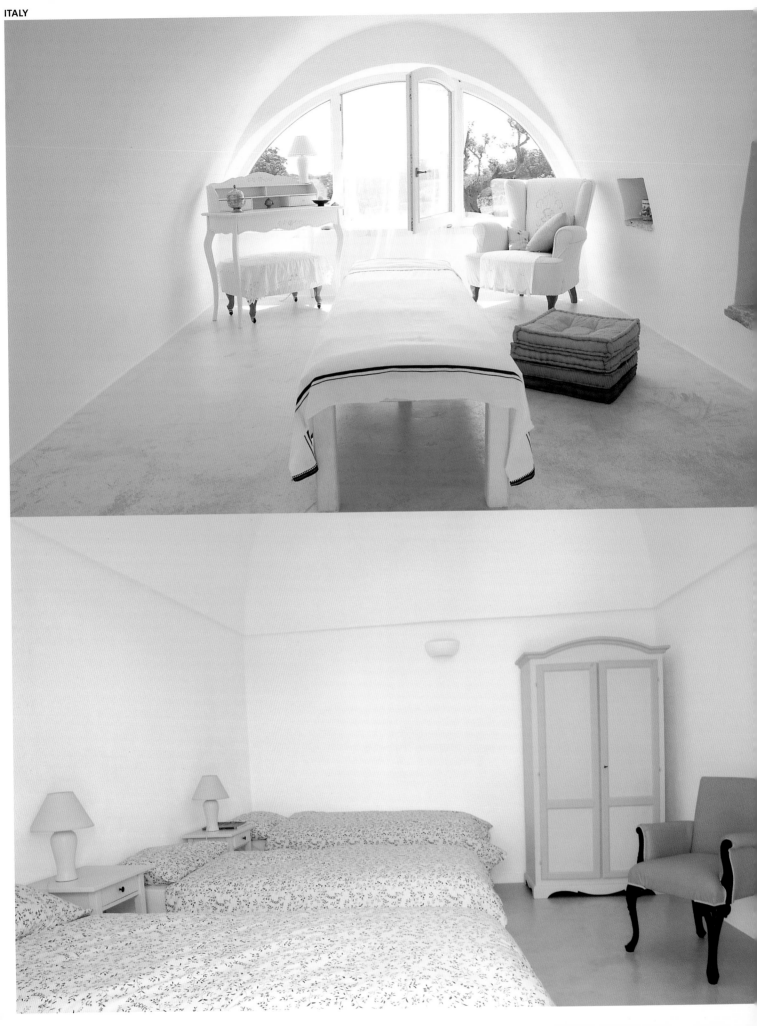

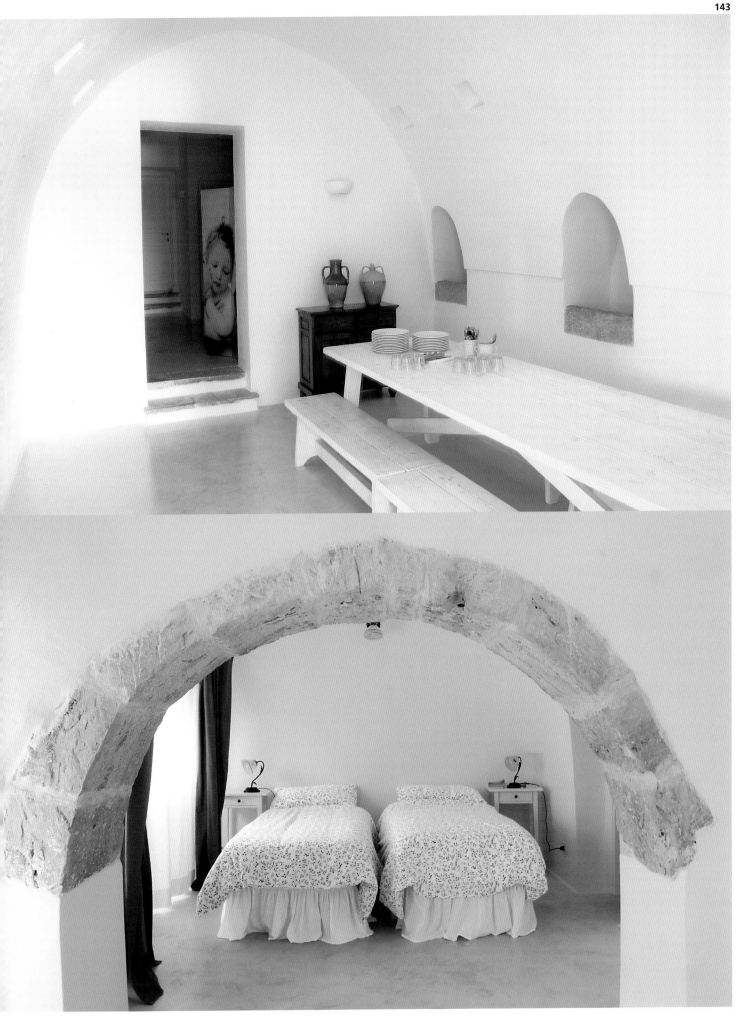

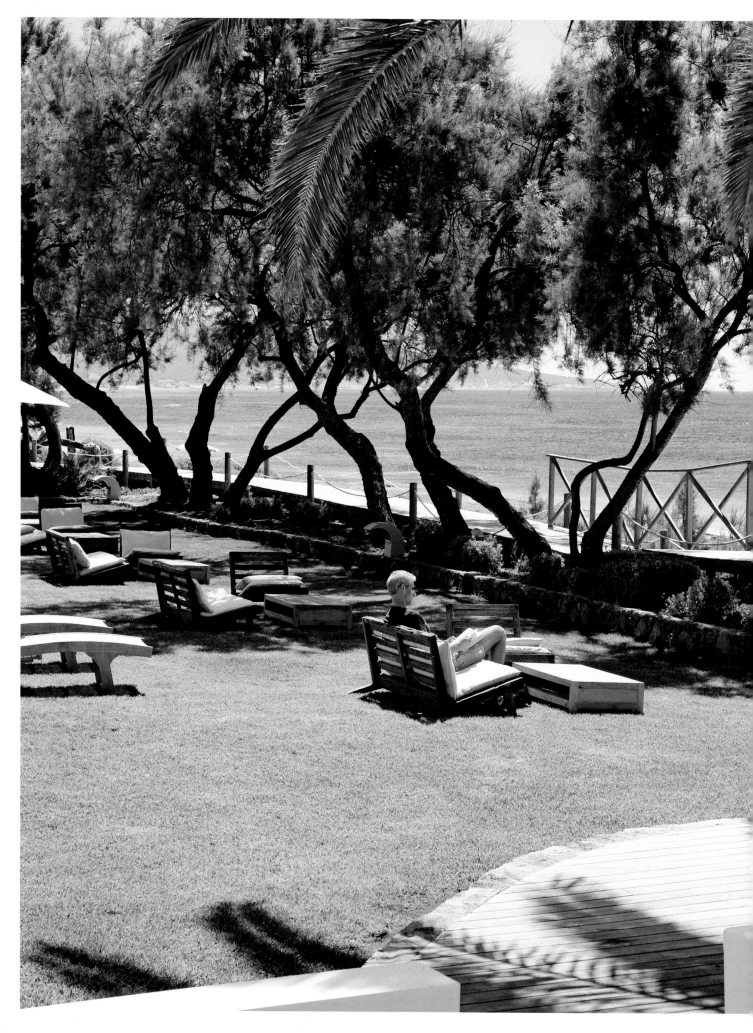

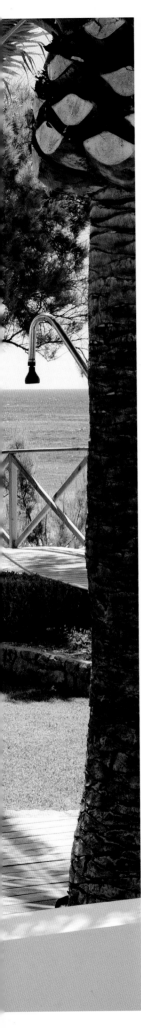

For all our appreciation of elaborate design, sometimes we simply want to walk along an unmade track to the beach, stay in an inconspicuous deluxe barrack and practise yoga to music—put on by Sundara from New York, one of the self-styled yoga teachers, to hot things up for her students, who have travelled from all over Europe. Ibiza is within spitting distance and yet far enough away not to interfere with its quieter little sister Formentera. Tiny enchanted fishing coves, unspoilt hinterland, transparent turquoise water and endless beaches onto which at most an old shoe is washed up from the mainland: even if word has long got around that Elle Macpherson secretly relaxes here—this Balearic island, which is on UNESCO's World Cultural Heritage list, is still a little Mediterranean treasure. The Romans knew that, and so did Bob Dylan; the resident bohemians know it, too, when after two hours of hefty Asana practice they wander over to the Blue Bar at the Playa Migjorn, where every evening cool DJs from Scotland spin discs as the sun goes down.

Books to pack: "It's Here Now (Are You?)" by Bhagavan Das and "Speaking with the Angel" edited by Nick Hornby

Formentera Yoga

Platja de Migjorn
Formentera, The Balearics
Spain
Tel. +34 606 117 373 and +44 7956 854 922
jill@formenterayoga.com
www.formenterayoga.com

Directions	Located 11 miles south of the island of Ibiza. Go by boat from Ibiza Old Town Port to La Savina Port Formentera; continue from there by taxi
Yoga	Restorative, Meditation, Vinyasa, Yin Yoga, Ashtanga, Dynamic Yoga, Jivamukti
Teachers	Jax May Lysycia, Bryan Kest, Liz Lark and others
Rooms	10 double rooms, five 3-bed rooms, 7 twin rooms and 2 suites for max. 40 people
Food	Vegetarian, Ayurvedic cuisine possible
Treatments	Facials, pedicure, massage
Leisure	Sailing, water-skiing, cookery courses, volleyball, cycling, swimming

Bei aller Liebe zu ausgetüfteltem Design: Manchmal ist einem einfach danach, auf einem ungeteerten Feldweg zum Strand zu laufen, in einer unaufdringlichen Luxusbaracke unterzukommen und bei Musik Yoga zu üben. Die legt Sundara aus New York auf, eine der selbsternannten Yoga-lehrerinnen, die ihren aus ganz Europa angereisten Schülern einheizt. Ibiza ist in Spuckweite und doch weit genug entfernt, um der ruhigeren kleinen Schwester Formentera nicht dazwischenzureden. Verträumte, winzige Fischerbuchten, unberührtes Hinterland, durchsichtiges, türkisfarbenes Wasser, endlose Strände, an die höchstens mal ein alter Schuh vom Festland angeschwemmt wird: Auch wenn sich längst herumgesprochen hat, dass Elle Macpherson hier heimlich entspannt, ist die balearische Insel, von der UNESCO zum Weltkulturerbe erklärt, noch immer ein kleiner Schatz im Mittelmeer. Das wussten die Römer, das wusste Bob Dylan, das weiß die Bohème, wenn sie nach zwei Stunden saftiger Asana-Übung zur Blue Bar an der Playa Migjorn schlendert, wo jeden Abend coole DJs aus Schottland zum Sonnenuntergang auflegen.

Reisebegleiter: »It's Here Now (Are You?)« von Bhagavan Das und »Speaking with the Angel« von Nick Hornby (Hrsg.)

Sans renier le goût du design raffiné, la simple envie vous prend parfois de marcher sur un chemin de campagne non goudronné menant à la plage, de loger dans une baraque luxueuse et de faire du yoga en musique. C'est cette musique que choisit Sundara de New York, l'une des professeurs de yoga autoproclamées, pour stimuler ses élèves venus de toute l'Europe. Ibiza est à deux pas et pourtant assez éloignée pour ne pas couvrir la voix de Formentera, la tranquille petite sœur plus tranquille. De minuscules criques de pêche romantiques, un arrière-pays encore intact, une eau transparente couleur turquoise, des plages à perte de vue où vient seulement, de temps à autre, échouer du continent une vieille chaussure : même si plus personne n'ignore qu'Elle Macpherson vient s'y reposer icognito, cette île des Baléares, inscrite au patrimoine mondial de l'UNESCO, demeure un petit joyau de la Méditerranée. Les Romains le savaient, de même que Bob Dylan, de même que les bohèmes de passage qui, après deux heures d'Âsana, flânent en direction du Blue Bar de la Playa Migjorn où, chaque soir, des DJ écossais branchés passent leurs disques face au coucher du soleil.

Livres à emporter : « It's Here Now (Are You?) » de Bhagavan Das et « Conversation avec l'ange » édité par Nick Hornby

Anreise	18 km südlich von der Insel Ibiza gelegen. Mit dem Boot von Ibiza Old Town Port zum La Savina Port von Formentera und von dort aus weiter mit dem Taxi
Yoga	Restorative, Meditation, Vinyasa, Yin Yoga, Ashtanga, Dynamic Yoga, Jivamukti
Lehrer	Jax May Lysycia, Bryan Kest, Liz Lark und andere
Zimmer	10 Doppelzimmer, 5 Dreibettzimmer, 7 Twins und 2 Suiten für insgesamt max. 40 Personen
Küche	Vegetarisch, ayurvedische Küche möglich
Anwendungen	Facials, Pediküre, Massage
Aktivitäten	Segeln, Wasserski, Kochkurse, Volleyball, Radfahren, Schwimmen

Accès	Situé à 18 km de l'île d'Ibiza. Accessible en bateau d'Ibiza Old Town Port à La Savina Port Formentera et, de là, transfert par taxi
Yoga	Restauratif, méditation, yoga dynamique, Vinyasa, Yin Yoga, Ashtânga, Dynamic Yoga, Jivamukti
Professeurs	Jax May Lysycia, Bryan Kest, Liz Lark et autres
Chambres	10 chambres doubles, 5 chambres à 3 lits, 7 doubles et 2 suites pour 40 personnes max.
Restauration	Cuisine végétarienne ayurvédique possible
Traitements	Soins du visage, pédicurie, massages
Activités	Voile, ski nautique, volley-ball, cyclisme, natation

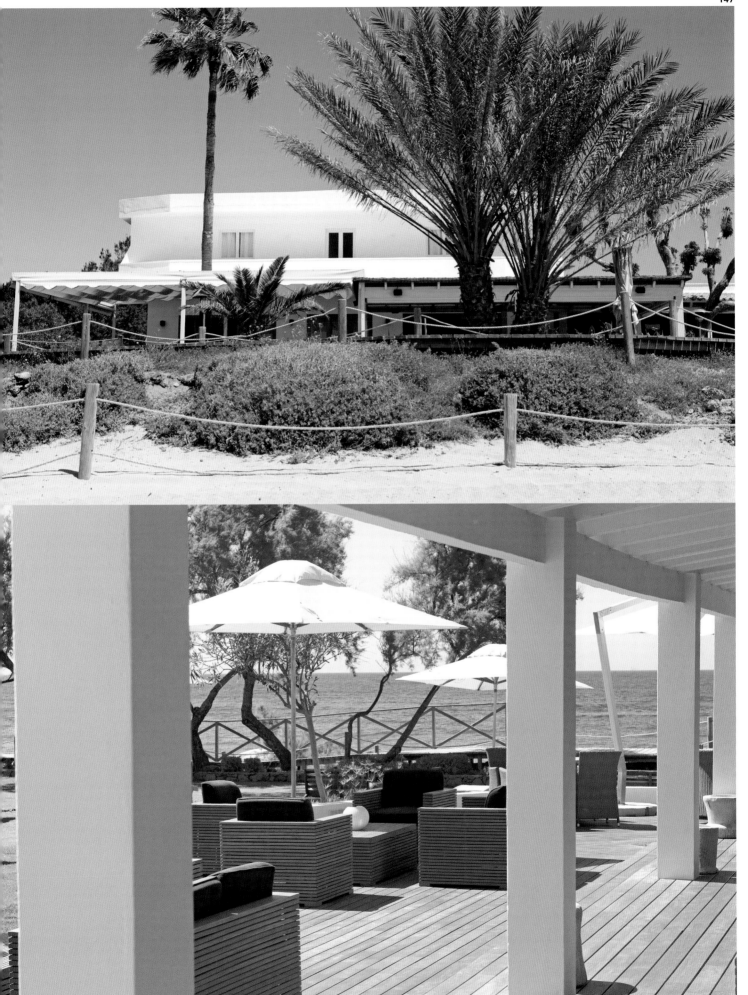

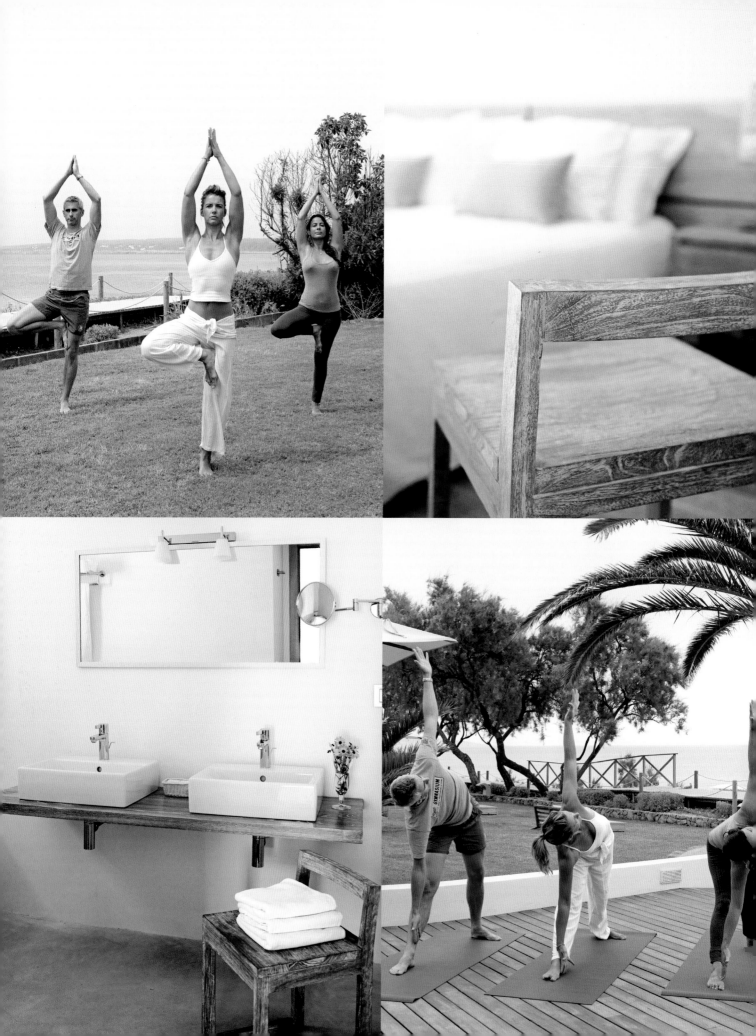

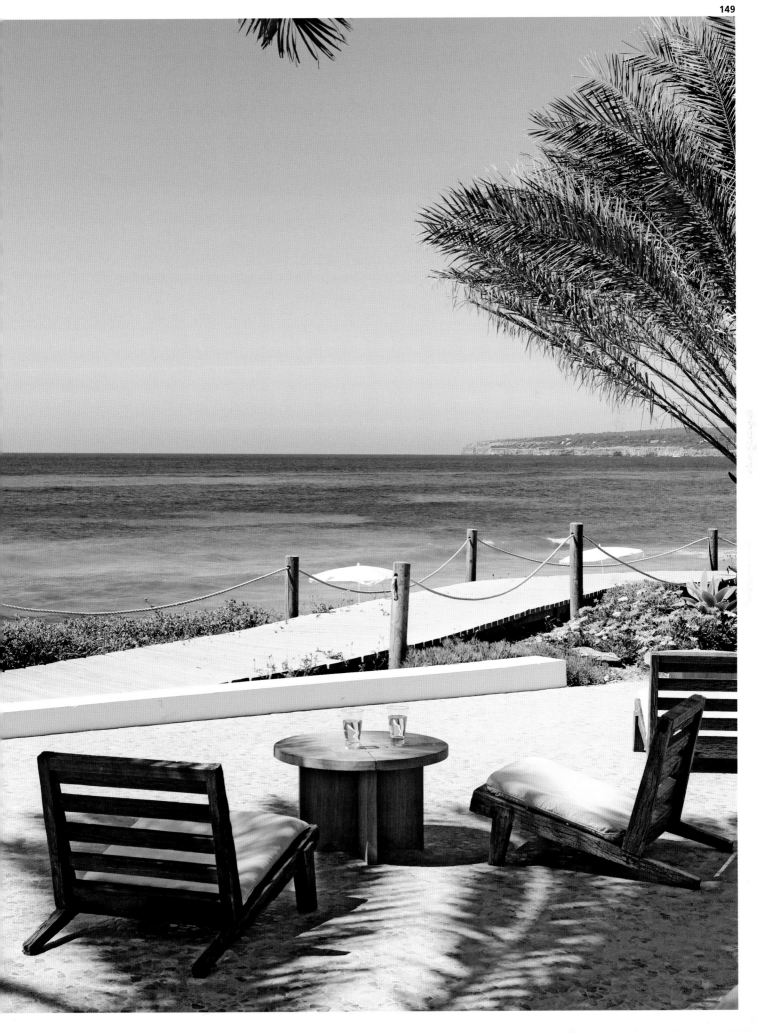

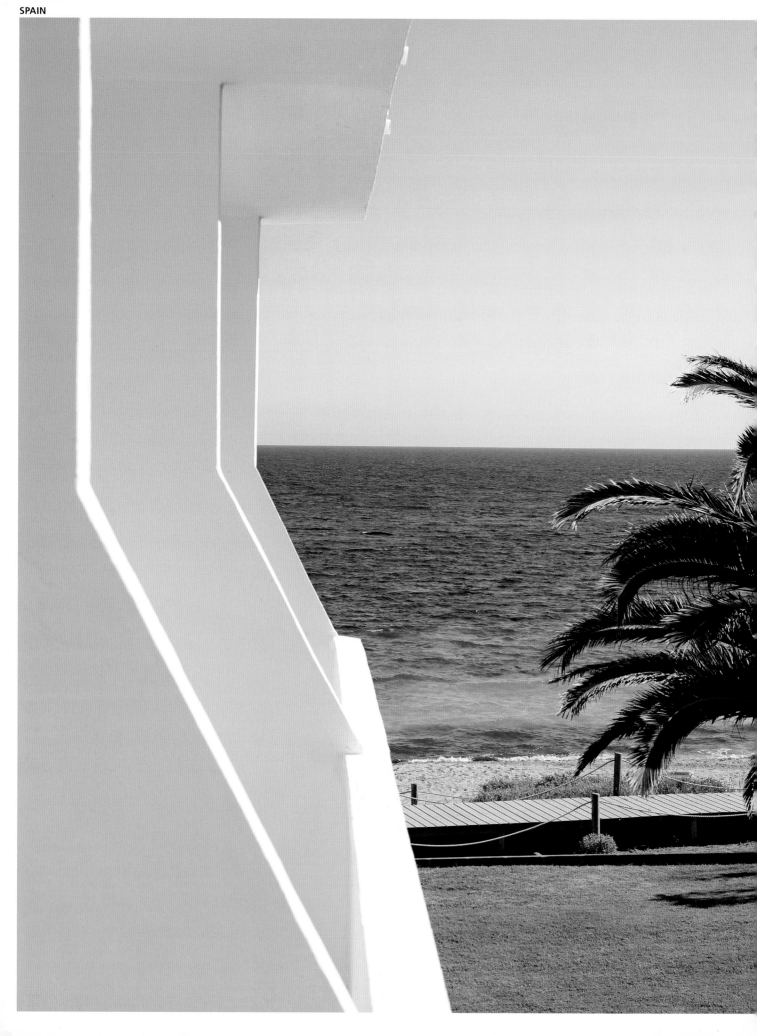

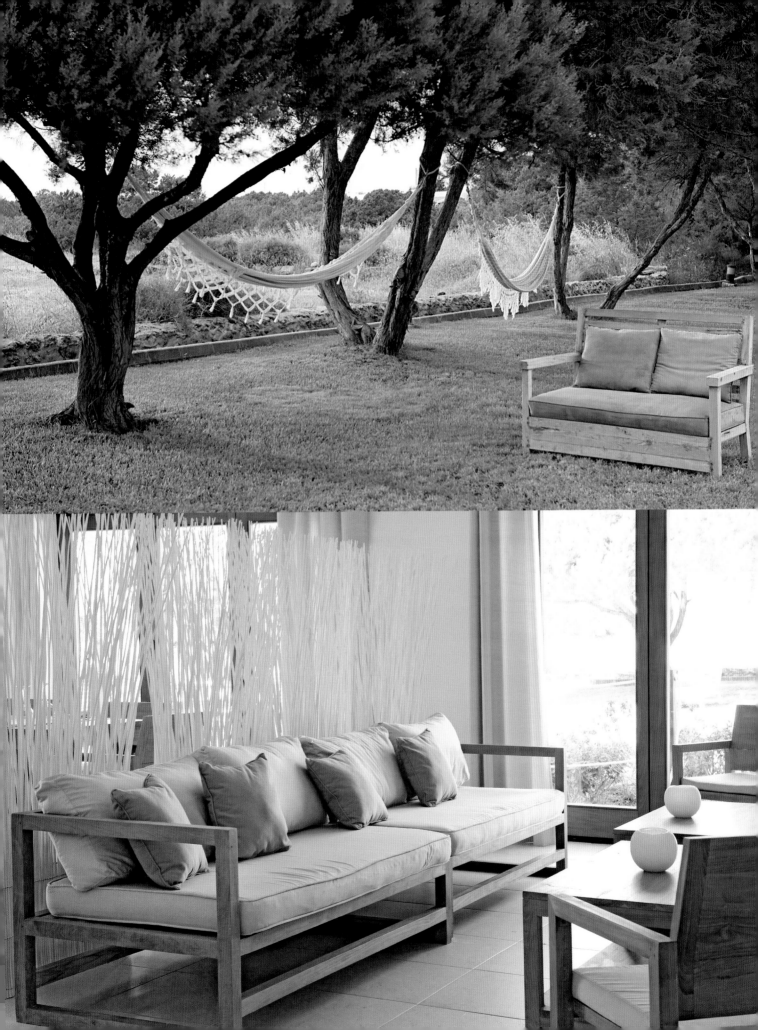

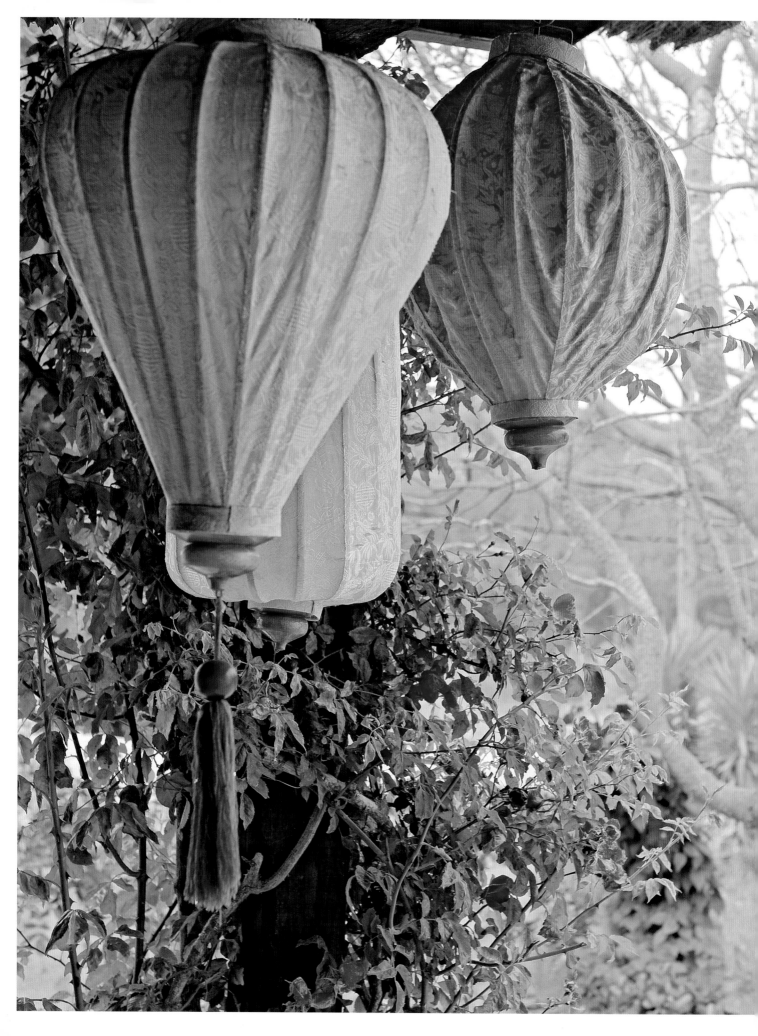

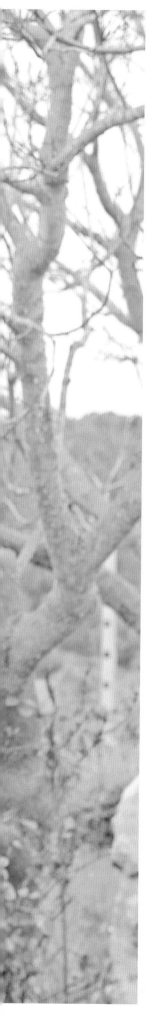

In the quiet north of the island, far from the English tourists who come to dance, stands a 400-year-old Ibizan finca, bedded in between orange and apricot groves. Nothing here is reminiscent of the hyped-up nervousness that Ibiza owes to its unique reputation as a party island. Ancient olive trees, brought here by the Phoenicians, entwine the white walls, along with mint and jasmine. The name Ibiza comes from the Phoenician god Bes, responsible for fertility, dance and music. Another derivation translates the original meaning as "island of perfumes". An intensive Hatha Yoga session, some craniosacral therapy and a long stroll across the neighboring fields while the almond trees are in bloom lift the spirits so far that the evening's programme of dance and music reveals its own unstoppable charm, and may even persuade you to set foot on the dance floor in one of the legendary clubs towards the end of the holiday after all. A leap into the delightful pool the next morning, and your spiritual peace is restored.

Books to pack: "The Yoga-Sûtra of Patañjali" by Georg Feuerstein and "On Love and Death" by Patrick Süskind

Ibiza Moving Arts

P.O. Box 144
07815 San Miguel, Ibiza
Spain
Tel. +34 971 324 275 and +34 637 269 884
info@ibizamovingarts.com
www.ibizamovingarts.com

Directions	15 1/2 miles from Ibiza Airport in the north of the island
Yoga	Hatha, Vinyasa Flow, Vijnana Yoga, meditation
Teachers	Clive Sheridan, Rebecca Parker, Sandra Morrel, Marte Kamzelas, Larah Baumann
Rooms	8 rooms for up to 18 people
Food	Mediterranean organic vegetarian cuisine
Treatments	Holistic massage, craniosacral therapy, Hawaiian healing bodywork, rebalancing, healing dance
Leisure	Swimming, hiking, sailing, diving, horseback riding, cycling, free climbing

Im ruhigen Norden der Insel, weit weg von den englischen Touristen, die zum Tanzen kommen, liegt eingewachsen zwischen Orangen- und Aprikosenhainen eine 400 Jahre alte ibizenkische Finca. Nichts erinnert hier an die überdrehte Nervosität, der Ibiza seinen einzigartigen Ruf als Partyinsel verdankt. Uralte Olivenbäume, von den Phöniziern hergebracht, Minze und Jasmin umranken das weiße Gemäuer. Der Name Ibiza geht zurück auf den phönizischen Gott Bes, verantwortlich für Fruchtbarkeit, Tanz und Musik. Eine andere Ableitung übersetzt die ursprüngliche Bedeutung als »Insel des Wohlgeruchs«. Während der Mandelblüte eine intensive Hatha-Yogastunde, eine Cranio-Sacral-Therapie und einen langen Spaziergang über die angrenzenden Felder zu machen, hebt die Stimmung so weit, dass die abendlichen Tanz- und Musikprogramme ihren eigenen ungebremsten Charme entfalten können und einen vielleicht sogar so weit bringen, gegen Ende der Ferien doch noch die Tanzfläche eines der legendären Clubs zu betreten. Ein Sprung in den entzückenden Pool am nächsten Morgen – und die Stille im Geist ist wiederhergestellt.

Reisebegleiter: »Patañjali: Das Yogasutra« von R. Sriram und »Über Liebe und Tod« von Patrick Süskind

Au nord de l'île, au calme, bien loin des touristes anglais qui viennent pour danser, entre les bosquets d'orangers et d'abricotiers se trouve enracinée depuis 400 ans une finca ibizienne. Ici, rien ne rappelle l'extrême fébrilité à laquelle Ibiza doit sa réputation exclusive d'île fêtarde. Les oliviers ancestraux, importés autrefois par les Phéniciens, la menthe et le jasmin recouvrent les murailles blanches. Le nom Ibiza remonte au dieu phénicien Bès, divinité de la fécondité, de la danse et de la musique. Une autre dérivation traduit le sens originel comme « île aux fragrances ». Au moment de la floraison de l'amandier, une heure intensive de Hatha-yoga, une thérapie cranio-sacrale et une longue promenade à travers les champs avoisinants vous mettent de si bonne humeur que les programmes de danse et de musique du soir peuvent déployer leur charme sans retenue et vous amener peut-être même, vers la fin des vacances, à risquer quelques pas sur la piste de danse d'un des clubs légendaires. Le lendemain, un plongeon dans la merveilleuse piscine et la paix de l'esprit est revenue.

Livres à emporter : « Yoga-Sutras de Patanjali » de Françoise Mazet et « Sur l'amour et la mort » de Patrick Süskind

Anreise	25 km vom Ibiza-Flughafen entfernt, im Norden der Insel gelegen
Yoga	Hatha, Vinyasa Flow, Vijnana Yoga, Meditation
Lehrer	Clive Sheridan, Rebecca Parker, Sandra Morrel, Marte Kamzelas, Larah Baumann
Zimmer	8 Zimmer für bis zu 18 Personen
Küche	Mediterrane biologisch-vegetarische Küche
Anwendungen	Holistische Massage, Cranio-Sacral-Therapie, Hawaiian Bodywork, Rebalancing, Healing Dance
Aktivitäten	Schwimmen, Wandern, Segeln, Tauchen, Reiten, Radfahren, Freeclimbing

Accès	Situé au nord de l'île, à 25 km de l'aéroport d'Ibiza
Yoga	Hatha, Vinyasa Flow, Vijnana yoga, méditation
Professeurs	Clive Sheridan, Rebecca Parker, Sandra Morrel, Marte Kamzelas, Larah Baumann
Chambres	8 chambres pouvant accueillir jusqu'à 18 personnes
Restauration	Cuisine méditerranéenne, bio-végétarienne
Traitements	Massage holistique, thérapie cranio-sacrale, bodywork réparateur hawaïen, rééquilibrant, danse guérisseuse
Activités	Natation, randonnées, voile, plongée, équitation, bicyclette, escalade

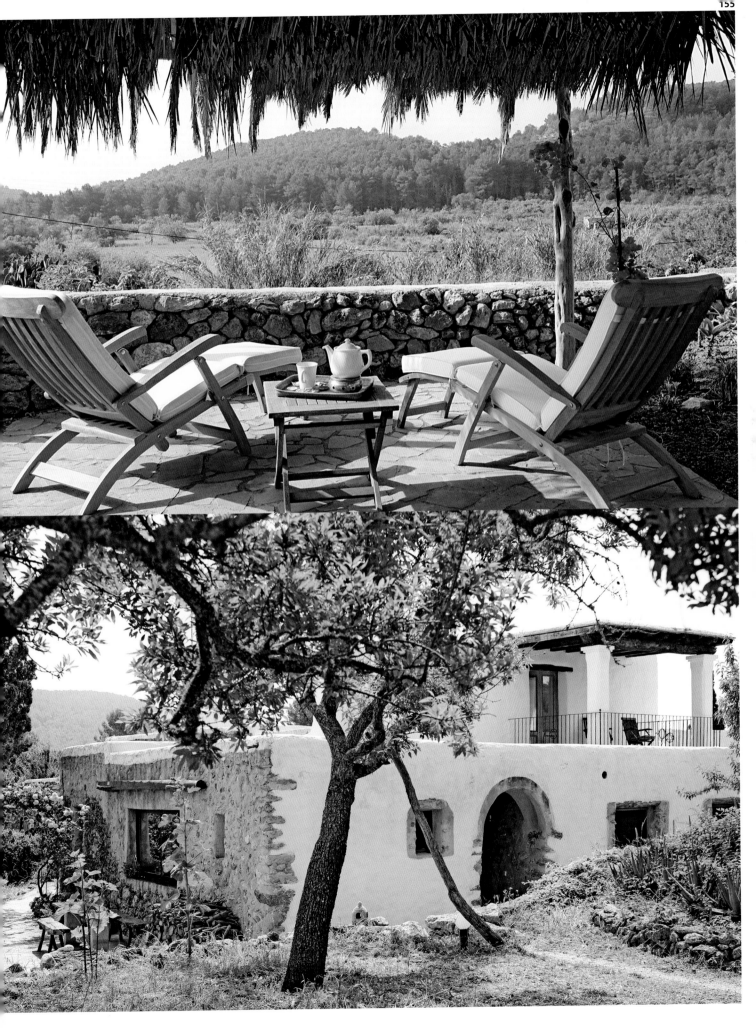

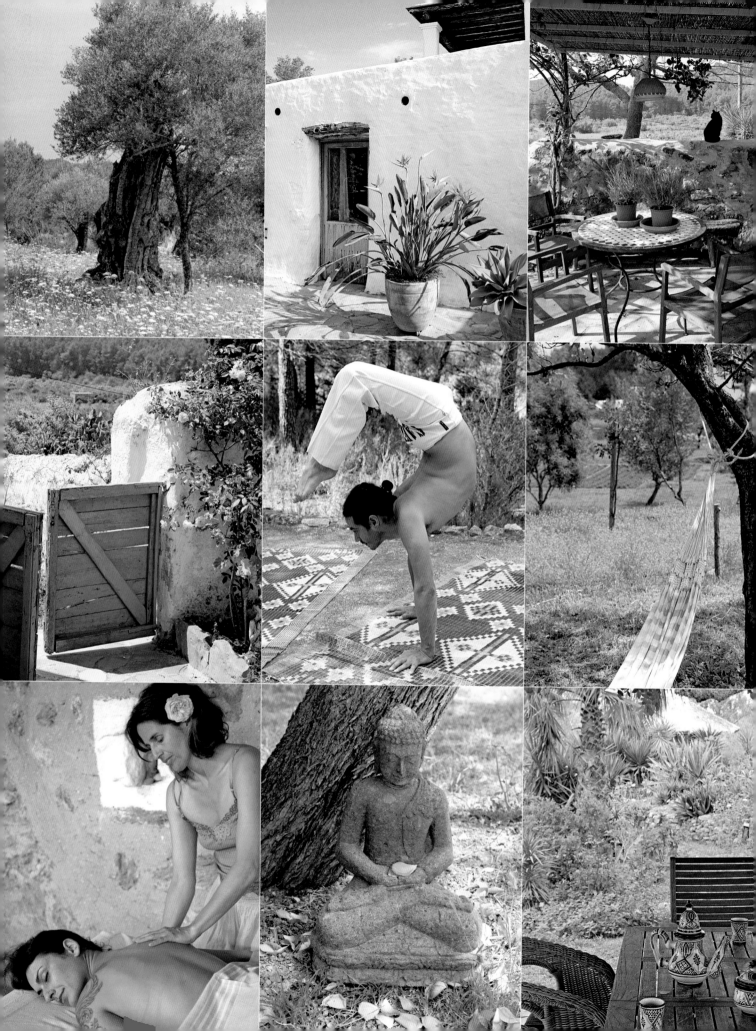

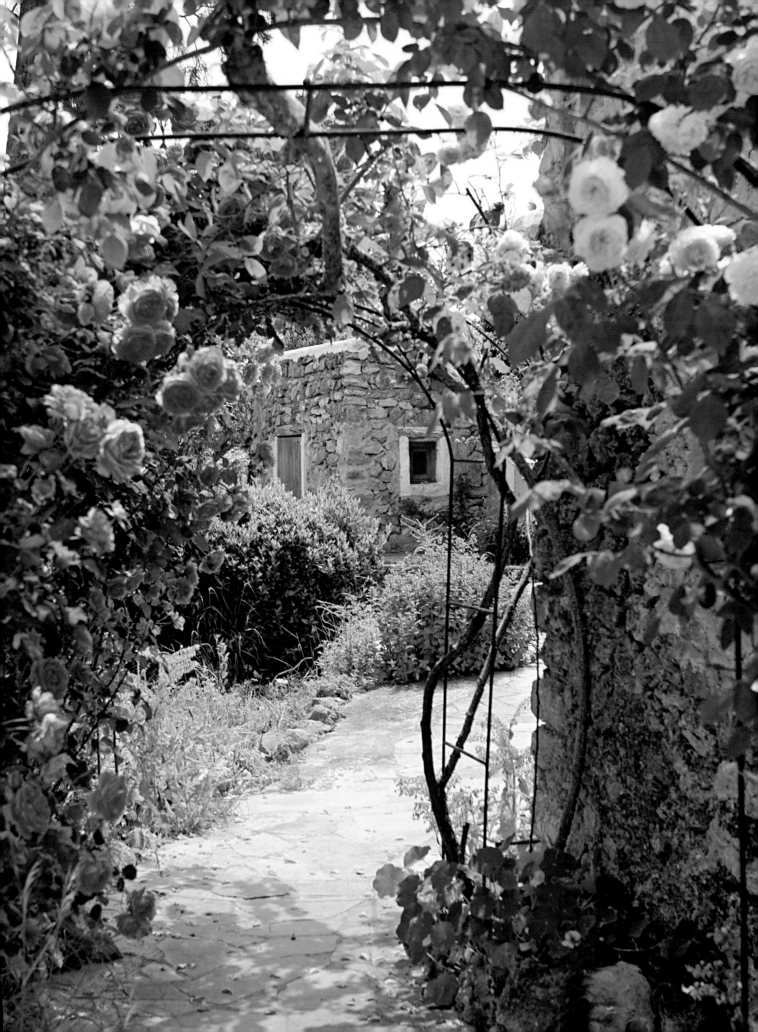

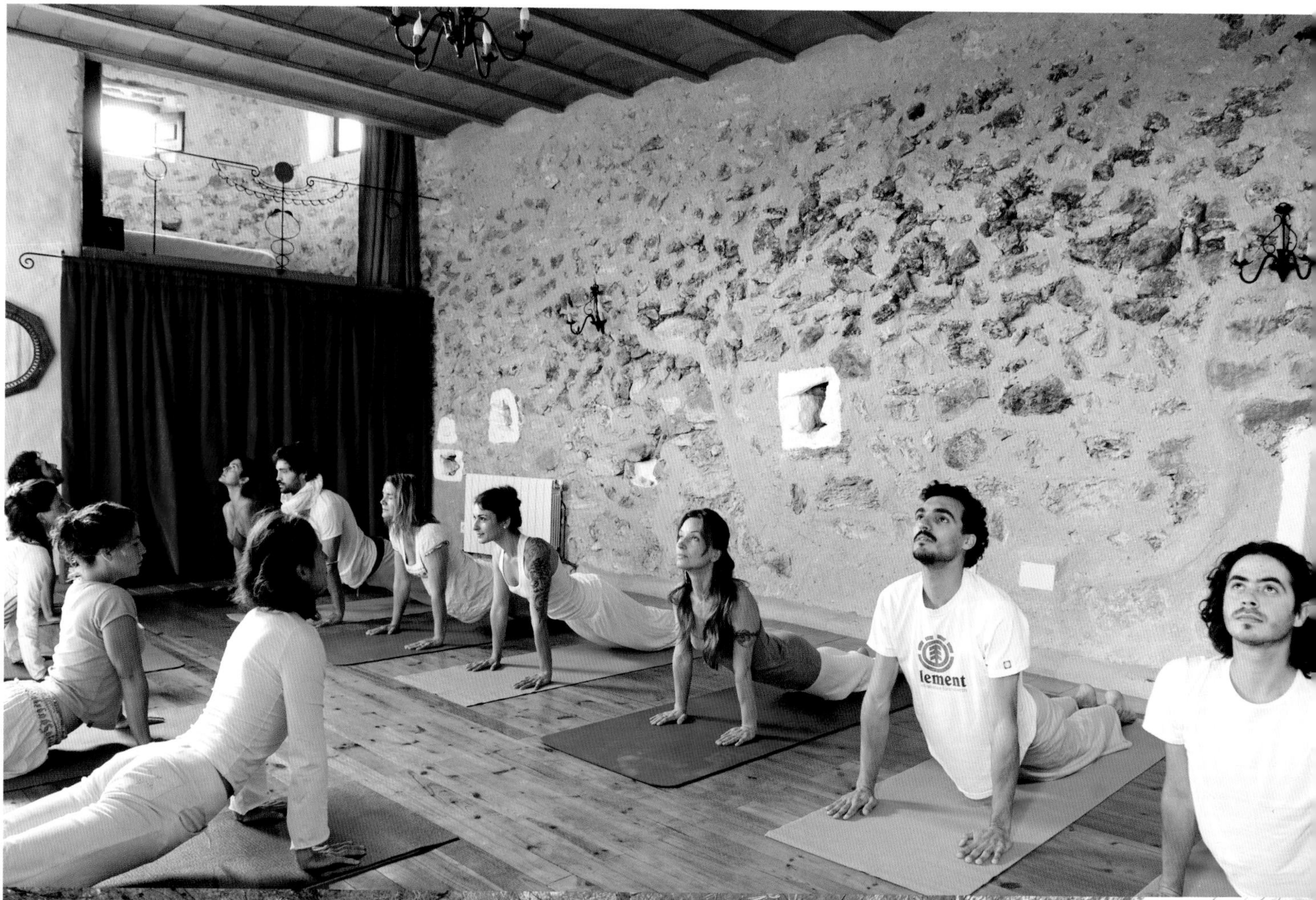
lement

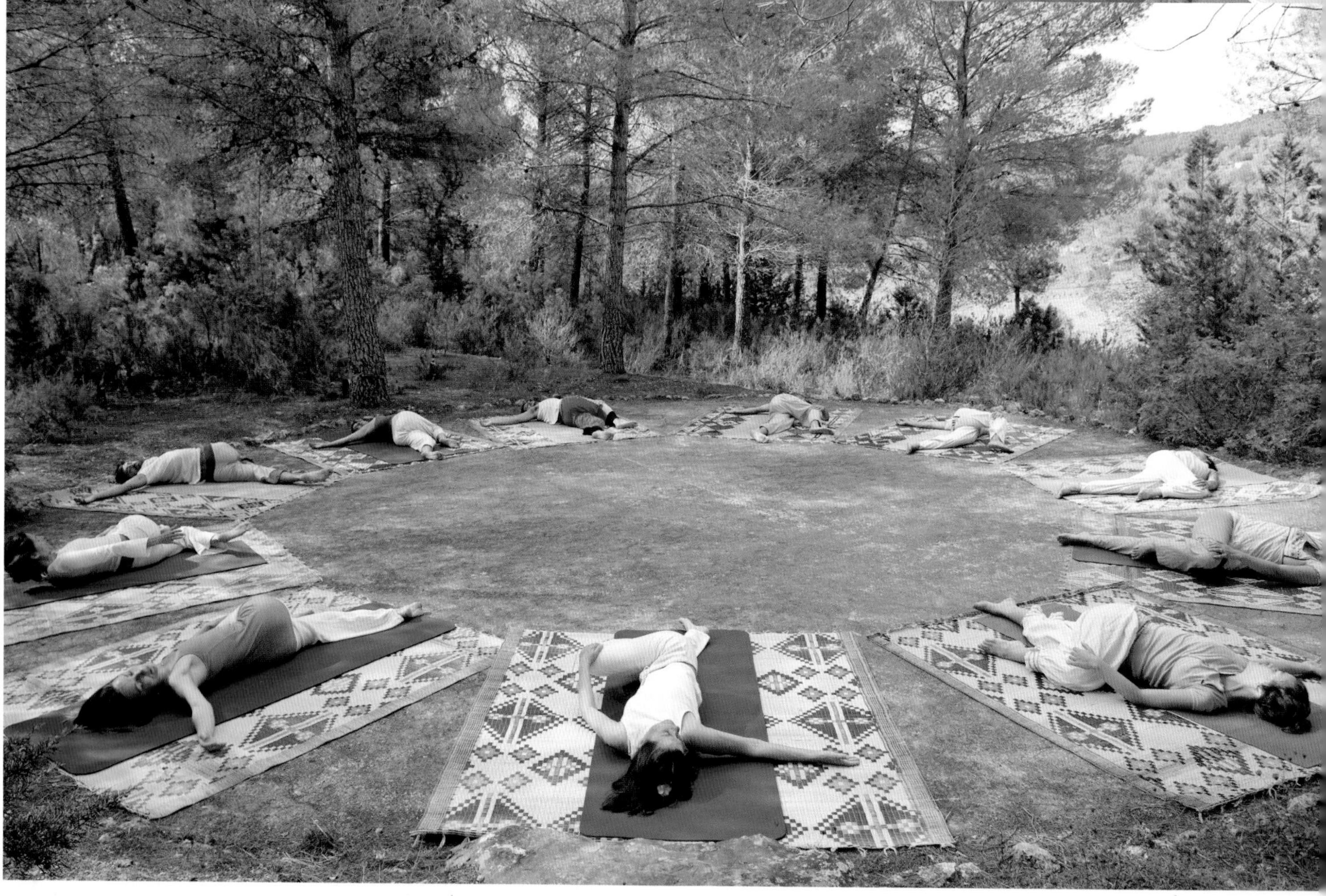

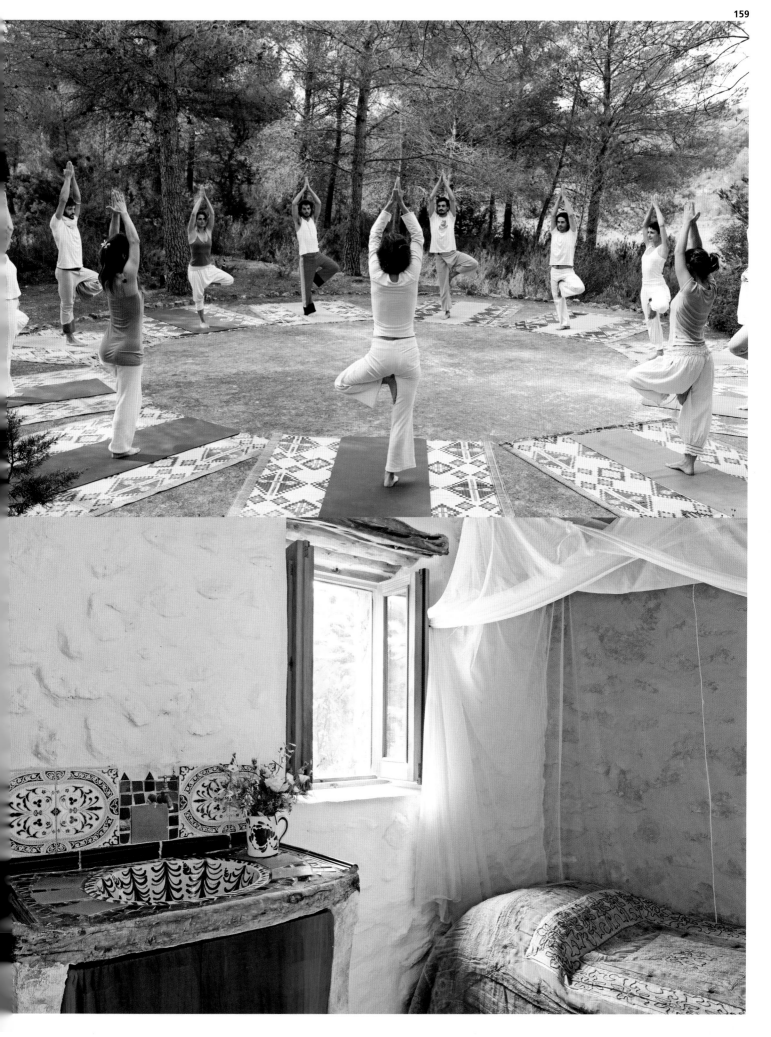

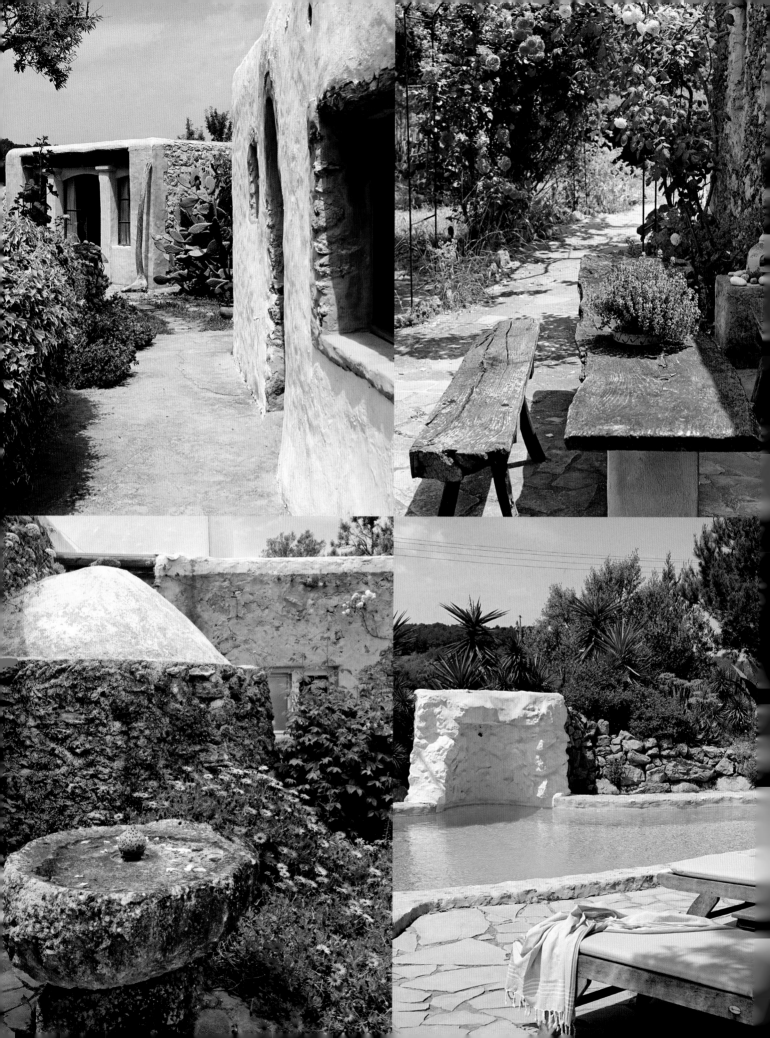

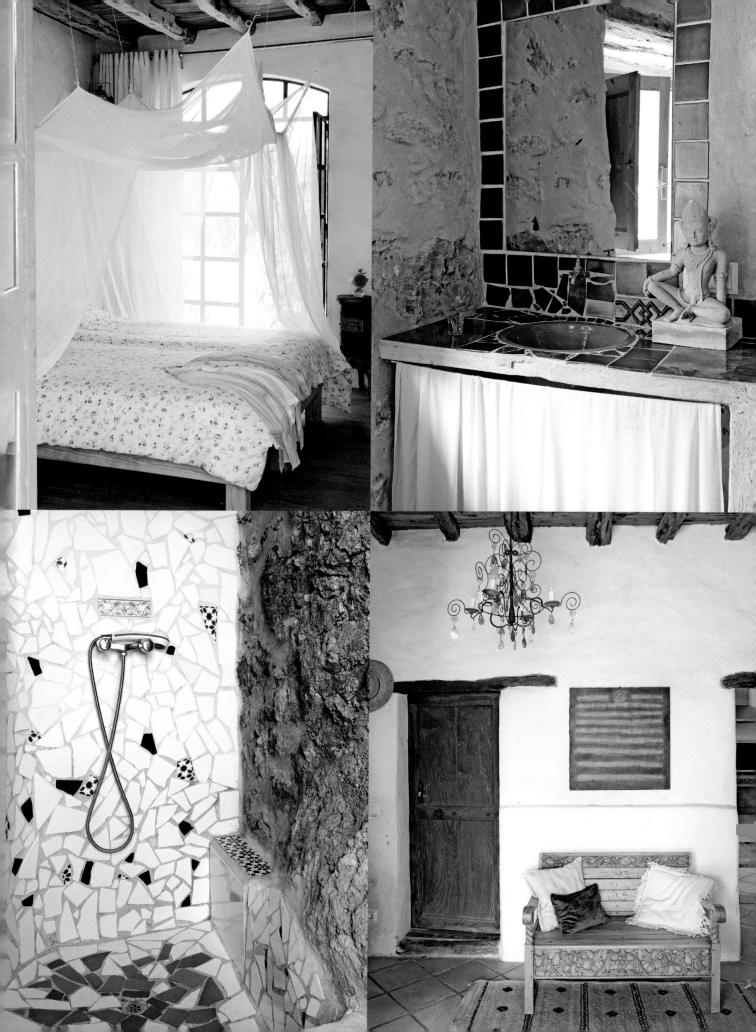

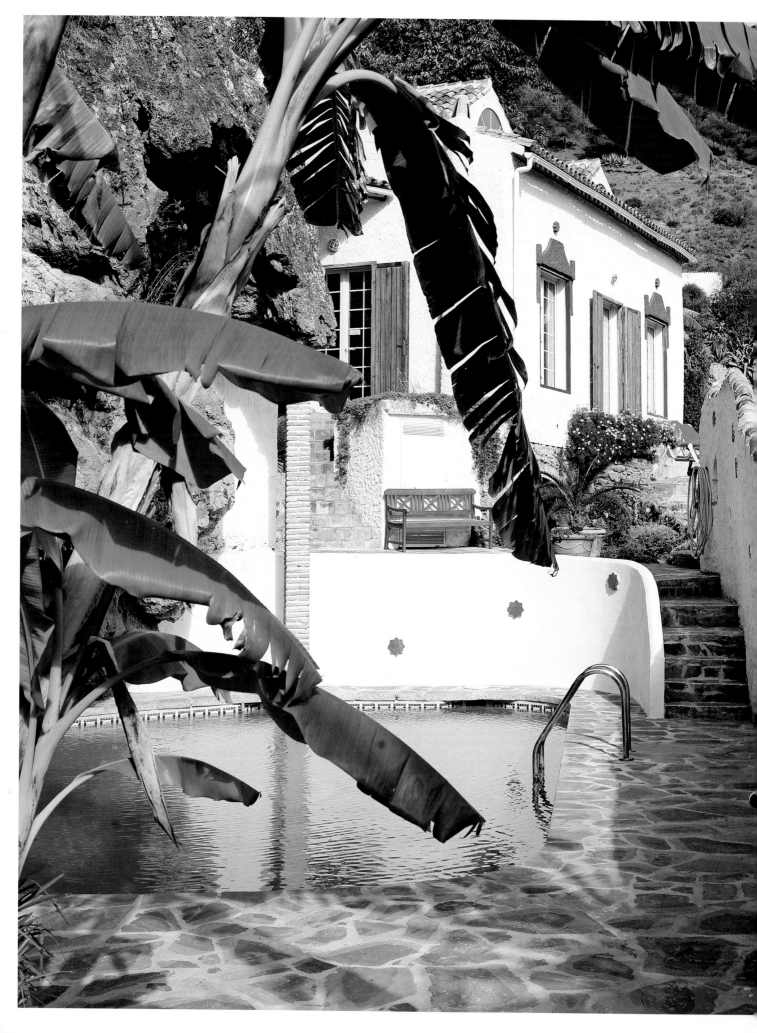

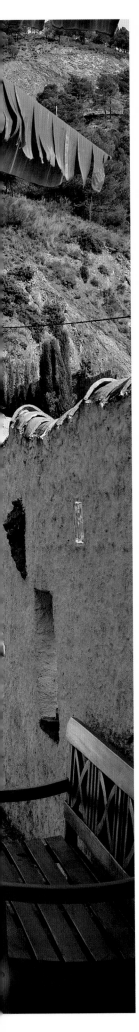

Whichever king it was that these two former mills belonged to, you can't feel sorry enough for him. Of course he would have felt pride and love for his land as he looked towards the horizon across the deep green Andalusian hills and the orange and avocado groves. But however rich he might have been, his was the fate of those born too soon. He was never to enjoy being taught by famous English gurus in the Yoga Shala carved into the mountain; he would never meditate in the cave in the rock, never swim by candlelight in the seawater pool. With the conversion work undertaken by the owners themselves, these mills, which lie at the source of one of the tributaries of the Rio Grande, attract an enthusiastic clientele from all over the world. The guests here are spoilt for choice: a trip between yoga lessons to Granada, Seville, Córdoba or Ronda, a trek through the breathtaking conservation area next door, or simply a hot stone massage in the shade. The place itself is a source for new ideas and a change in perspective.

Books to pack: "Health, Healing & Beyond: Yoga and the Living Tradition of Krishnamacharya" by T. K. V. Desikachar and "Raquel, the Jewess of Toledo" by Lion Feuchtwanger

Molino del Rey

Valle de Jorox
Alozaina-Málaga 29567
Spain
Tel. +34 952 480 009
molinodelrey@hotmail.com
www.molinodelrey.com

Directions	30 miles west of Malaga Airport
Yoga	Ashtanga, Kundalini, Vinyasa Flow, Iyengar
Teachers	Simon Low, James Jewell, Arien & Mirjam van Erkelens, Joanna Najduch, Evita Lindblom, Fenella Lindsell, Gerry Kielty, Ulrike Helund, Andrea Kwiatkowski
Rooms	Total of 22 beds, 10 twins and 2 single. All en-suite with air-conditioning and tea facilities
Food	Vegetarian; specialities are chocolate muffins, Spanish tortilla, paella
Treatments	Dry skin brushing, hot stone massage, Hawaiian massage, Swedish massage, Thai massage, Chavutti Thirumal massage, Japanese facial massage, Indian head massage
Leisure	Hiking, meditation cave, saltwater pool, excursions to Ronda, Seville, Marbella etc.

Welchem König diese beiden ehemaligen Mühlen auch immer gehört haben mögen, man kann ihn gar nicht genug bedauern. Sicherlich blickte er mit Stolz über die tiefgrünen Hügel Andalusiens, die Orangen- und Avocadohaine zum Horizont und liebte sein Land, doch so reich er auch gewesen sein mochte, ihn ereilte das Schicksal des zu früh Geborenen. Nie kam er in den Genuss, in der in den Berg hineingehauenen Yoga-Shala von berühmten englischen Gurus unterrichtet zu werden, in der Höhle im Fels zu meditieren oder im Seewasserpool bei Kerzenlicht zu schwimmen. Diese von den Besitzern eigenhändig umgebauten Mühlen, die an der Quelle eines der Seitenflüsse des Rio Grande liegen, ziehen ein begeistertes Publikum aus der ganzen Welt an, das die Qual der Wahl hat: ein Ausflug zwischen den Yogastunden nach Granada, Sevilla, Córdoba oder Ronda oder doch lieber eine Wanderung durch das angrenzende atemberaubende Naturschutzgebiet oder einfach eine Heiße-Stein-Massage im Schatten. Der Platz selbst wird zur Quelle neuer Ideen und ermöglicht einen Perspektivwechsel.

Reisebegleiter: »Yoga. Gesundheit von Körper und Geist: Leben und Lehren Krishnamacharyas« von T. K. V. Desikachar und »Die Jüdin von Toledo« von Lion Feuchtwanger

Quel que soit le roi à qui ces deux anciens moulins aient pu appartenir, on ne pourra jamais le plaindre assez. Certes, son regard glissait fièrement sur les collines d'un vert profond de l'Andalousie, les orangers et avocatiers se profilant à l'horizon et il aimait son pays, pourtant aussi riche qu'il ait pu être, le fait d'être né trop tôt lui fut fatal. Jamais ne put se délecter de l'enseignement d'un célèbre guru anglais dans la yoga-shala implantée sur la montagne, d'une méditation au cœur d'une caverne ou d'un bain d'eau de mer en piscine, à la lueur de bougies. Ces moulins, situés à la source d'un affluent du Rio Grande et transformés grâce au travail personnel des propriétaires, attirent du monde entier un public enthousiaste qui n'a que l'embarras du choix : entre les séances de yoga faire une excursion à Grenade, Séville, Cordoue ou Ronda ou plutôt une randonnée à travers la réserve naturelle avoisinante, d'une beauté époustouflante, ou simplement profiter d'un massage aux pierres chaudes à l'ombre. L'endroit lui-même, induisant un changement de perspective, devient source d'idées nouvelles.

Livres à emporter : « Le yoga du yogi : L'héritage de T. Krishnamacharya » de Kausthub Desikachar et « La Juive de Tolède » de Lion Feuchtwanger

Anreise	50 km westlich vom Flughafen Malaga entfernt
Yoga	Ashtanga, Kundalini, Vinyasa Flow, Iyengar
Lehrer	Simon Low, James Jewell, Arien & Mirjam van Erkelens, Joanna Najduch, Evita Lindblom, Fenella Lindsell, Gerry Kielty, Ulrike Hedlund, Andrea Kwiatkowski
Zimmer	Insgesamt 22 Betten, 10 Doppelzimmer und 2 Einzelzimmer, jeweils mit Bad, Klimaanlage und Teekocher
Küche	Vegetarisch, Spezialitäten sind Schokoladenmuffins, spanische Tortilla, Paella
Anwendungen	Bürstenmassage, Heiße-Steine-Massage, Hawaiianische Massage, Thai-Massage, Chavutti-Thirumai-Massage, Japanische Gesichtsmassage, Indische Kopfmassage, Schwedische Massage
Aktivitäten	Wandern, Meditationshöhle, Salzwasserpool, Ausflüge nach Ronda, Sevilla, Marbella etc.

Accès	A 50 km à l'ouest de l'aéroport de Malaga
Yoga	Ashtânga, Kundalini, Vinyasa Flow, Iyengar
Professeurs	Simon Low, James Jewell, Arien et Mirjam van Erkelens, Joanna Najduch, Evita Lindblom, Fenella Lindsell, Gerry Kielty, Ulrike Hedlund, Andrea Kwiatkowski
Chambres	22 lits répartis dans 10 chambres doubles et 2 individuelles ; suites avec air conditionné et service à thé
Restauration	Végétarienne, spécialités : muffins au chocolat, tortillas espagnoles, paëlla
Traitements	Gommage pour peaux sèche, massage facial japonais, massage aux pierres chaudes, massage hawaïen, suédois, thaï et Charutti Thirumal, massage crânien indien
Activités	Randonnées, caverne de méditation, piscine d'eau salée, excursions à Ronda, Séville, Marbella, etc.

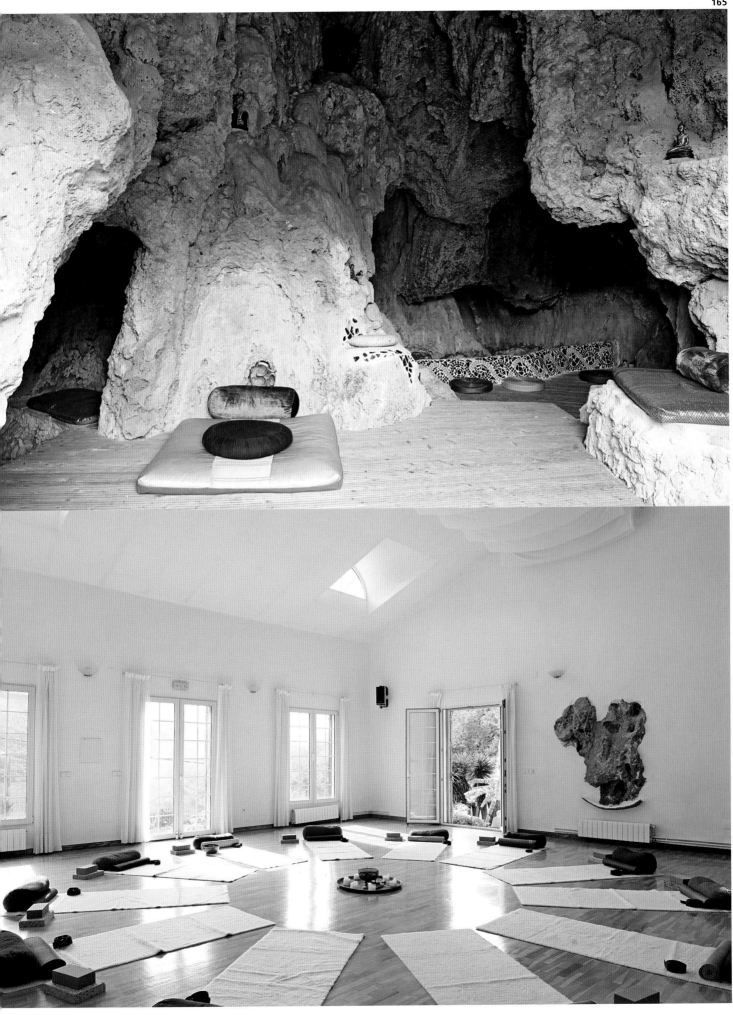

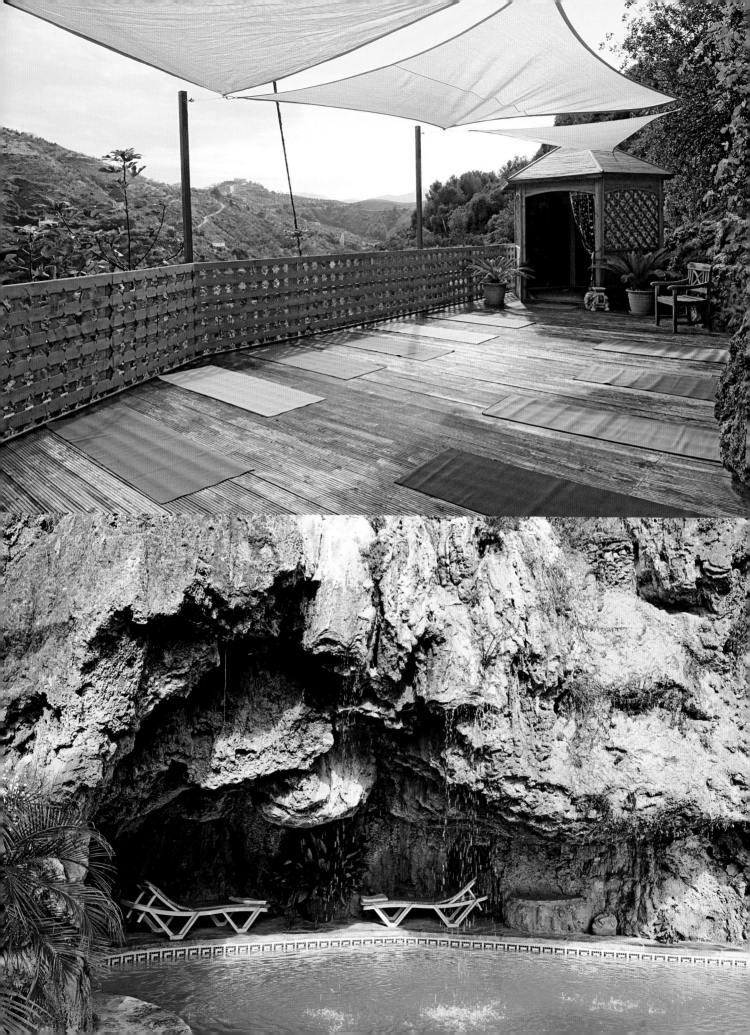

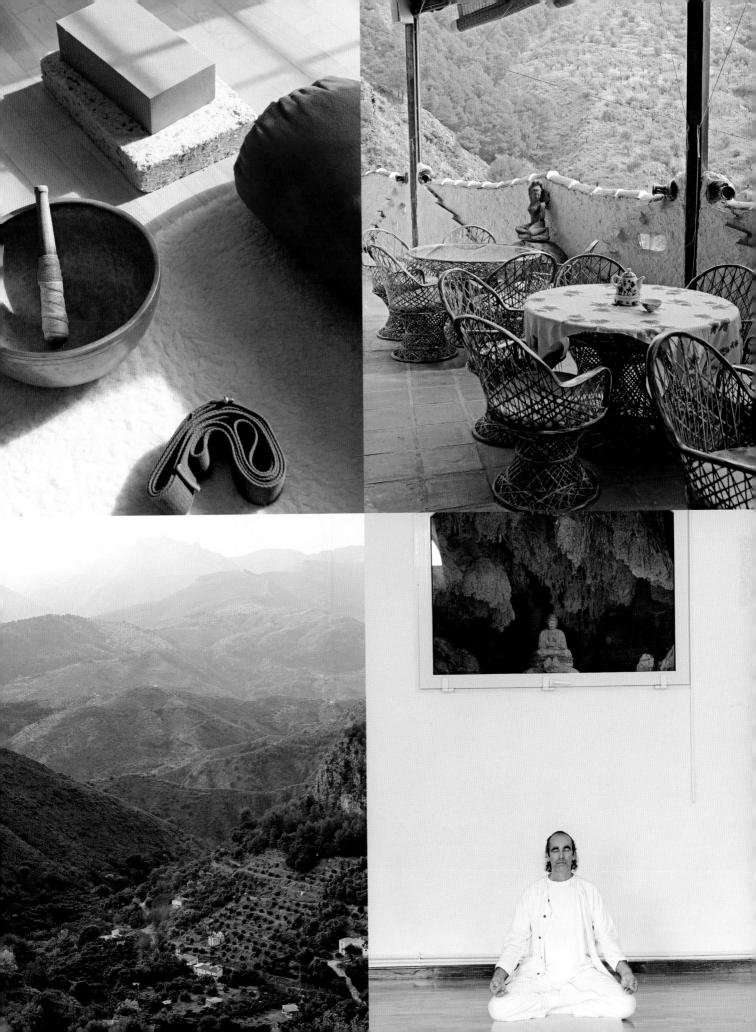

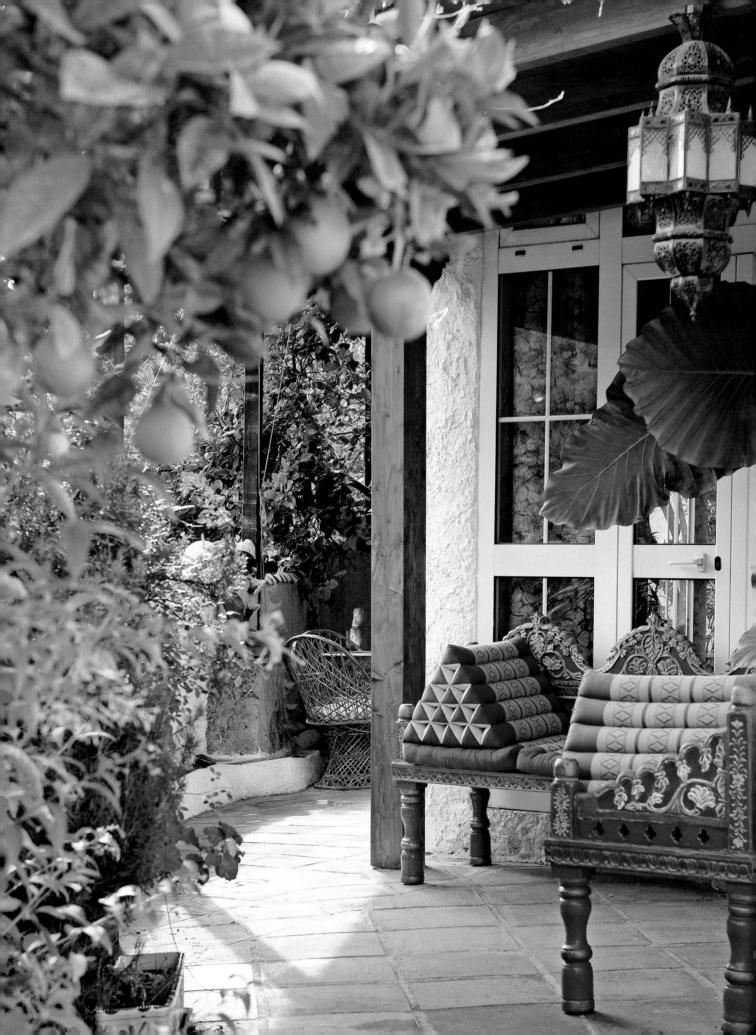

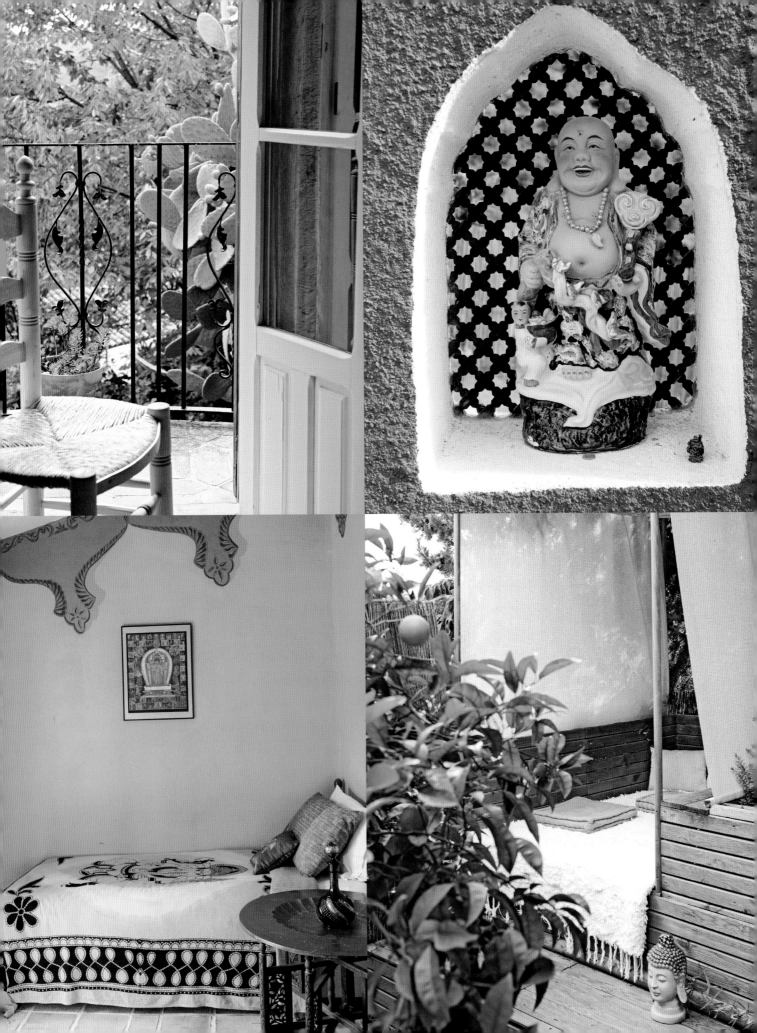

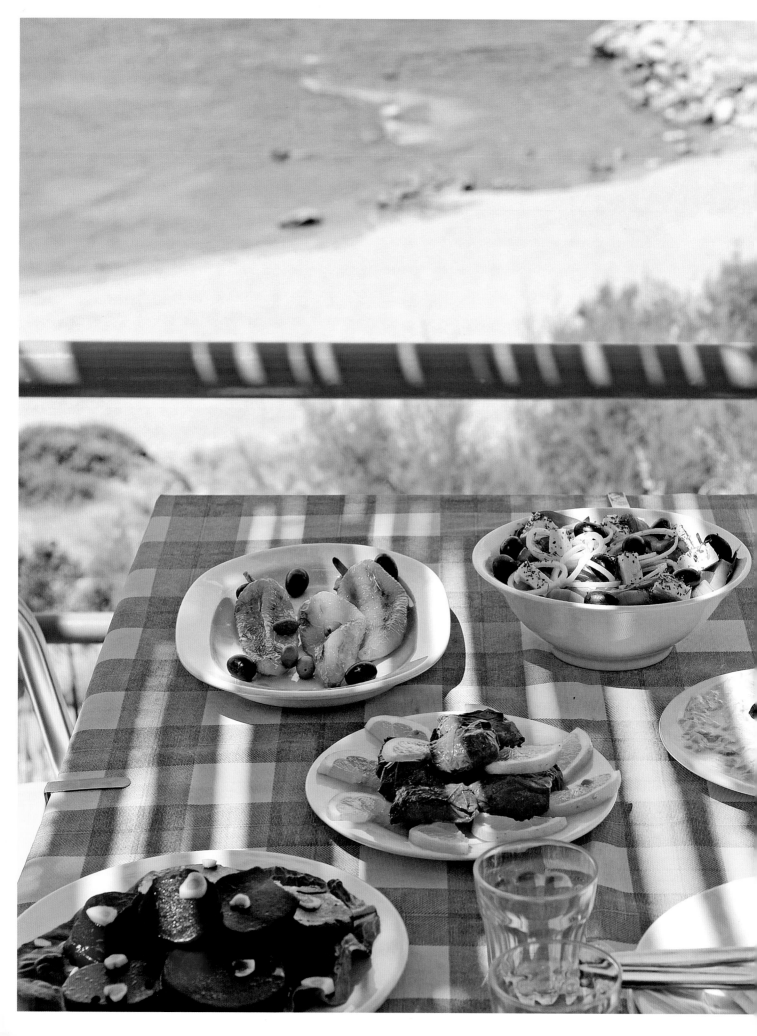

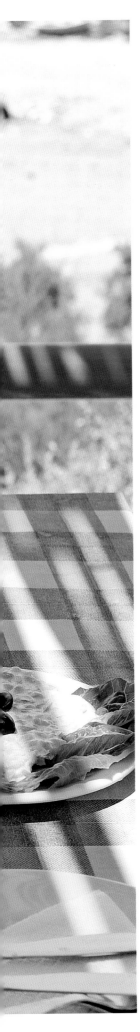

Far up on a cliff behind a high mountain chain, on which goats live an arduous life between dusty foliage and bristly bushes, stands Pavlos's guest house, a little oasis of humanity. "Handstand," orders the Greek yoga teacher Petros in a light Bavarian accent and all at once, to the sound of Moby, the world stands on its head: the endless expanse of the Libyan Sea and the three rocks that give the region its name. No wonder that one of the most popular places for Vinyasa Yoga in Europe has developed here. The tiny tavern with check tablecloths, the terrace grown over with oleander bushes, deep-red geraniums and palm trees, the bright yoga room and the small comfortable rooms with their light-blue varnished doors is run by Pavlos and his family. If Prometheus had not set light to the common giant fennel that also grows here and thus, against the will of Zeus, given the people fire, it would surely have been Pavlos—you couldn't wish for a more attentive host. After working up a sweat during a yoga session, an extended stroll along the long solitary bay and an evening meditation session, there awaits baked fennel, stuffed vine leaves, sweet pita with pears, pomegranate and figs. It can even happen that Petros reaches for the guitar after dinner, and everybody starts to dance.

Books to pack: "The Odyssey" by Homer and "Gods and Heroes: Myths and Epics of Ancient Greece" by Gustav Schwab

Kretashala

Pavlos Kakogiannakis, Triopetra
74100 Rethymnon, Crete
Greece
Tel. +49 89 333 295
info@kretashala.de
www.kretashala.de

Directions	Located in the west of the south coast of Crete, about 2 hrs from Heraklion Airport
Yoga	Jivamukti, Anusara, Ashtanga, Kirtan, Nada Yoga
Teachers	Petros Haffenrichter, Gabriela Bozic, Antje Schäfer, Mark Whitwell, Bryan Kest, Dave Stringer
Rooms	21 rooms for max. 45 guests
Food	Vegetarian, authentic Cretan cuisine
Treatments	Massages, Thai massage, Shiatsu
Leisure	Hiking, swimming, walks along the beach

Hinter einer hohen Bergkette, auf der Ziegen ein mühseliges Leben zwischen staubigen Kräutern und borstigen Sträuchern führen, liegt hoch oben auf einem Kliff Pavlos' Pension, eine kleine Oase der Menschlichkeit. »Handstand« befiehlt Petros, der griechische Yogalehrer, in leichtem Bayerisch, und auf einmal steht die Welt zum Sound von Moby auf dem Kopf: die unendliche Weite der Libyschen See und die drei Felsen, die der Gegend den Namen gaben. Kein Wunder, dass sich dies zu einer der beliebtesten Adressen für Vinyasa Yoga in Europa entwickelt hat. Die winzige Taverne mit ihren karierten Tischdecken, der von Oleanderbüschen, tiefroten Geranien und Palmen bewachsenen Terrasse, dem lichten Yogaraum und den gemütlichen, kleinen Zimmern mit ihren hellblau lackierten Türen wird von Pavlos und seiner Familie geführt. Hätte nicht Prometheus das hier ebenfalls wachsende gemeine Steckenkraut entflammt und so den Menschen gegen den Willen von Zeus Feuer geschenkt, wäre es wohl Pavlos gewesen. Fürsorglicher kann man sich einen Wirt nicht wünschen. Nach schweißtreibenden Yogastunden, ausgedehnten Spaziergängen durch die lang gestreckte, einsame Bucht und einer Abendmeditation gibt es gebackenen Fenchel, gefüllte Weinblätter, süße Pita mit Birnen, Granatäpfeln und Feigen. Es kann einem sogar passieren, dass Petros danach zur Gitarre greift und alle anfangen zu tanzen.

Reisebegleiter: »Die Odyssee« von Homer und »Sagen des klassischen Altertums« von Gustav Schwab

Derrrière une haute chaîne de montagnes, là où les chèvres mènent une vie rude entre herbes poussiéreuses et buissons épineux, tout en haut d'une falaise, est perchée la pension Pavlos, un petit havre d'humanité. « Faites le poirier », ordonne Petros, le professeur de yoga grec, avec un léger accent bavarois et, tout à coup, sur la musique de Moby, le monde est à l'envers : l'espace infini de la mer Lybienne et les trois rochers qui ont donné leur nom à la région. Rien d'étonnant que l'une des adresses les plus prisées du yoga Vinyasa en Europe ait pris ici son essor. La minuscule taverne avec ses nappes à carreaux, sa terrasse envahie de buissons de laurier rose, de géraniums rouge foncé et de palmiers, sa salle de yoga baignée de lumière et ses petites chambres confortables aux portes laquées en bleu clair est dirigée par Pavlos et sa famille. Si Prométhée n'avait pas allumé la férule commune, qui pousse ici aussi, et ainsi, contre la volonté de Zeus, apporté le feu aux hommes, c'est bien Pavlos qui s'en serait chargé. Impossible de trouver un hôtelier plus attentionné. Après les séances de yoga sudorifiques, les longues promenades sur l'immense crique solitaire et la méditation, place aux fenouils au four, aux feuilles de vigne farcies, à la pita sucrée aux poires, aux pommes et aux figues. Il peut même arriver que Pavlos prenne ensuite sa guitare et que tous se mettent à danser.

Livres à emporter : « L'Odyssée » d'Homère et « Légendes de l'Antiquité classique » de Gustav Schwab

Anreise	Im Westen der Südküste von Kreta gelegen, etwa 2 Std. vom Flughafen Heraklion entfernt
Yoga	Jivamukti, Anusara, Ashtanga, Kirtan und Nada Yoga
Lehrer	Petros Haffenrichter, Gabriela Bozic, Antje Schäfer, Mark Whitwell, Bryan Kest, Dave Stringer
Zimmer	21 Zimmer für max. 45 Gäste
Küche	Vegetarisch, authentische kretische Küche
Anwendungen	Massage, Thai-Massage, Shiatsu
Aktivitäten	Wandern, Schwimmen, Strandspaziergänge

Accès	Situé à l'ouest de la côte sud de la Crète, à environ 2 h de l'aéroport d'Héraklion
Yoga	Jivamukti, Anusara, Ashtânga, Kirtan et Nada Yoga
Professeurs	Petros Haffenrichter, Gabriela Bozic, Antje Schäfer, Mark Whitwell, Bryan Kest, Dave Stringer
Chambres	21 chambres pour 45 personnes max.
Restauration	Cuisine végétarienne, cuisine crétoise régionale authentique
Traitements	Massage, massage thaïlandais, shiatsu
Activités	Randonnées, natation, promenades sur la plage

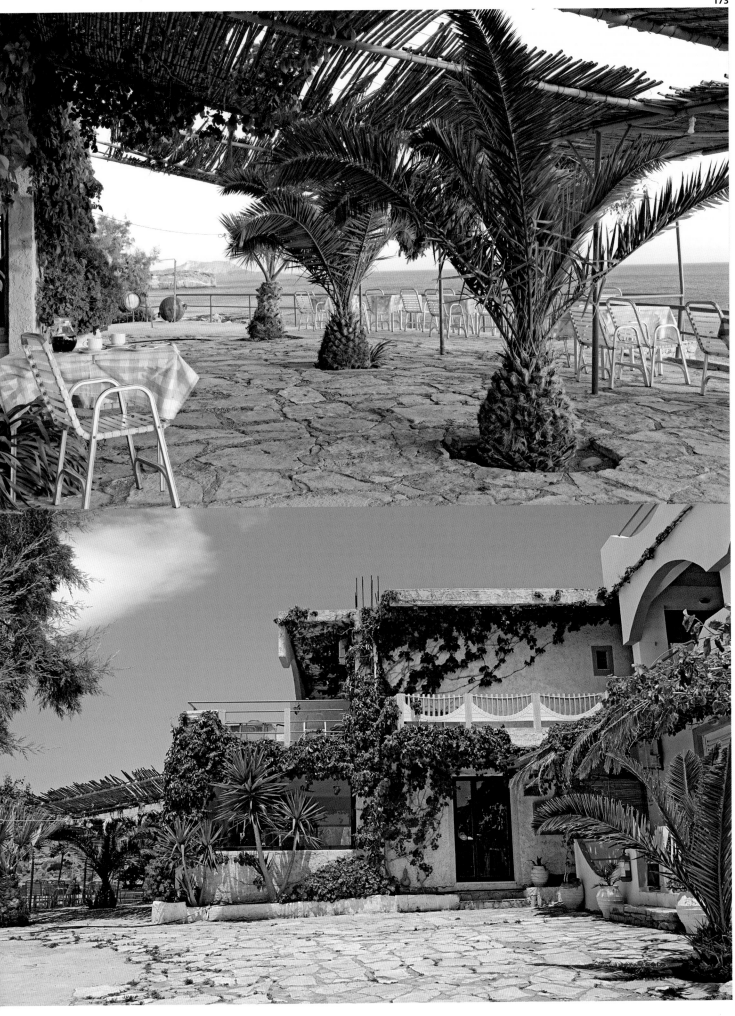

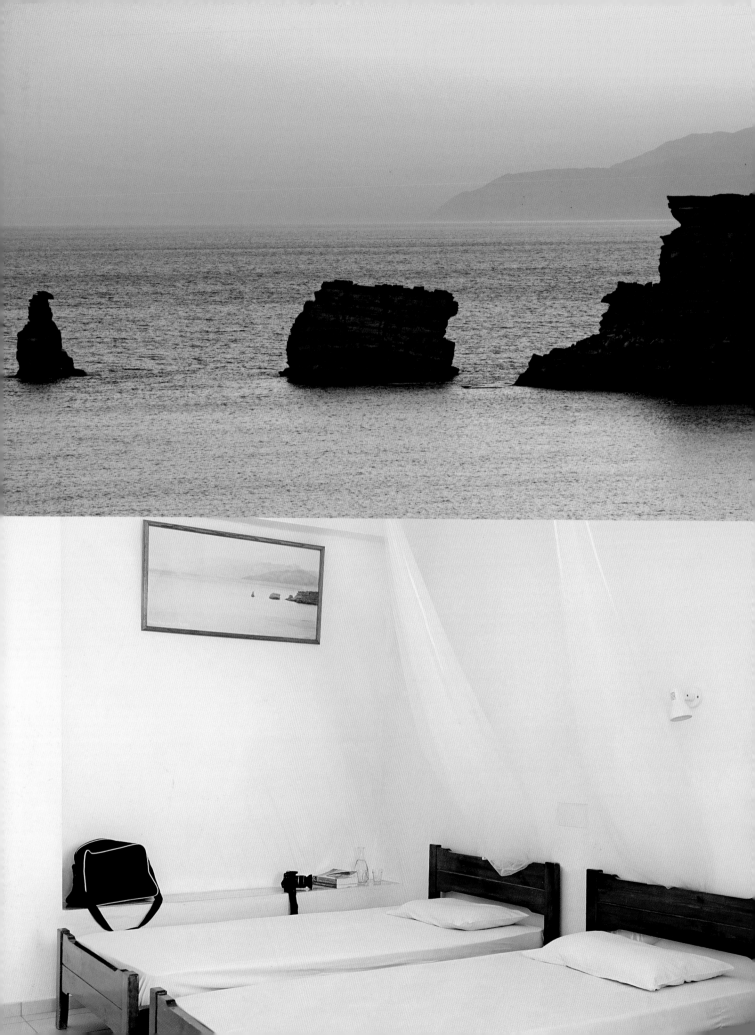

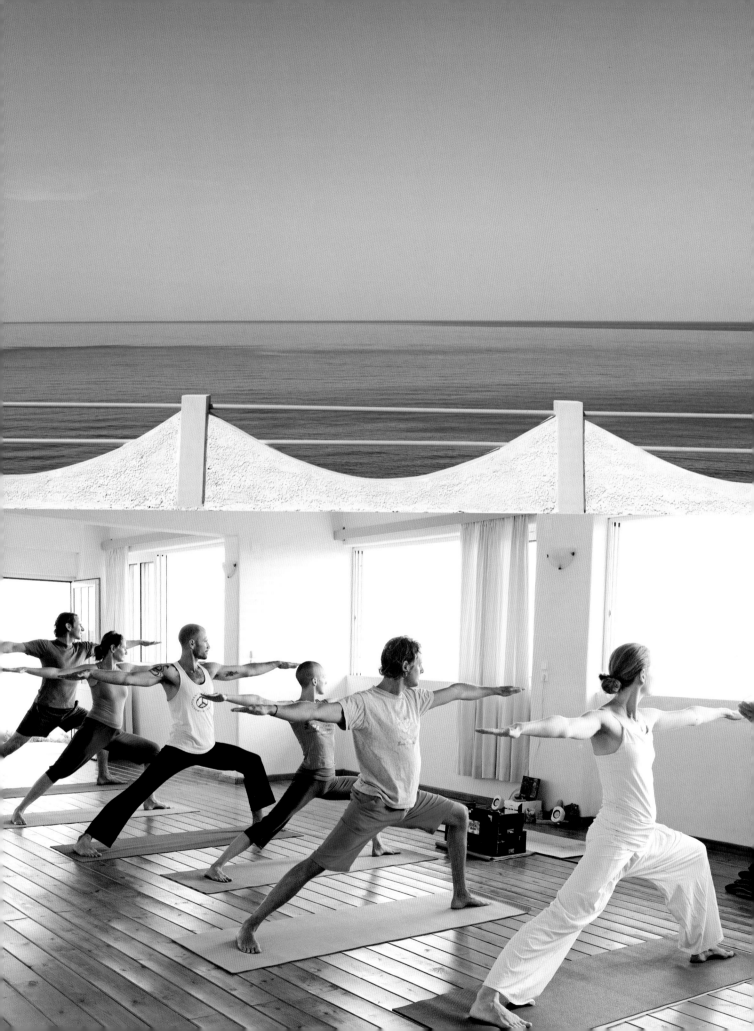

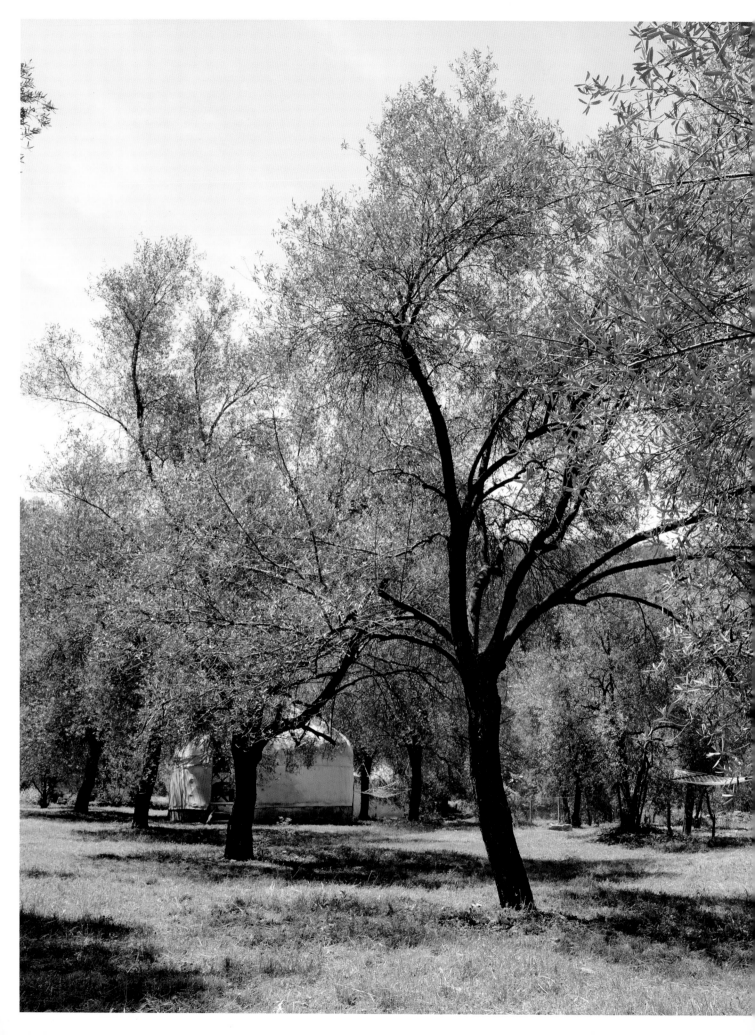

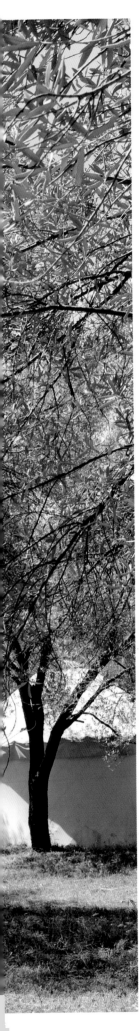

Ashtanga in the Mysore style is, as everybody knows, no picnic. By the tenth jump back into Chaturanga Dandasana at the latest, the arms are trembling, the thighs hurt and the Achilles tendon is sending distress signals. Or maybe not. Because those who are guided through Pattabhi Jois's Primary Series will in the end love the köşk, as the wonderfully pretty wooden summer pavilion where the sessions take place is called. Indeed, this small charming retreat, built in the midst of olive groves, is firmly in British and Turkish hands. Almost all the teachers come from Triyoga, the famous yoga school in London's Primrose Hill, London Bikram College and Jivamukti Berlin, and they return year after year. Is it because of the broad hammocks that invite you to take extended lunch breaks under the fig trees, or the delicious lovingly prepared meals, attended by all at a long table in the open air, or the yurts, round comfortable tents from which you can look at the stars in the sky whilst falling asleep under mosquito nets? Or is it just that in this peaceful valley, as the name Huzur Vadisi translates, with a view of the turquoise-coloured sea, a peace of mind sets in through which that slight ache in the legs and those tensed-up stomach muscles are—how do we put it in the rational world?—"transcended" towards a general feeling of bliss.

Books to pack: "Stillness Speaks: Whispers of Now" by Eckhart Tolle and "Memed, My Hawk" by Yaşar Kemal

Huzur Vadisi

Gökçeovacık
Göcek 48310, Fethiye
Turkey
Tel. +90 252 644 0008 (summer only)
and +44 759 148 1074
huzvad@gmail.com
www.huzurvadisi.com

Directions	Located in the southwest of Turkey, 40 min from the next airport, Dalaman
Yoga	Hatha, Sivananda, Scaravelli, Jivamukti, Vinyasa, Bikram, Ashtanga
Teachers	Simon Low, Michele Pernetta, Katy Appleton, Anja Kuhnel, Dechen Thurman, Hilary Menting-Brown, Gary Carter
Rooms	12 yurts, 1 cottage, 1 summer house for max. 30 guests
Food	Predominantly vegetarian Turkish dishes; vegan, fish or meat on request
Treatments	Massage, Turkish bath
Leisure	Swimming pool, day trips, boat trips

Ashtanga im Mysore-Stil zu üben, ist, wie jeder weiß, kein Zuckerschlecken. Spätestens beim zehnten Zurückspringen in Chaturanga Dandasana zittern die Arme, schmerzen die Oberschenkel, meldet sich die Achillessehne. Oder nicht. Denn wer durch Pattabhi Jois' Primary Series begleitet wird, liebt am Ende den Köşk, wie der wunderhübsche, aus Holz gebaute Sommerpavillon heißt, in dem geübt wird. Überhaupt ist dieses kleine charmante Retreat, mitten in einen Olivenhain gebaut, fest in britischer und türkischer Hand. Fast alle Lehrer kommen von Triyoga, der berühmten Londoner Yogaschule in Primrose Hill, sowie vom London Bikram College und von Jivamukti Berlin, und sie kehren jedes Jahr hierher zurück. Liegt es an den breiten Hänge-matten, die unter Feigenbäumen zu ausgedehnten Mittags-pausen einladen? An den köstlichen, liebevoll zubereiteten Mahlzeiten, zu denen sich alle an einem langen Tisch im Freien einfinden? An den Jurten, den komfortablen runden Zelten, in denen man unter Moskitonetzen liegend die Sterne am Himmel sehen kann? Oder einfach daran, dass sich in diesem »friedlichen Tal«, wie Huzur Vadisi übersetzt heißt, mit Blick auf die türkisfarbene türkische See, ein Seelenfrieden einstellt, der das leichte Ziehen in den Beinen und die angekurbelten Bauchmuskeln – wie sagt man in der rationalen Welt – »transzendiert«? Was bleibt, ist ein gene-relles Summen der Glückseligkeit.

Reisebegleiter: »Stille spricht: Wahres Sein berühren« von Eckhart Tolle und »Der Baum des Narren« von Yaşar Kemal

Comme chacun sait, la pratique de l'Ashtânga dans le style Mysore n'est vraiment pas du gâteau. Au plus tard au dixième saut en arrière dans un Chaturanga Dandasana, les bras tremblent, les cuisses sont douloureuses, le tendon d'Achille se fait sentir. Ou non. Car celui qui effectue les séries pri-maires de Pattabhi Jois' finit par aimer le « köşk », comme on appelle le ravissant pavillon d'été construit en bois dans lequel on s'entraîne. Cette petite et charmante oasis bâtie au cœur d'un bosquet d'oliviers est une petite enclave anglo-turque. Presque tous les professeurs sont issus de Triyoga, la fameuse école de yoga de la Primrose Hill à Londres, du London Bikram College et de Jivamukti à Berlin, et-ils reviennent tous les ans. Cela tient-il aux larges hamacs qui, sous les figuiers, invitent à des siestes prolongées ? Aux succulents repas concoctés avec amour, pour lesquels tout le monde se réunit autour d'une longue table en plein air ? Aux yourtes, ces confortables tentes rondes, où l'on peut, sous les moustiquaires, contempler la nuit les étoiles au fir-mament ? Ou simplement à ce que, dans cette vallée paisible (traduction littérale de Huzur Vadisi), les yeux posés sur la mer Egée de couleur turquoise, la paix s'installe en vous qui – comme on le dit dans le monde rationnel – « trans-cende » les petites crampes dans les jambes et les muscles abdominaux stimulés jusqu'à ce qu'il ne reste qu'un bruisse-ment de béatitude.

Livres à emporter : « Quiétude : A l'écoute de sa nature essen-tielle » d'Eckhart Tolle et « Mémed le faucon » de Yaşar Kemal

Anreise	Im Südwesten der Türkei, 40 min vom Flughafen Dalaman entfernt
Yoga	Hatha, Sivananda, Scaravelli, Jivamukti, Vinyasa, Bikram, Ashtanga
Lehrer	Simon Low, Michele Pernetta, Katy Appleton, Anja Kuhnel, Dechen Thurman, Hilary Menting-Brown, Gary Carter
Zimmer	12 Jurten, 1 Hütte, 1 Sommerhaus für max. 30 Gäste
Küche	Überwiegend türkisch-vegetarisch; vegan, Fisch oder Fleisch auf Anfrage
Anwendungen	Massage, türkisches Bad
Aktivitäten	Schwimmbad, Ausflüge, Bootsfahrten

Accès	Situé au sud-ouest de la Turquie, à 40 min de l'aéroport le plus proche à Dalaman
Yoga	Hatha, Sivananda, Scaravelli, Jivamukti, Vinyasa, Bikram, Ashtânga
Professeurs	Simon Low, Michele Pernetta, Katy Appleton, Anja Kuhnel, Dechen Thurman, Hilary Menting-Brown, Gary Carter
Chambres	12 yourtes, 1 cottage, un pavillon d'été pour 30 personnes max.
Restauration	Cuisine essentiellement turque et végétarienne ; végétalienne, poisson ou viande sur demande
Traitements	Massage, bain turc
Activités	Piscine, excursions, promenades en bateau

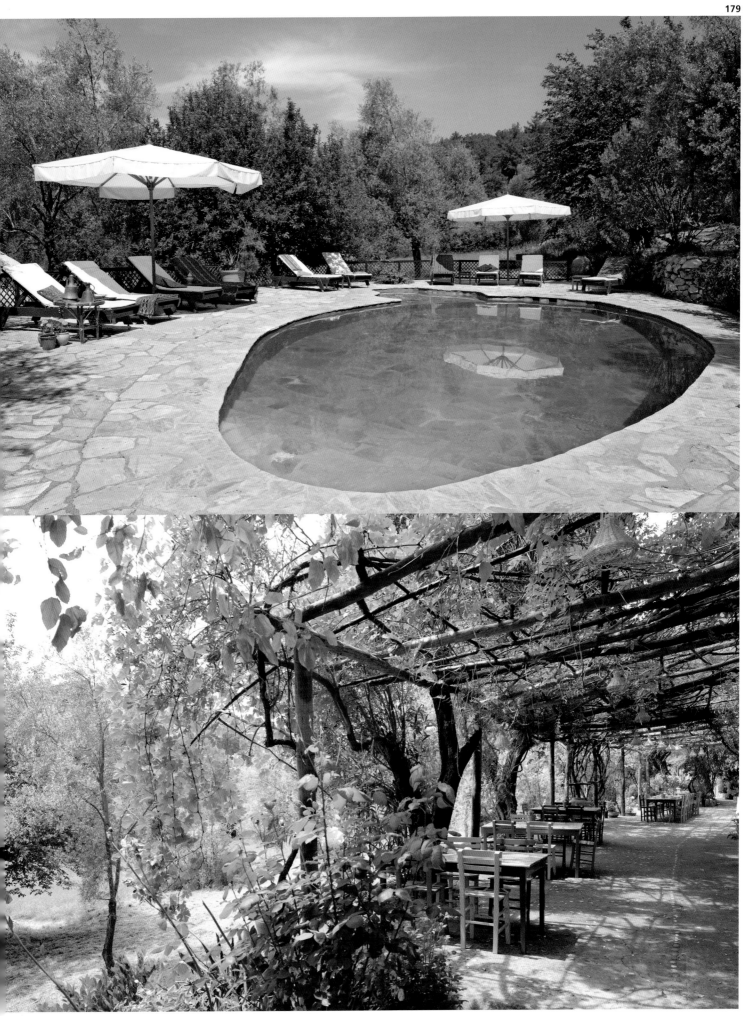

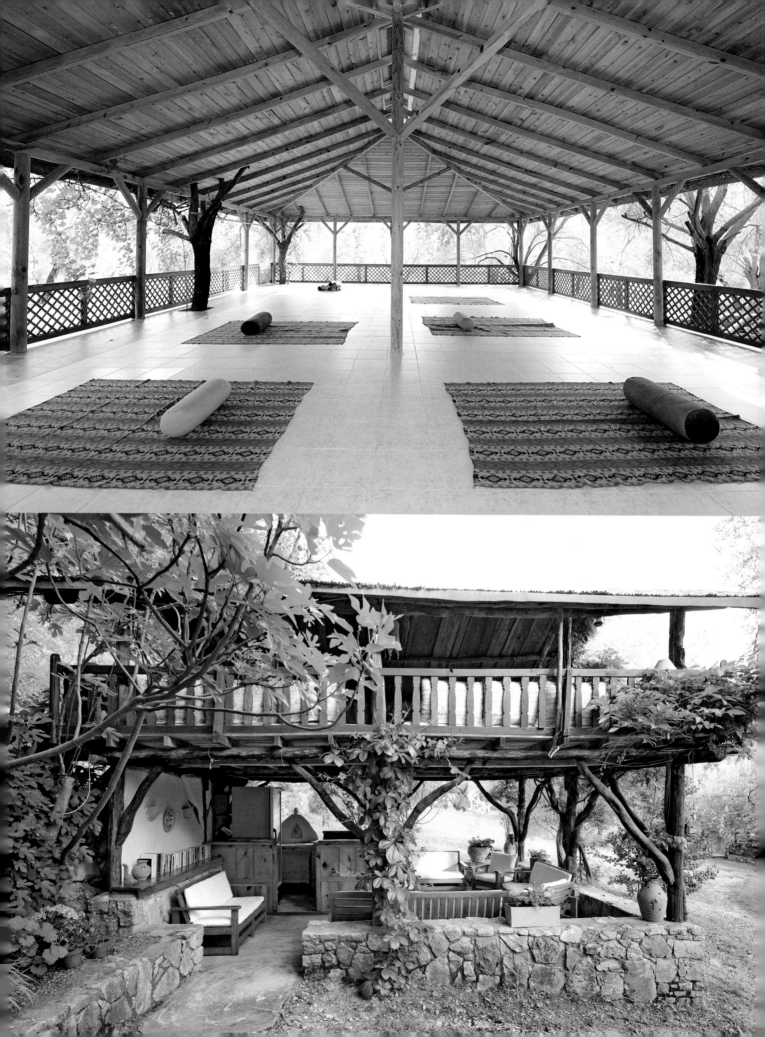

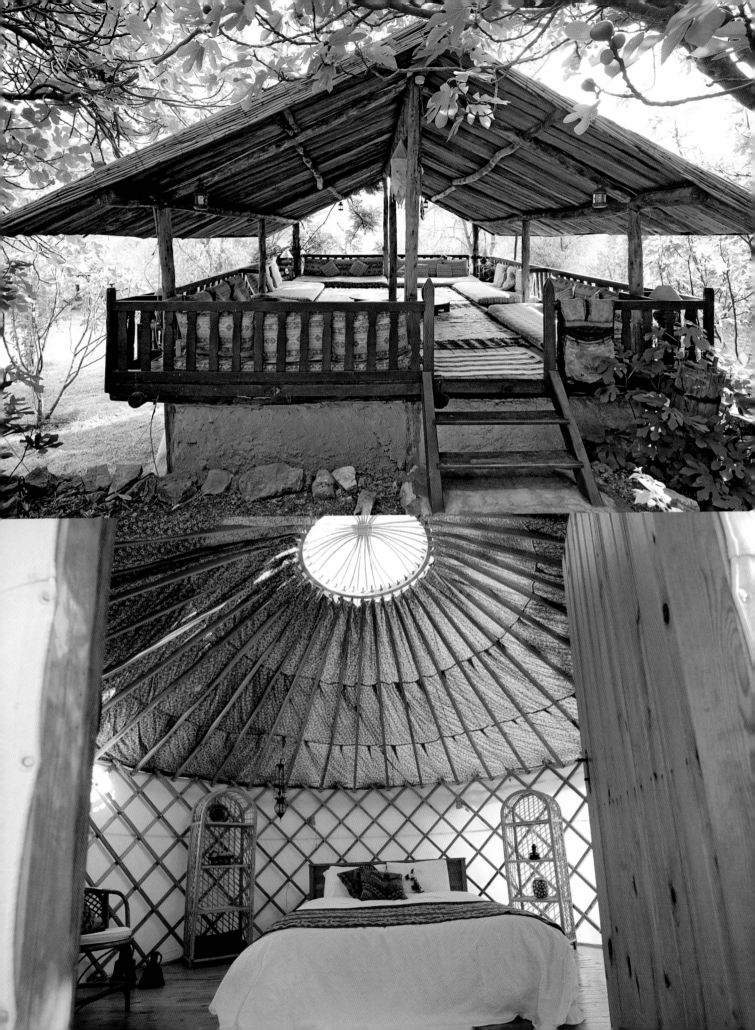

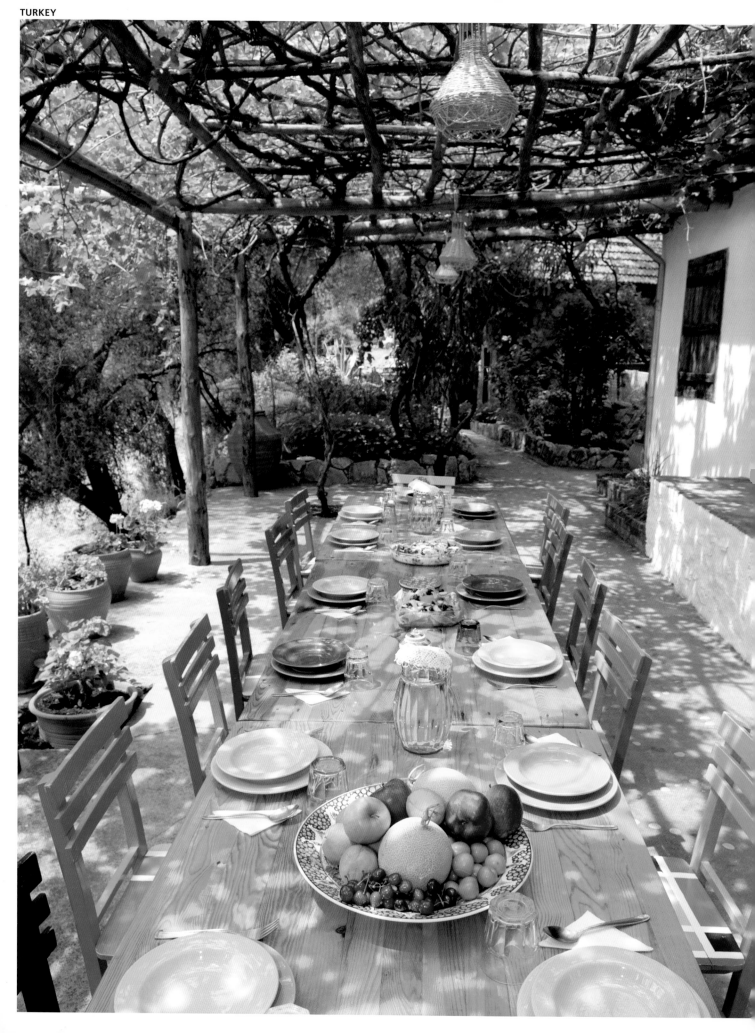

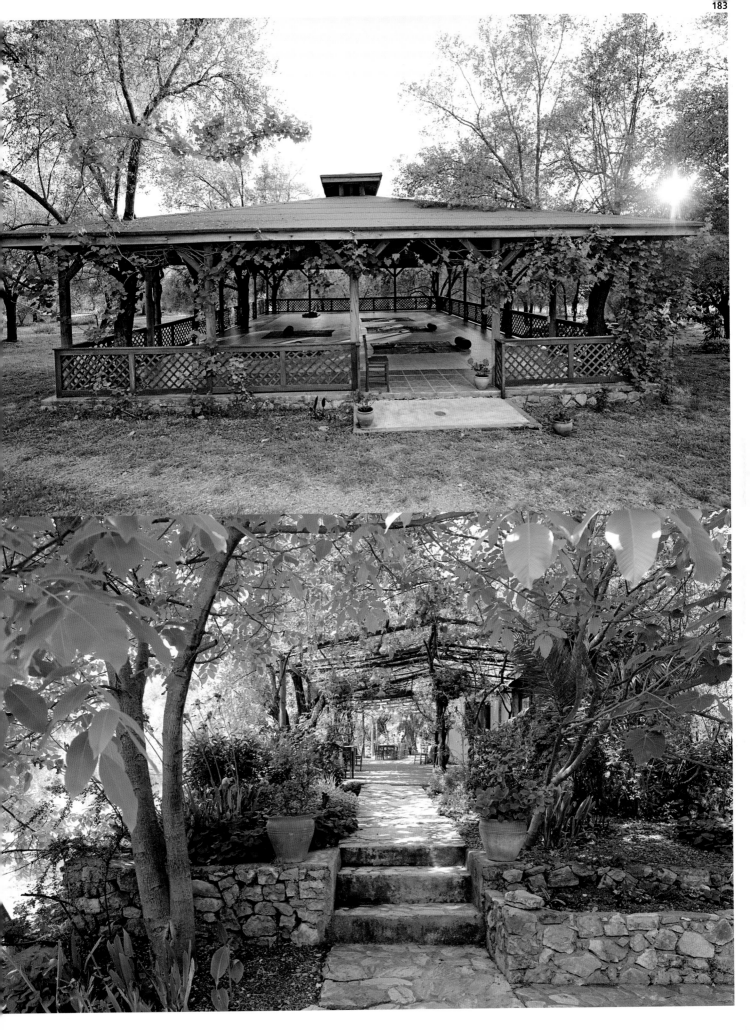

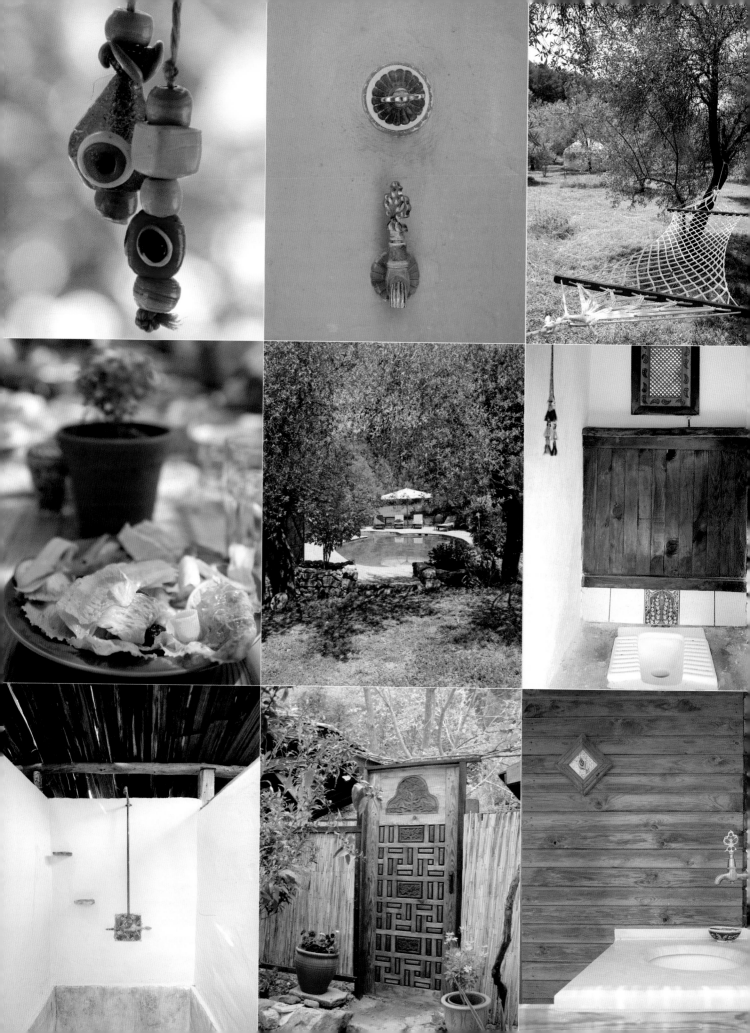

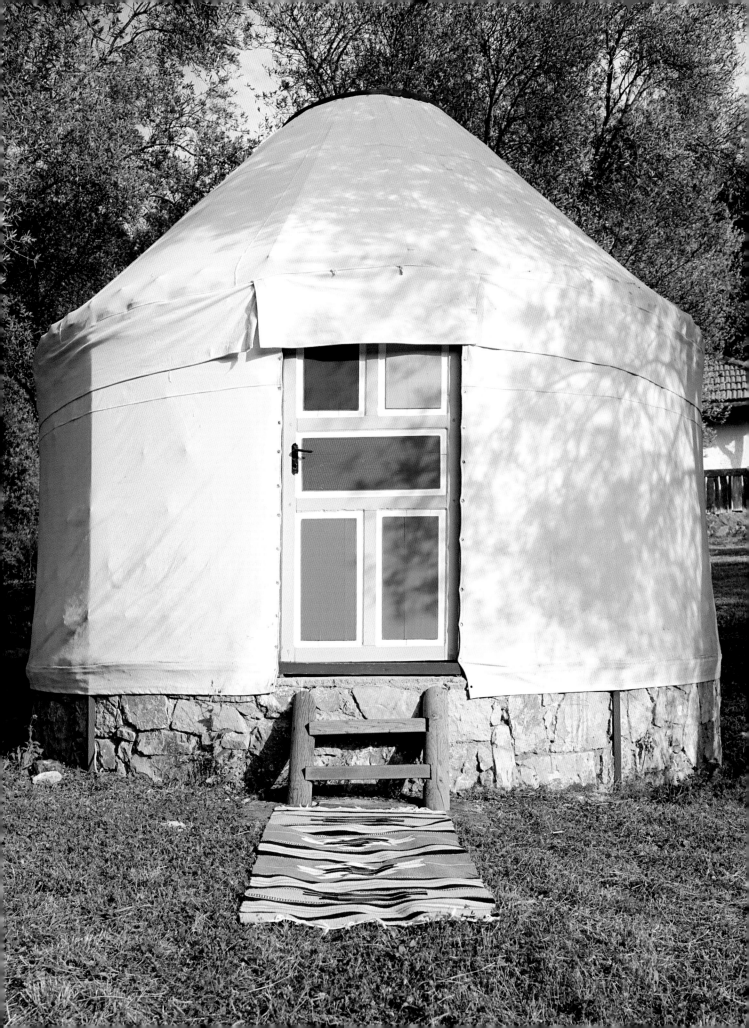

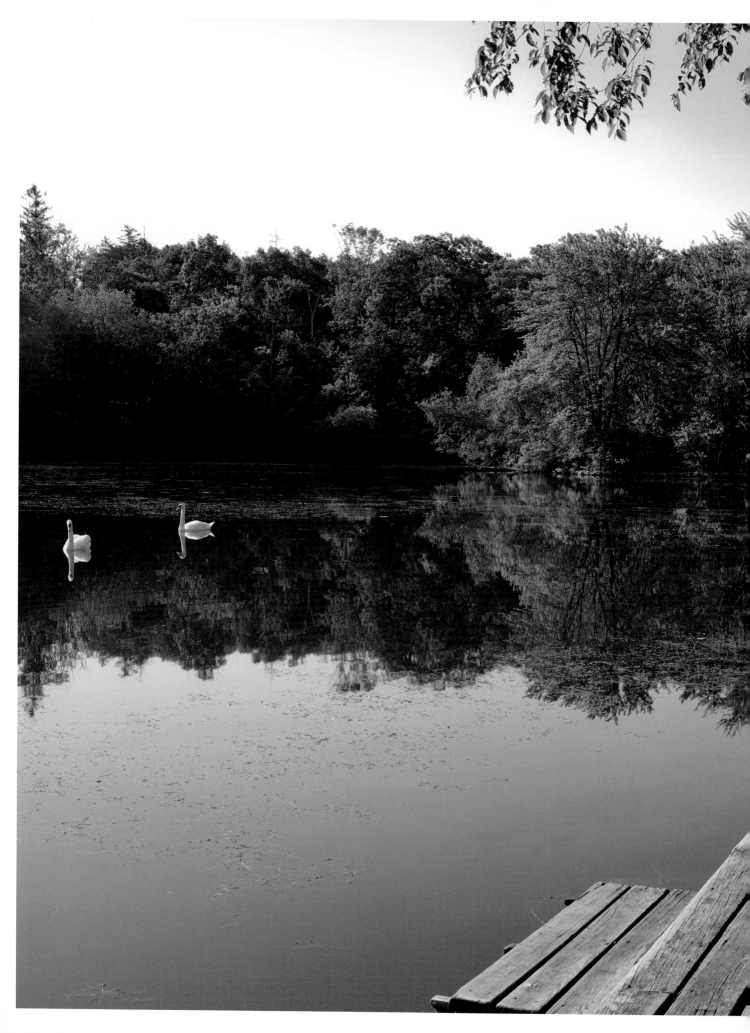

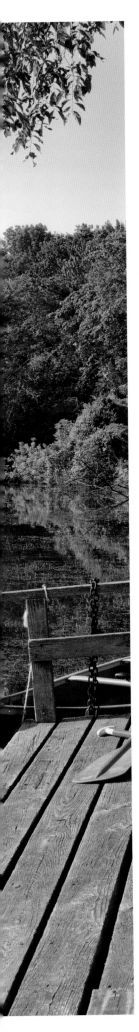

It is barely two hours from Park Avenue, but here at the foot of the Catskill Mountains even the leaves under your feet rustle more peacefully than they do in New York. It is easy to imagine that this ashram was once ultra fashionable, back in the days when girls in miniskirts sat in the grass between the pretty white wooden houses and learnt how to meditate from the Indian neurosurgeon and Sanskrit scholar Rammurti S. Mishra. Roe deer are still to be seen in the early-morning mist on the hill above the little lake, and the oddball old ladies who teach Sanskrit here and run the place wear little white dresses that swing when they dance. At least two daily sessions of Hatha Yoga and Sanskrit are included in the price. The weekend programme must be paid for separately, but it's worth it. When stars like Ruth Lauer-Manenti of Jivamukti, New York, are doing the teaching, the students, running with sweat, stagger afterwards with shining eyes down to the water. At other weekends, under the strict supervision of Joan Suval, no word may be spoken; a week later in Laraaji Nadananda's Laughter Workshop everyone is bent double in mirth for hours. The better end of the New York esoteric scene is regularly seen here, and people come from the entire East Coast to this mountain country to find themselves again amongst deep forests and hidden watercourses. Because, in spite of the ban on alcohol and tobacco and alongside a tender hint of nostalgia, one thing dominates here above all else: the spirit of enlightenment, which welcomes every guest into the constantly self-renewing community.

Books to pack: "The Textbook of Yoga Psychology" by Rammurti S. Mishra and "Glamorama" by Bret Easton Ellis

Ananda Ashram

Yoga Society of New York
13 Sapphire Road
Monroe, NY 10950
USA
Tel. +1 845 782 5575
Fax +1 845 774 7368
ananda@anandaashram.org
www.anandaashram.org

Directions	About 1 1/2 hrs north of New York
Yoga	Hatha, Vinyasa, Ashtanga, Jivamukti
Teachers	Joan Suval, Ma Bhaskarananda, David Michael Hollander, Krishna Das, Shyam Das, Julie Kirkpatrick
Rooms	Three guest houses with a total of 45 beds, 6-bed rooms and 2-bed rooms, camping possible in summer
Food	Predominantly vegetarian, with a fantastic breakfast buffet
Treatments	Ayurvedic facial and massage, Swedish massage, Shiatsu, foot reflexology massage, aromatherapy, Raindrop Technique, relaxation training, sauna
Leisure	Meditation, Kathak dance, hiking, swimming, tabla and sitar lessons

Es sind nicht mal zwei Stunden von der Park Avenue, aber hier am Fuße der Catskill Mountains raschelt selbst das Laub unter den Füßen friedlicher als in New York. Man kann es sich gut vorstellen, dass der Ashram früher todschick war, als Mädchen in Miniröcken im Gras zwischen den hübschen, weißen Holzhäusern saßen und von dem indischen Neurochirurgen und Sanskritgelehrten Rammurti S. Mishra lernten, wie man meditiert. Noch immer stehen morgens im Frühnebel Rehe auf dem Hügel oberhalb des kleinen Sees, und die schrulligen älteren Damen, die hier Sanskrit unterrichten und den Laden schmeißen, tragen weiße Kleidchen, die beim Tanzen schwingen. Täglich mindestens zweimal Hatha Yoga und Sanskrit sind im Preis inbegriffen; das Wochenendprogramm muss extra bezahlt werden, lohnt sich aber. Wenn Stars wie Ruth Lauer-Manenti von Jivamukti New York, unterrichten, taumeln die Schüler hinterher schweißüberströmt mit glänzenden Augen hinunter zum Wasser. An anderen Wochenenden darf unter der strengen Aufsicht von Joan Suval kein Wort gesprochen werden, während sich eine Woche später im Lach-Workshop von Laraaji Nadananda alle stundenlang vor Lachen biegen. Die bessere New Yorker Esoterikszene lässt sich regelmäßig sehen, und von der ganzen Ostküste kommen Menschen, um in der idyllischen Berglandschaft zwischen tiefen Wäldern und versteckten Wasserläufen wieder zu sich zu finden. Denn trotz Alkohol- und Tabakverbot herrscht hier neben einem zärtlichen Hauch von Nostalgie vor allem eins: der Geist der Aufklärung, der jeden Gast herzlich in die immer nachwachsende Gemeinde aufnimmt.

Reisebegleiter: »The Textbook of Yoga Psychology« von Rammurti S. Mishra und »Glamorama« von Bret Easton Ellis

Park Avenue n'est qu'à deux heures à peine, mais ici, au pied des montagnes Catskill, même le feuillage bruisse plus doucement sous les pas qu'à New York. Il est aisé d'imaginer que l'âshram fut, à une époque, du dernier chic, lorsque des filles en minijupe, assises dans l'herbe entre les jolies maisons de bois blanc, apprenaient la méditation de Rammurti S. Mishra, neurochirugien indien et spécialiste du sanskrit. Comme autrefois, sur la colline dominant le petit lac, les biches se promènent dans la brume matinale et même les vieilles dames excentriques qui enseignent ici le sanskrit et tiennent boutique, portent des petites robes blanches qui volent quand elles dansent. Au moins deux séances d'Hatha-yoga et de sanskrit par jour sont incluses dans le prix. Le programme du week-end doit être payé en plus, mais il en vaut la peine. Quand des stars, comme Ruth Lauer-Manenti du centre new-yorkais Jivamukti, enseignent, les élèves, en nage et les yeux brillants, la suivent en titubant jusque dans l'eau. Pendant d'autres week-ends, sous la surveillance rigoureuse de Joan Suval, il est interdit de parler et, une semaine plus tard, tous se tordent de rire des heures durant dans l'atelier du rire de Laraaji Nadananda. La fine fleur de la scène ésotérique new-yorkaise fait régulièrement irruption ici, et les adeptes viennent de toute la côte est pour se retrouver avec eux-mêmes dans ce cadre idyllique de montagnes entre forêts profondes et torrents sauvages. Car, malgré l'interdiction d'alcool et de tabac, il règne surtout le souffle de la révélation, teinté de nostalgie, et chaque hôte est accueilli chaleureusement dans la communauté sans cesse renouvelée.

Livres à emporter : « The Textbook of Yoga Psychology » de Rammurti S. Mishra et « Glamorama » de Bret Easton Ellis

Anreise	Etwa 1,5 Std. nördlich von New York
Yoga	Hatha, Vinyasa, Ashtanga, Jivamukti
Lehrer	Joan Suval, Ma Bhaskarananda, David Michael Hollander, Krishna Das, Shyam Das, Julie Kirkpatrick
Zimmer	3 Gästehäuser mit insgesamt 45 Betten
Küche	Überwiegend vegetarisch, fantastisches Frühstücksbüfett
Anwendungen	Ayurvedische Facials und Massagen, Schwedische Massage, Shiatsu, Fußreflexzonen-Massage, Aromatherapie, Raindrop Technique, Entspannungstraining, Eukalyptus-Sauna
Aktivitäten	Meditation, Kathak-Tanz, Wandern, Schwimmen, Unterricht in Tabla und Sitar

Accès	Situé à environ 1 h 30 au nord de New York
Yoga	Hatha, Vinyasa, Ashtânga, Jivamukti
Professeurs	Joan Suval, Ma Bhaskarananda, David Michael Hollander, Krishna Das, Shyam Das, Julie Kirkpatrick
Chambres	3 maisons d'hôtes avec en tout 45 lits
Restauration	Végétarienne, fantastique buffet au petit-déjeuner
Traitements	Soins du visage et massage ayurvédiques, massage suédois, shiatsu, réflexologie plantaire, aromathérapie, technique Raindrop, relaxation, sauna à l'eucalyptus
Activités	Méditation, danse kathak, randonnées, natation, cours de tablâ et de sitar

Ananda Ashram

YOGA SOCIETY OF NEW YORK, INC.

—— EST. 1958 ——

ENTRANCE

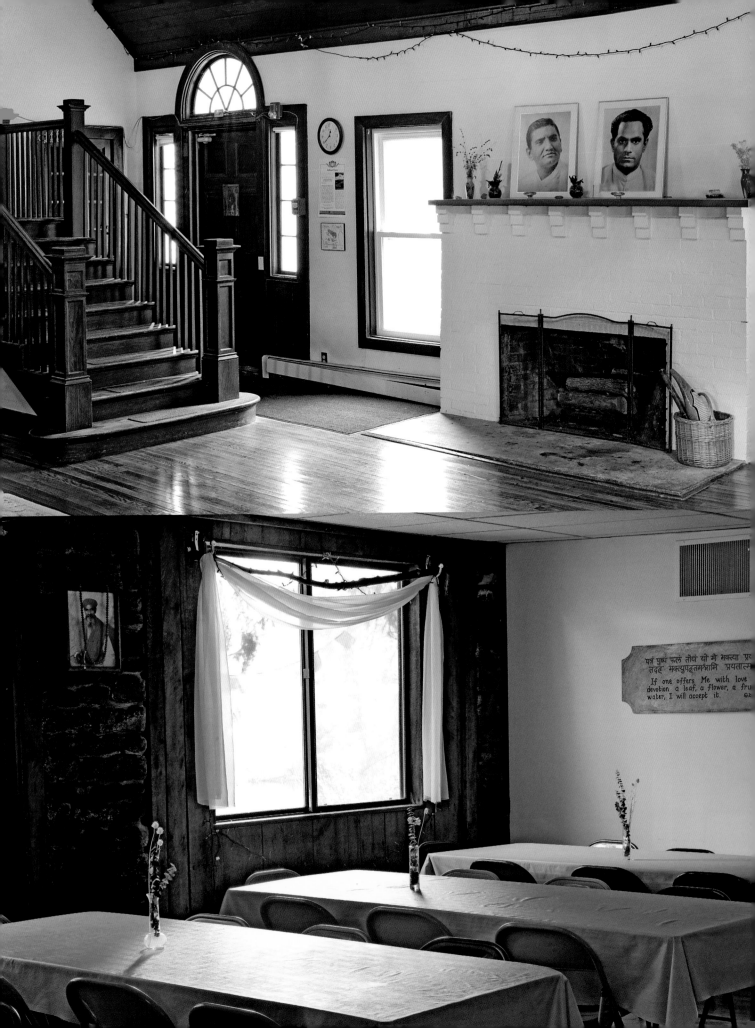

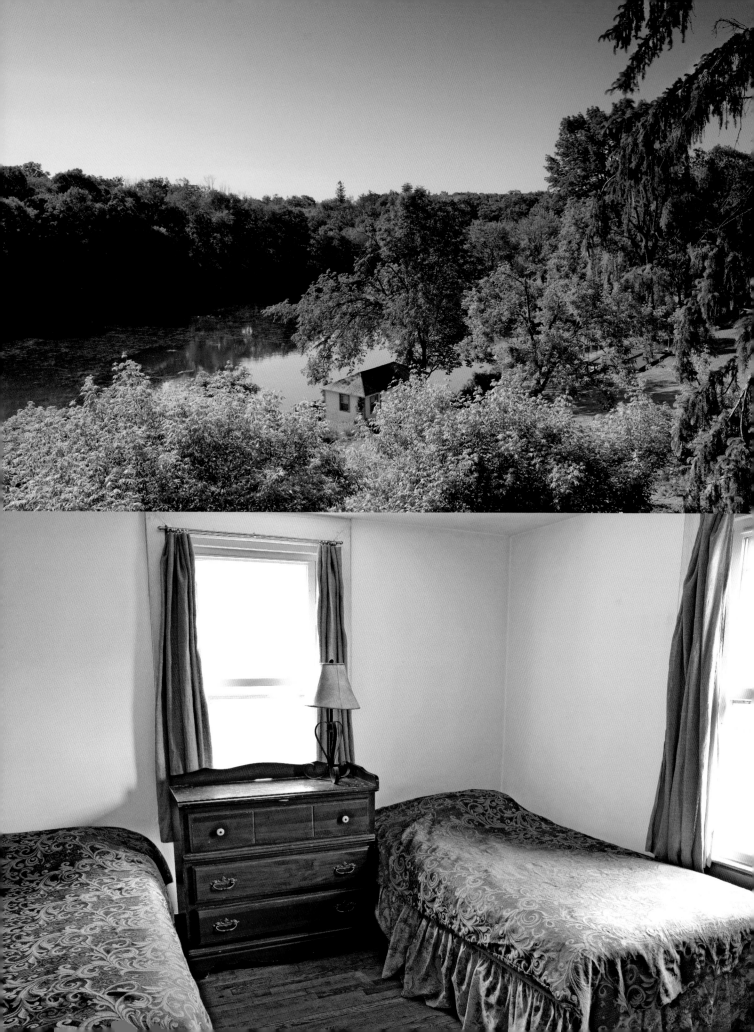

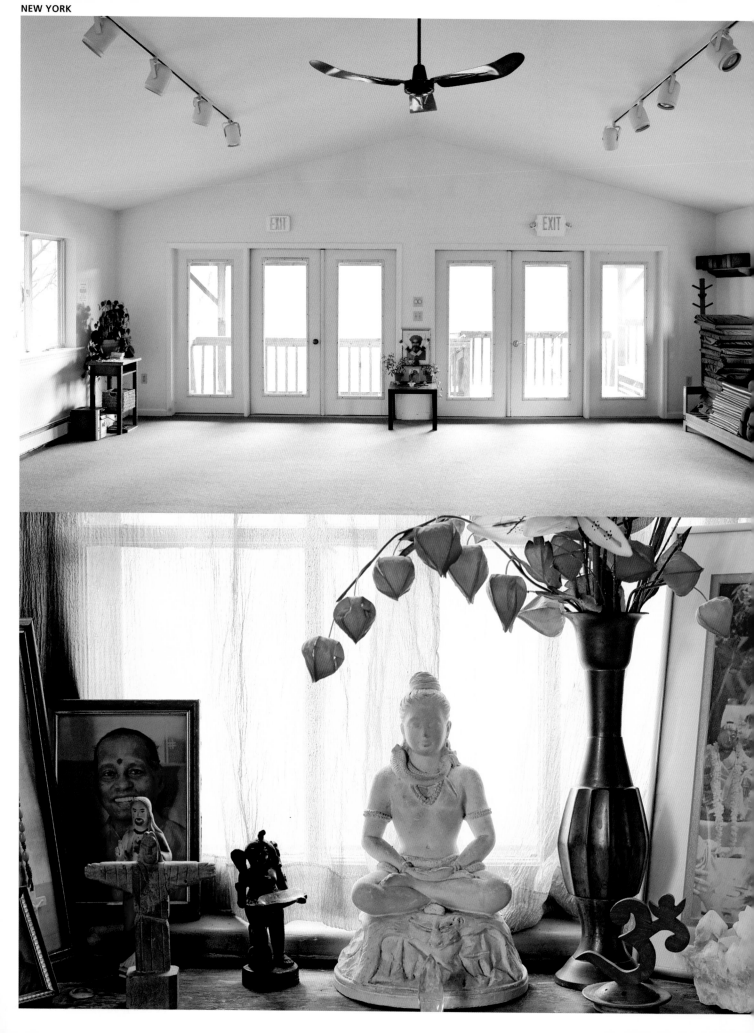

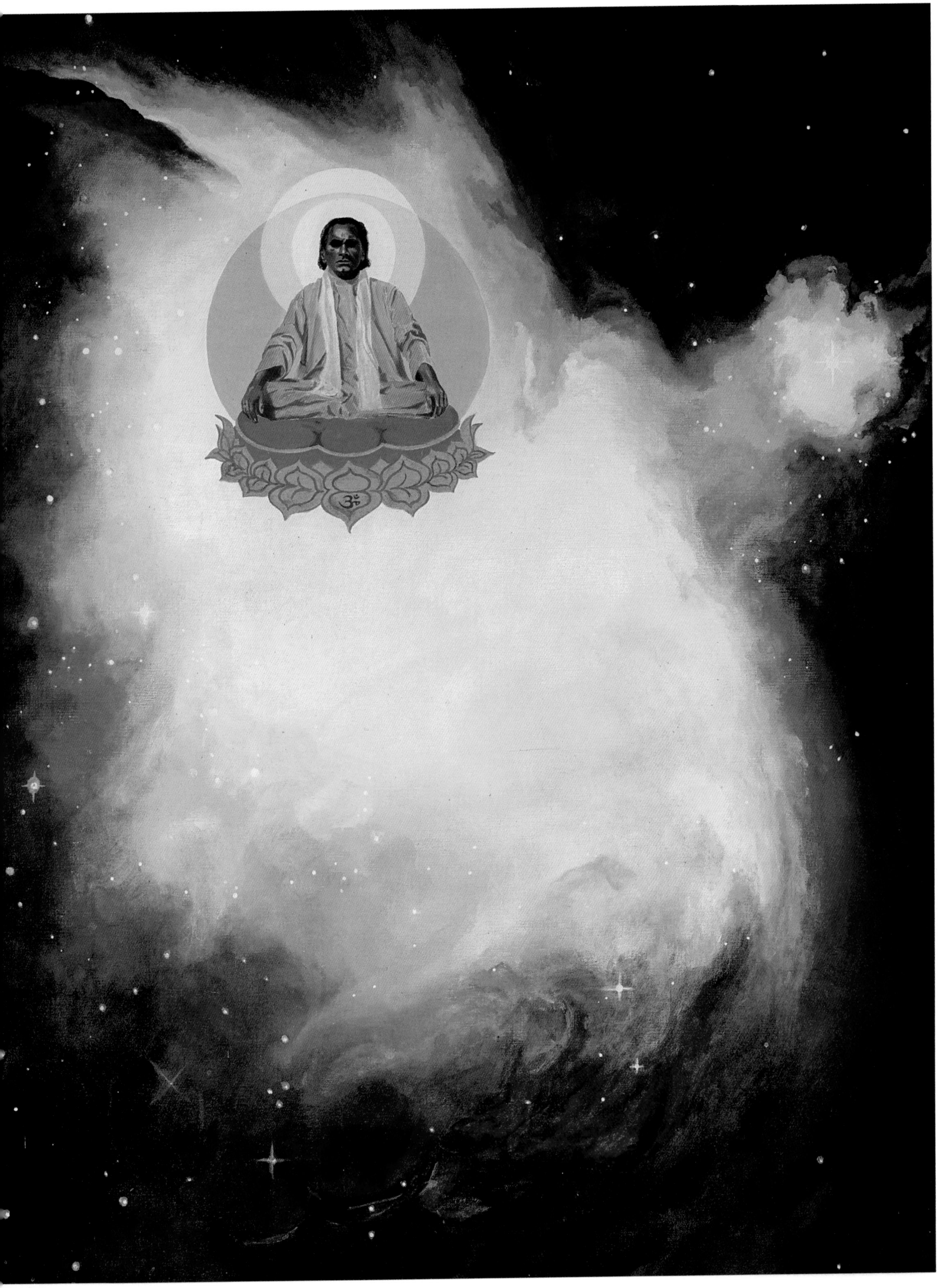

What happens when a former revue girl from Las Vegas, in her own opinion too old to become a cowgirl or an astronaut, becomes a yoga teacher instead? After having taught her legendary morning sessions in New York's "OM" yoga center Susan "Lip" Orem decided to go freelance, painted a house in the country lilac and invited her teachers. Since then, stars of the New York yoga scene like Genny Kapuler and Rodney Yee have been holding highly sought-after familial workshops here, in which the "Susan Sarandon of Yoga" still serves her own blueberry pancakes with bacon on a Sunday and likes to open a bottle of red wine in the evenings. Delightful little rooms with names such as "Ponderosa", "Westwing" or "Betty Ford Clinic", a wild garden with a maze and a pond that has been left to nature serve to underline the individual under-statement of this retreat. Only the excellently appointed yoga room gives away something about the outstanding quality of the yoga taught here without the customary pathos but instead with plenty of dry humor. Where else can you spend a weekend hidden away in Delaware County practising yoga and tasting wine with characters straight out of a Woody Allen film?

Books to pack: "When Things Fall Apart" by Pema Chödrön and "The Art of Happiness" by the Dalai Lama

Heathen Hill Yoga

810 Heathen Hill Road
Franklin, NY 13775
USA
Tel. +1 607 829 5328
info@heathenhillyoga.net
www.heathenhillyoga.net

Directions	About 150 miles northwest of Manhattan, in the heart of the northern Catskill Mountains, a 3-hr drive from Manhattan—the next airport is Albany
Yoga	Hatha, Ashtanga, Vinyasa, Iyengar
Teachers	Rodney Yee, Genny Kapuler
Rooms	2 single rooms, five 2-bed rooms, camping
Food	Grown on site; eggs from Heathen Hill hens
Leisure	Hot tub, swimming, badminton, bocce, hiking

Nicht auszudenken, was passiert, wenn ein ehemaliges Revue-Girl aus Las Vegas, nach eigenen Aussagen zu alt, um Cowgirl oder Astronaut zu werden, Yogalehrerin wird. Nach ihren legendären Vormittagsstunden im New Yorker Yogacenter »OM« beschloss Susan »Lip« Orem, sich selbstständig zu machen, strich ein Haus auf dem Land lila und lud ihre Lehrer ein. Seitdem halten hier Stars der New Yorker Yogaszene wie Genny Kapuler oder Rodney Yee heiß begehrte, familiäre Workshops ab, bei denen die »Susan Sarandon des Yoga« sonntags noch immer eigenhändig Blaubeerpfannkuchen mit Speck serviert und abends gerne eine Flasche Rotwein öffnet. Entzückende kleine Zimmer mit Namen wie »Ponderosa«, »Westwing« oder »Betty Ford Clinic«, ein wilder Labyrinthgarten und ein naturbelassener Teich unterstreichen das individuelle Understatement dieses Retreats. Nur der erstklassig ausgerüstete Yogaraum verrät etwas über die herausragende Qualität des Yoga, das hier ohne das übliche Pathos, dafür mit viel trockenem Humor unterrichtet wird. Wo sonst kann man an einem Wochenende versteckt in Delaware County mit Charakteren wie aus einem Woody-Allen-Film »Yoga & Wine Tasting« machen?

Reisebegleiter: »Wenn alles zusammenbricht« von Pema Chödrön und »Die Regeln des Glücks« des Dalai Lama

Que croyez-vous qu'il arrive lorsqu'une ancienne danseuse de revue de Las Vegas, se jugeant trop vieille pour devenir cow-girl ou astronaute, devient professeur de yoga ? Après avoir donné les légendaires séances du matin au centre de yoga new-yorkais « OM », Susan « Lip » Orem décida de se mettre à son compte, repeignit une maison de campagne en violet et invita ses professeurs. Depuis, des stars du yoga new-yorkais comme Genny Kapuler und Rodney Yee organisent des stages conviviaux et fort prisés au cours desquels la « Susan Sarandon du yoga » sert en personne, le dimanche, ses crêpes aux myrtilles et lardons, débouchant volontiers une bouteille de vin rouge le soir. D'adorables petites chambres aux noms de « Ponderosa », « Westwing » ou encore « Betty Ford Clinic », un jardin-labyrinthe romantique et un étang laissé dans son état naturel soulignent le caractère individuel de ce lieu de méditation. Seule la salle de yoga, dotée d'un équipement haut de gamme, laisse deviner la qualité exceptionnelle du yoga enseigné ici, sans le pathos habituel mais avec une bonne portion d'humour pince-sans-rire. Où sinon ici peut-on le temps d'un week-end, bien caché, s'adonner au « Yoga and Wine Tasting » (yoga et dégustation de vin) avec des personnages tout droit sortis d'un film de Woody Allen ?

Livres à emporter : « Quand tout s'effondre » de Pema Chödrön et « L'Art du bonheur » du Dalaï Lama

Anreise	Etwa 250 km nordwestlich von Manhattan im Herzen der nördlichen Catskill Mountains, 3 Std. Fahrzeit von Manhattan – der nächste Flugplatz ist Albany
Yoga	Hatha, Ashtanga, Vinyasa, Iyengar
Lehrer	Rodney Yee, Genny Kapuler
Zimmer	2 Einzelzimmer, 5 Zweibettzimmer, Camping
Küche	Aus eigenem Anbau, Eier von Heathen-Hill-Hühnern
Aktivitäten	Hot Tub, Schwimmen, Badminton, Boccia, Wandern

Accès	Situé à environ 250 km au nord-ouest de Manhattan au cœur des montagnes Catskill, à 3 h de route de Manhattan – l'aéroport le plus proche est Albany
Yoga	Hatha, Ashtânga, Vinyasa, Iyengar
Professeurs	Rodney Yee, Genny Kapuler
Chambres	2 chambres simples, 5 chambres à deux lits, camping
Restauration	Produits cultivés sur place, œufs des poules d'Heathen Hill
Activités	Jacuzzi, natation, badminton, boules, randonnées

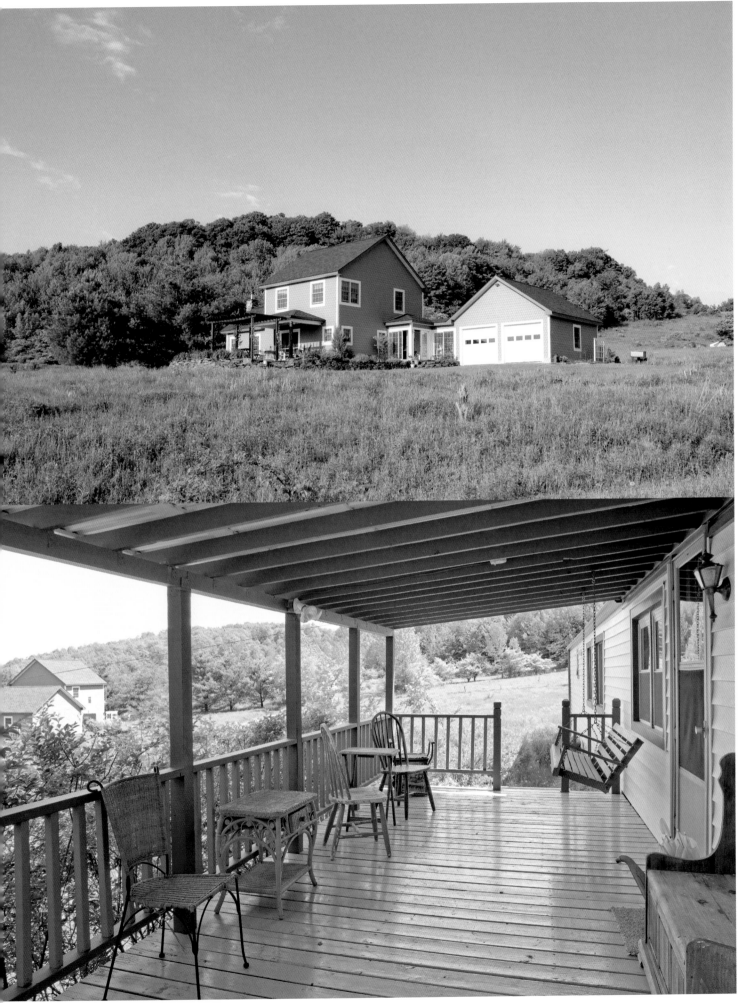

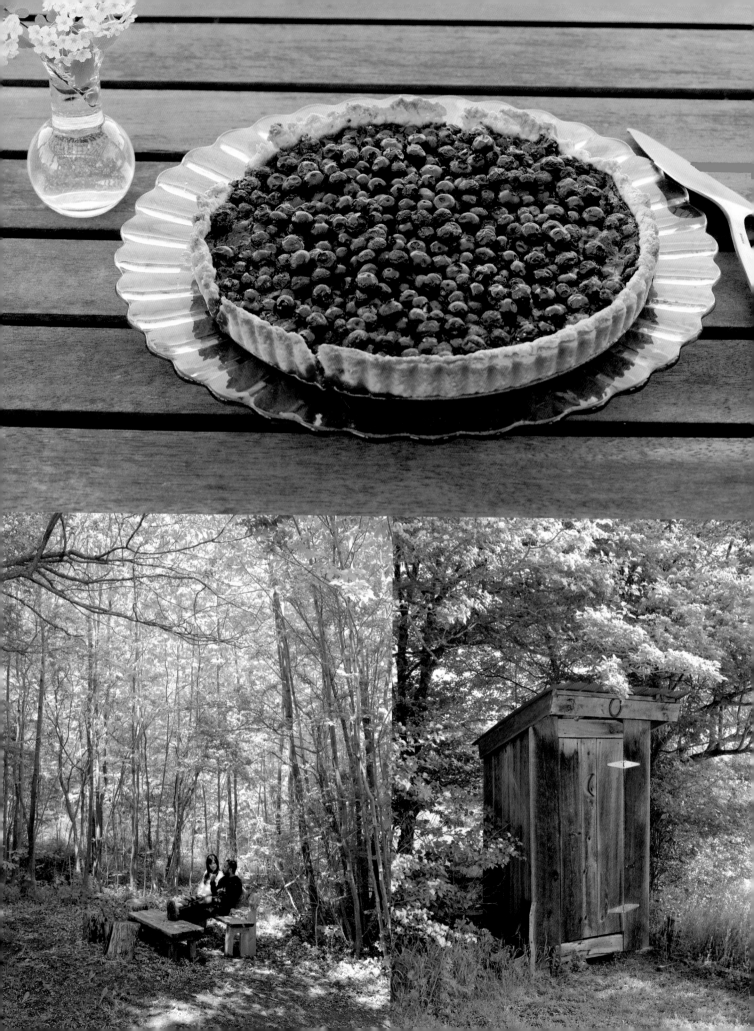

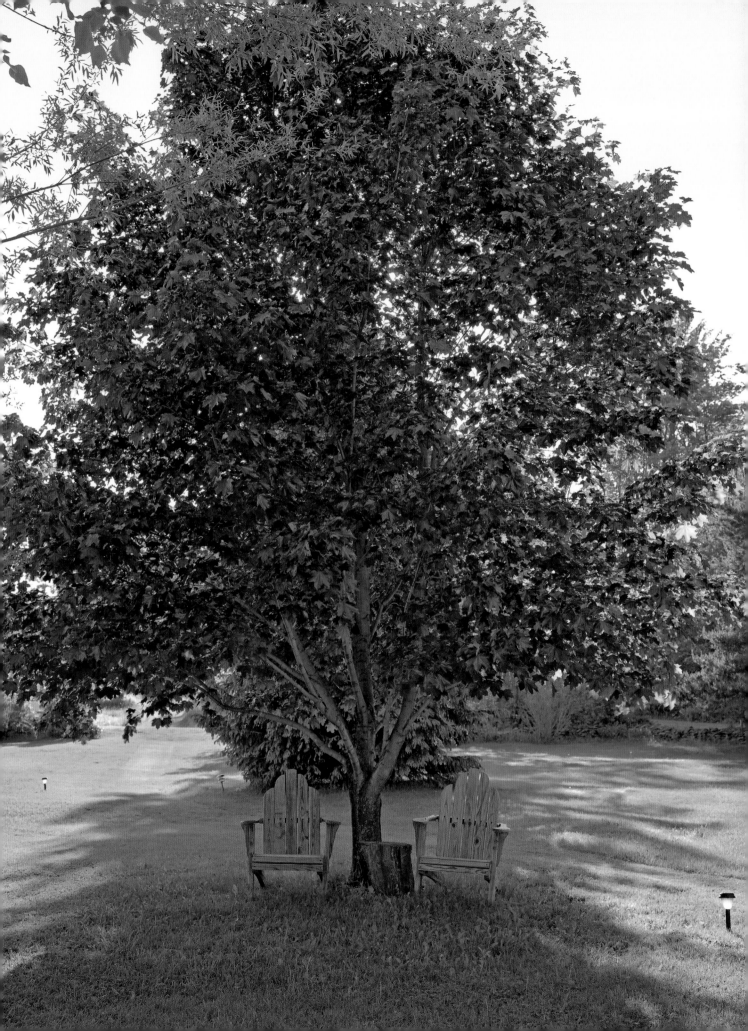

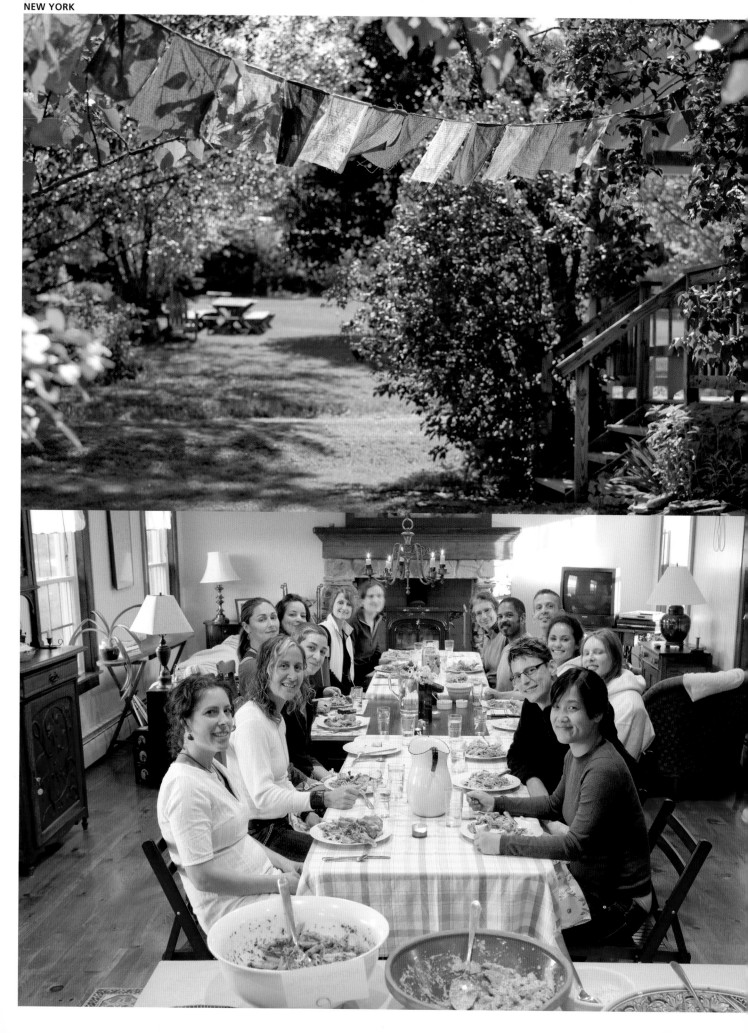

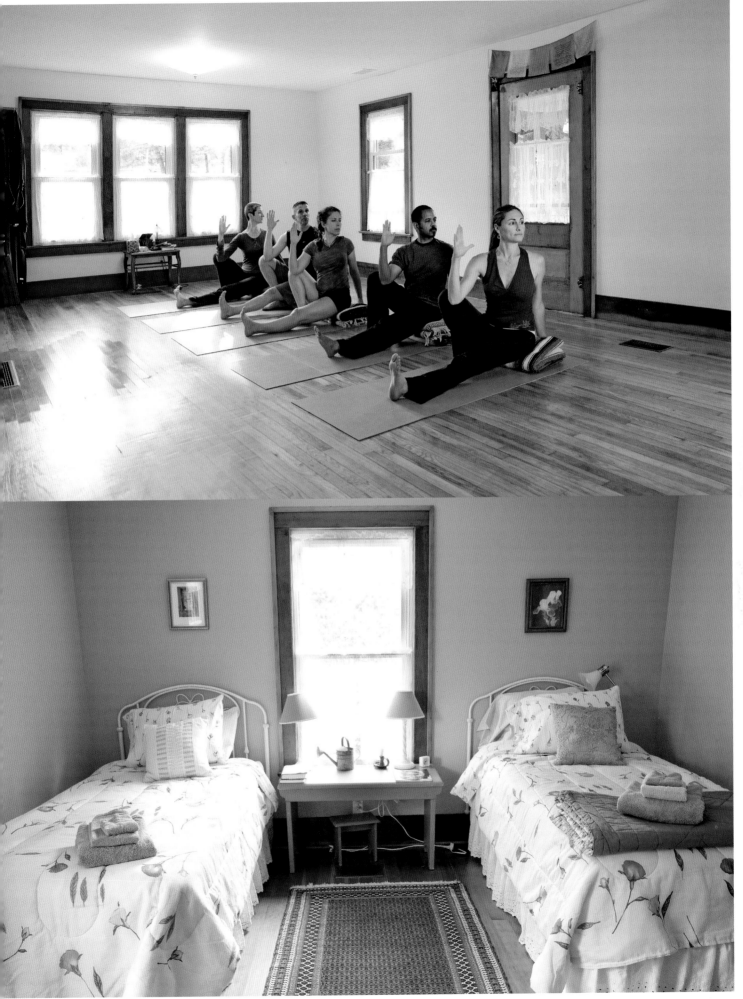

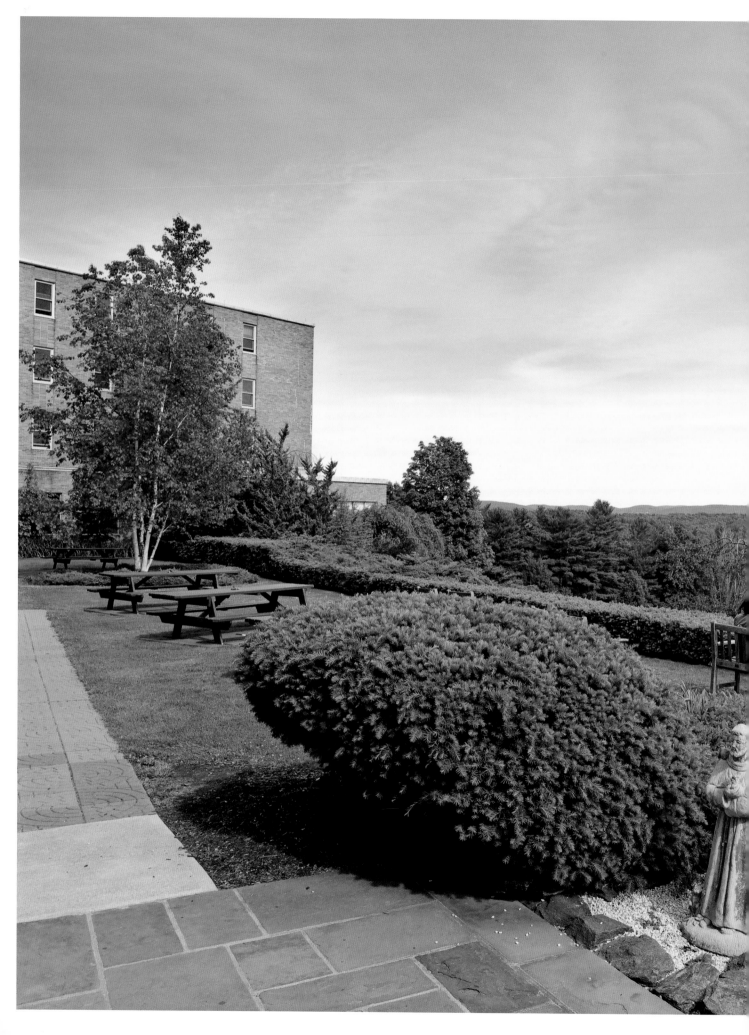

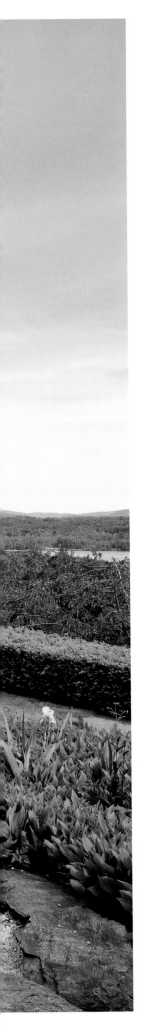

In Sanskrit, *kripalu* means compassionate, and you can indeed feel some sympathy for those who have to choose just one of the countless workshops in the Kripalu Center for Yoga and Health. Every year over 10,000 guests come to this brick complex, built by Jesuits in the charming meadows of the Berkshires. It may not be easy to decide upon the right path to enlightenment, but at this New Age university you can at least be sure that the courses on offer undergo careful scrutiny—almost 90 per cent of those who wish to teach here are turned down. Kripalu was born from a marriage of the spirited 1960s youth movement and a 5,000 year-old yoga tradition. Yogi Amrit Desai, who founded the institution in 1966, failed spectacularly to live up to his own requirement for celibacy and had to take his leave of the campus, forcing the ashram community to move beyond its traditional paradigm. Restructuring as a retreat center, Kripalu has transformed into a nonprofit educational organization dedicated to helping people realise their full potential as they learn to apply the principles of yoga on and off the mat.

Books to pack: "On Love and Loneliness" by Jiddu Krishnamurti and "The Road to Wellville" by T. C. Boyle

Kripalu Center

P.O. Box 309
Stockbridge, MA 01262
USA
Tel. +1 866 200 5203
Fax +1 413 448 3384
guestservices@kripalu.org
www.kripalu.org

Directions	About 150 miles north of New York, 45 min away from Albany Airport (airport transfer by arrangement); charter buses from Penn Station in New York City
Yoga	Hatha, Ashtanga, Sivananda, Iyengar, Anusara, Vinyasa
Teachers	Elena Brower, Krishna Das, Ana Forrest, David Frawley, Amy Ippoliti, Tias Little, David Nichtern, Sarah Powers, Shiva Rea, Robert Thurman, Patricia Walden
Rooms	Dormitory, double and single rooms, max. 475 guests
Food	Regional, organic whole foods
Treatments	More than 30 different healing therapies
Leisure	Swimming, hiking, Yoga training courses, massage courses

Kripalu bedeutet auf Sanskrit barmherzig, und Mitleid kann man tatsächlich mit denen bekommen, die eine Wahl unter den unzähligen Workshops dieses Center für Yoga und Gesundheit treffen müssen. Über 10 000 Gäste kommen pro Jahr in diesen Backsteinkomplex, den Jesuiten 1957 in die lieblichen Wiesen der Berkshires bauten. Es ist nicht einfach, sich für den richtigen Weg zur Erleuchtung zu entscheiden, aber an dieser New-Age-Universität darf man zumindest sicher sein, dass das Angebot sorgfältig überprüft wird: Fast 90 Prozent derer, die hier unterrichten wollen, werden abgelehnt. Kripalu-Yoga ist durch die Verbindung der Jugendbewegung der 1960er mit einer 5000 Jahre alten Yogatradition entstanden. Yogi Amrit Desai, der die Einrichtung 1966 gründete, scheiterte spektakulär am eigenen Anspruch aufs Zölibat und musste den Campus verlassen, was wiederum die Ashram-Gemeinschaft dazu zwang, ihre Traditionen zu überdenken. Mittlerweile hat sich das Kripalu zu einem spirituellen Zentrum gewandelt: In dieser Non-Profit-Einrichtung wird Yoga als Mittel zur Selbstfindung und Selbstheilung gelehrt – mit und ohne Matte.

Reisebegleiter: »Über die Liebe« von Jiddu Krishnamurti und »Willkommen in Wellville« von T. C. Boyle

Kripalu signifie « charitable » en sanskrit et l'on peut, en effet, être pris de pitié pour ceux qui doivent choisir l'un des innombrables stages du centre yoga-santé Kripalu. Plus de 10 000 visiteurs viennent chaque année dans ce complexe construit en briques par des jésuites, en 1957, dans les prairies ondoyantes du Berkshire. Il n'est certes pas aisé de choisir la voie qui mène à la révélation, mais à cette université du New Age l'on peut être au moins certain que le choix proposé fait l'objet d'un examen minutieux. Presque 90 pour cent des personnes désirant enseigner ici sont refusées. Kripalu est né de la rencontre entre le mouvement libertaire des années 1960 et la tradition du yoga, vieille de 5000 ans. Le yogi Amrit Desai, fondateur de cette institution en 1966, se heurta avec fracas à sa propre exigence de célibat et dut quitter le campus, et l'ashram dépassa, par la force des choses, son paradigme originel. Remodelé en lieu de retraite spirituelle, Kripalu s'est mué en institution éducative à but non lucratif dédiée à aider les gens à s'accomplir pleinement, en appliquant les principes du yoga, sur les tapis et en dehors.

Livres à emporter : « De l'amour et de la solitude » de Jiddu Krishnamurti et « Aux bons soins du docteur Kellogg » de T. C. Boyle

Anreise	Etwa 250 km nördlich von New York, 45 min vom Flughafen Albany; Charterbusse ab Penn Station in New York City
Yoga	Hatha, Ashtanga, Sivananda, Iyengar, Anusara, Vinyasa
Lehrer	Elena Brower, Krishna Das, Ana Forrest, David Frawley, Amy Ippoliti, Tias Little, David Nichtern, Sarah Powers, Shiva Rea, Robert Thurman, Patricia Walden
Zimmer	Schlafsaal, Doppel- und Einzelzimmer, max. 475 Gäste
Küche	Regional-biologische Vollwertküche
Anwendungen	Mehr als 30 verschiedene Heiltherapien
Aktivitäten	Schwimmen, Wandern, Yoga-Trainings- und Massagekurse

Accès	Situé à environ 250 km au nord de New York, à 45 min de l'aéroport d'Albany Bus charter depuis Penn Station New York City
Yoga	Hatha, Ashtânga, Shivananda, Iyengar, Anusara, Vinyasa
Professeurs	Elena Brower, Krishna Das, Ana Forrest, David Frawley, Amy Ippoliti, Tias Little, David Nichtern, Sarah Powers, Shiva Rea, Robert Thurman, Patricia Walden
Chambres	Dortoir et chambres doubles ou simples pour 475 personnes max.
Restauration	Cuisine bio et régionale aux aliments complets
Traitements	Plus de 30 soins thérapeutiques différents
Activités	Natation, randonnées, cours d'entraînement au yoga et cours de massage

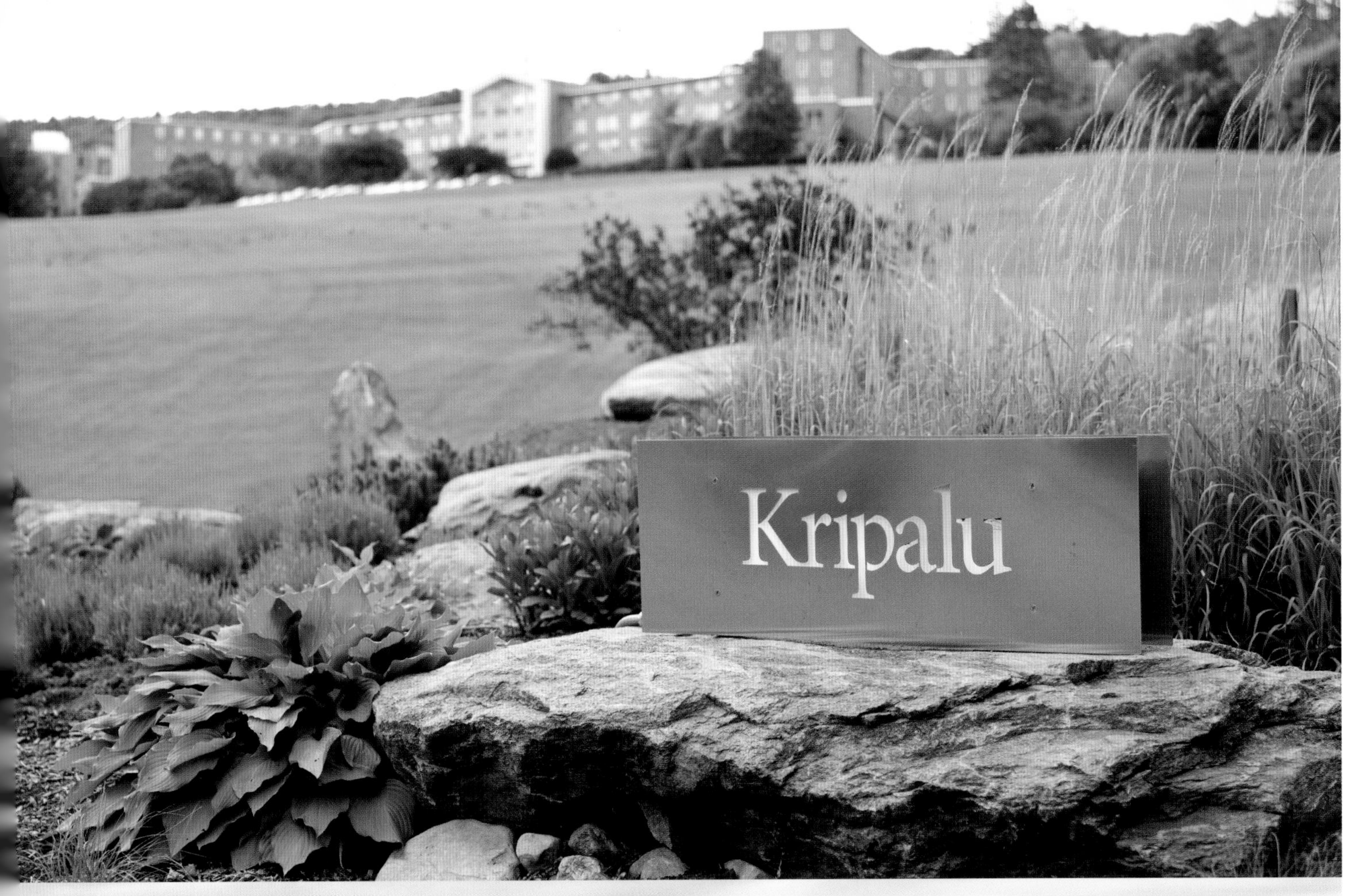
Kripalu

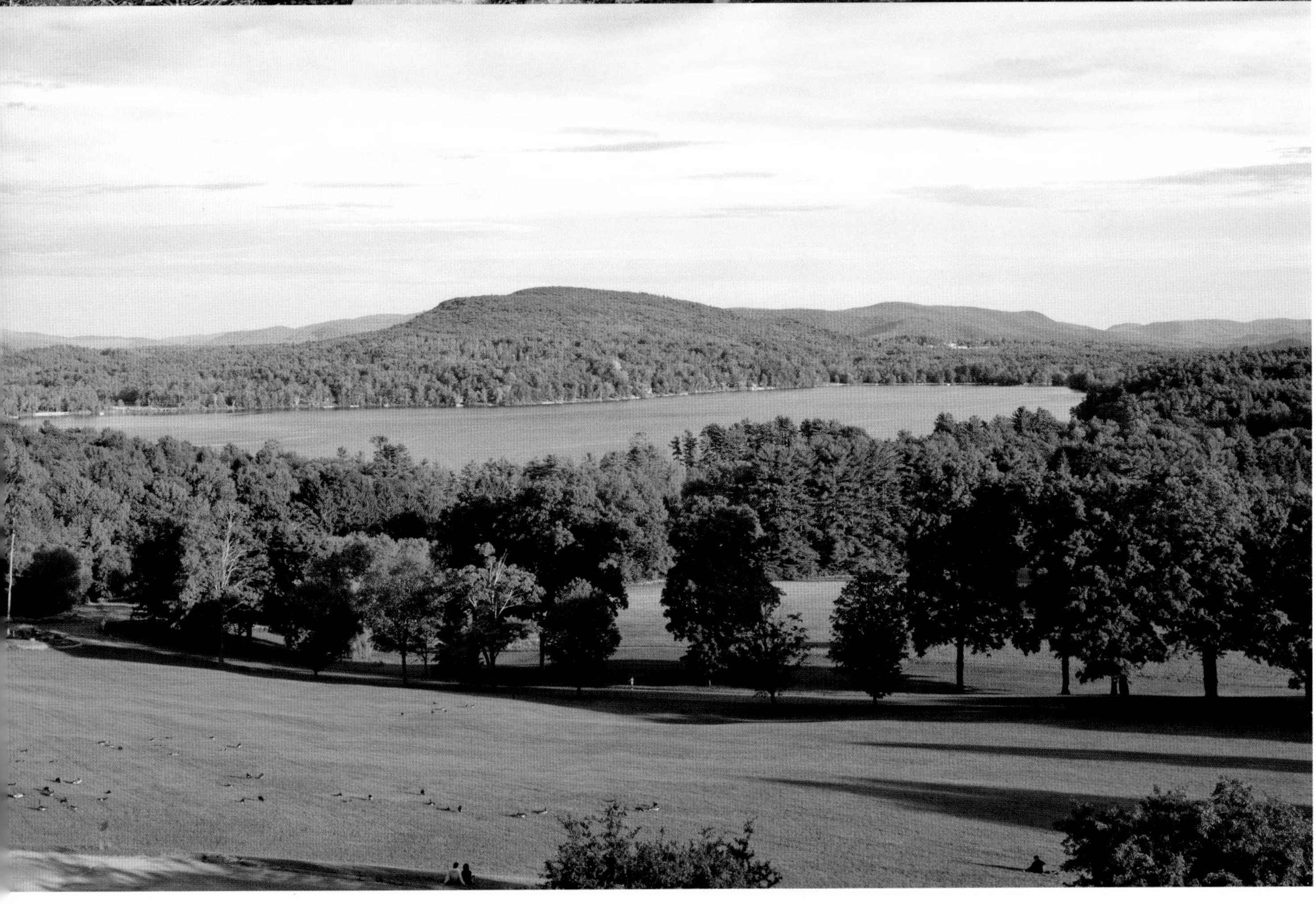

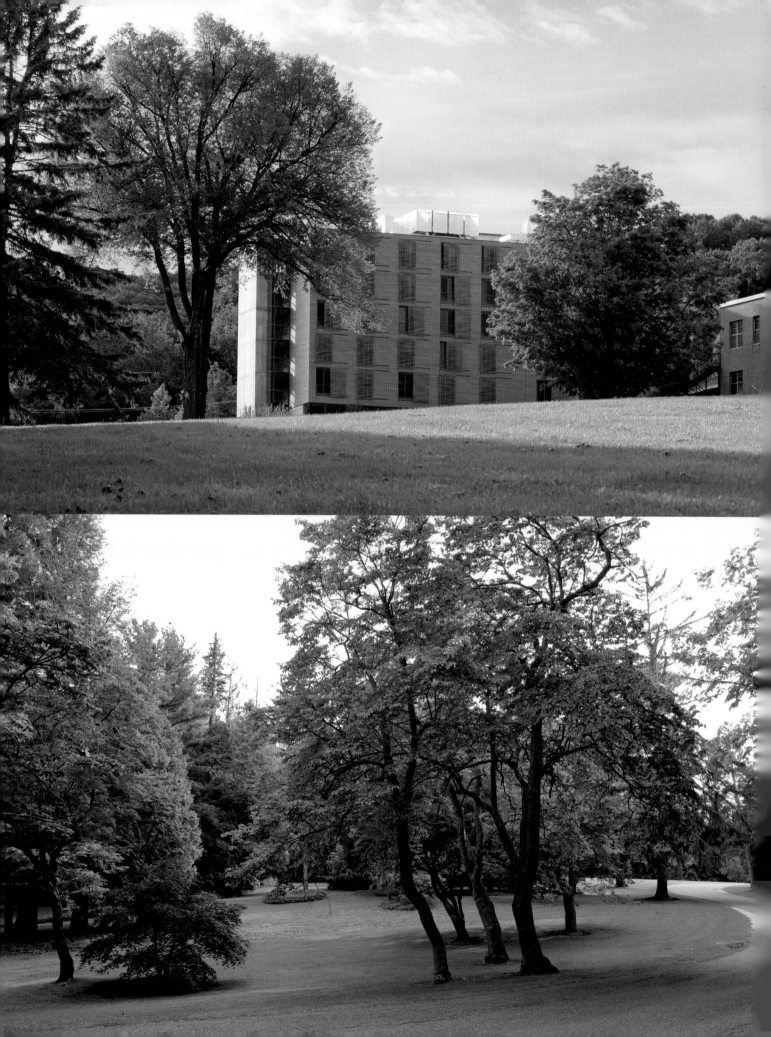

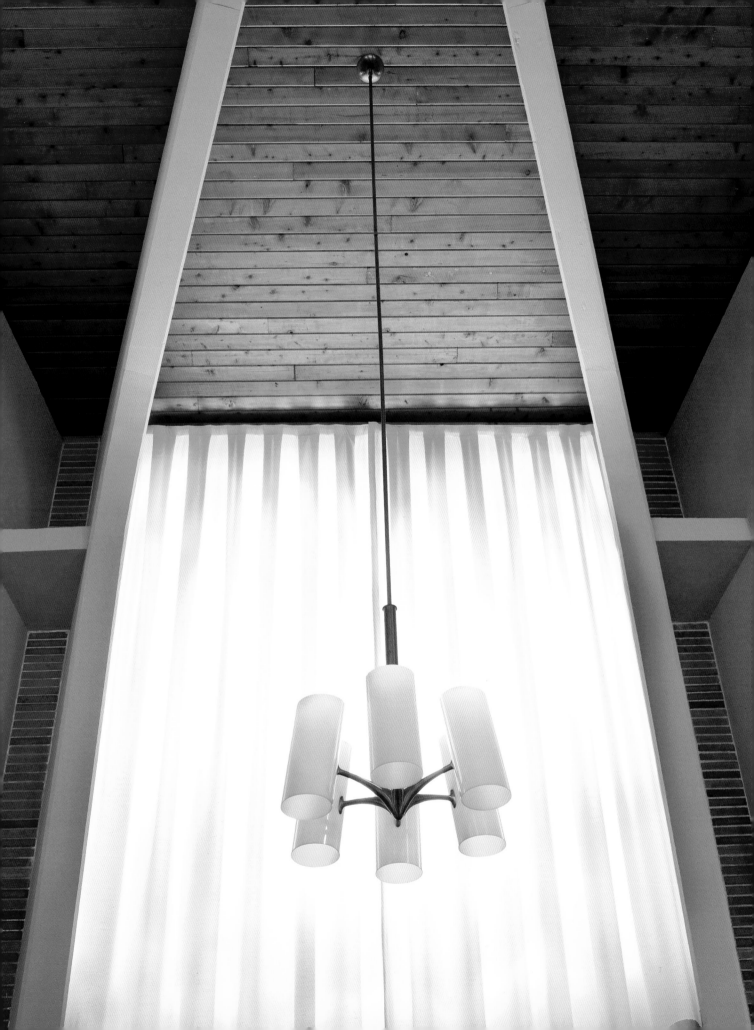

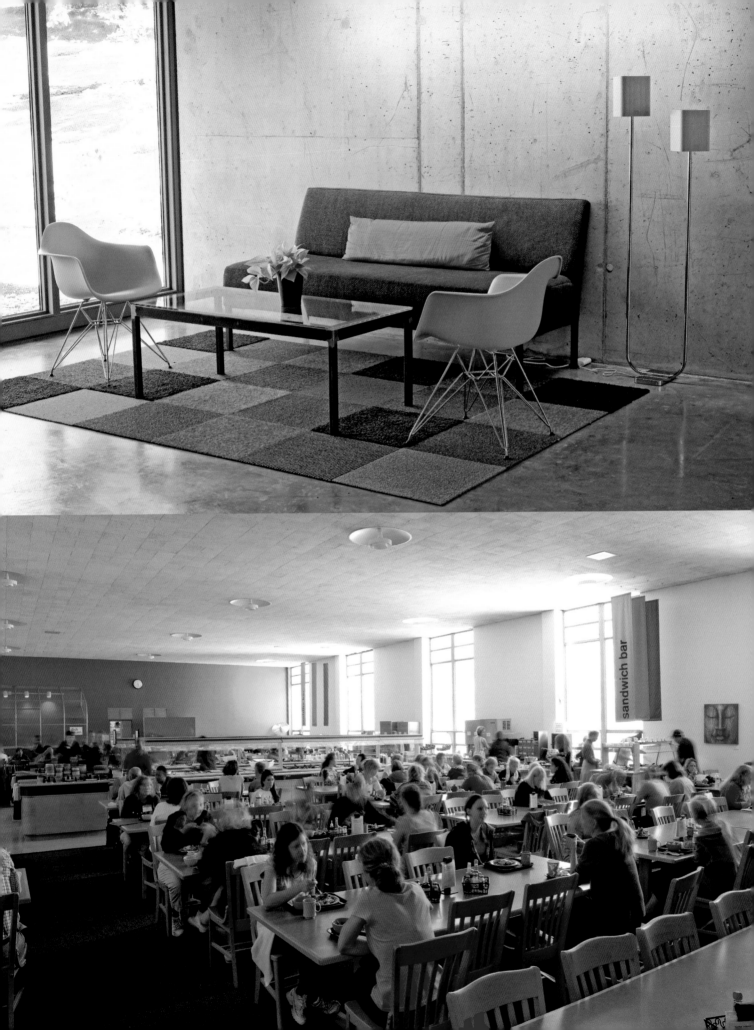

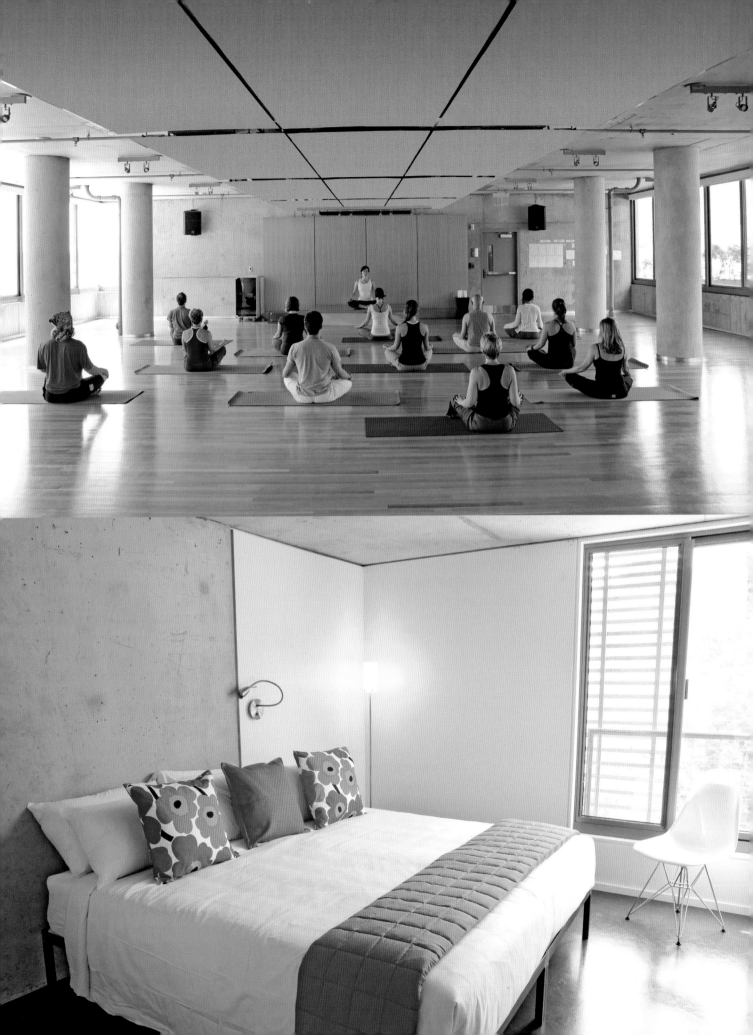

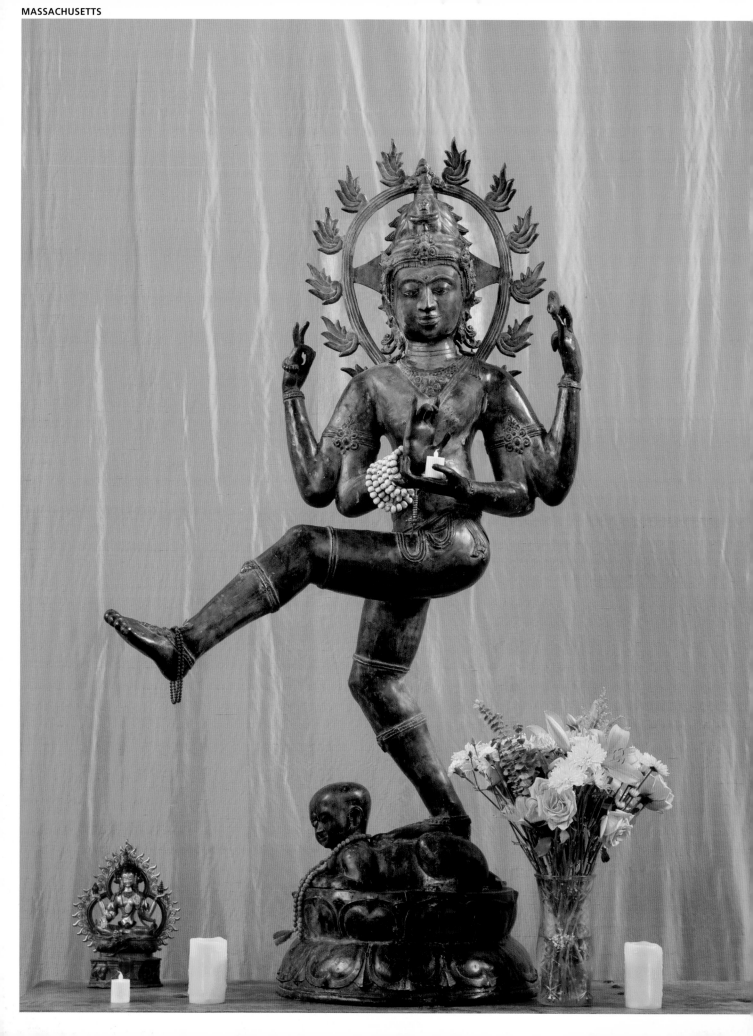

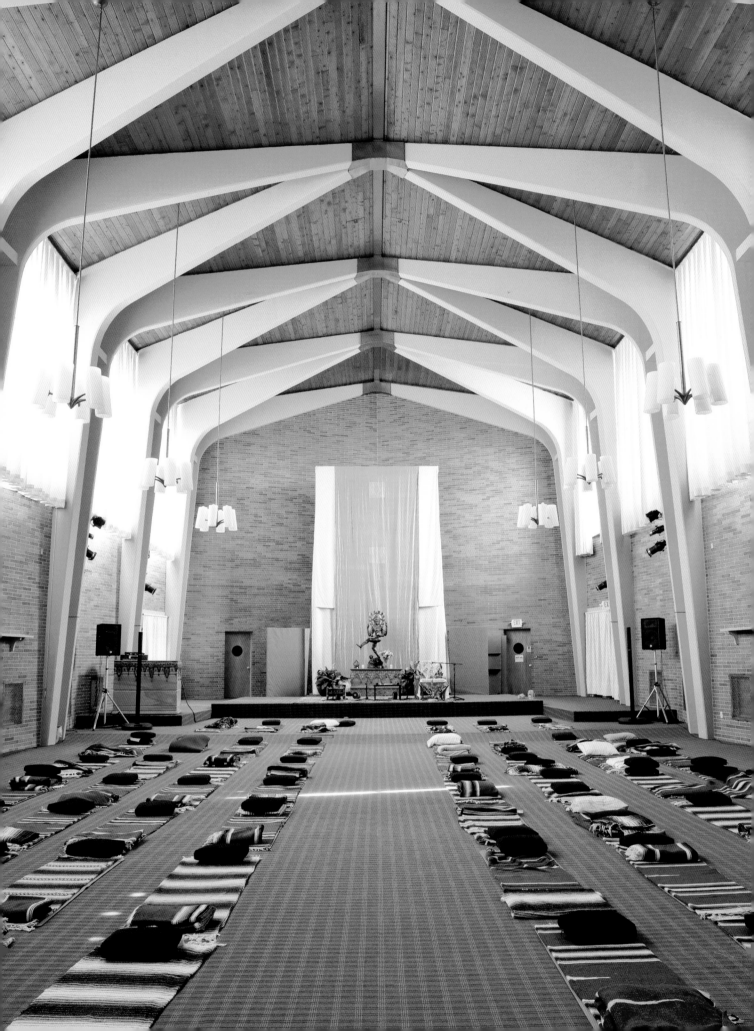

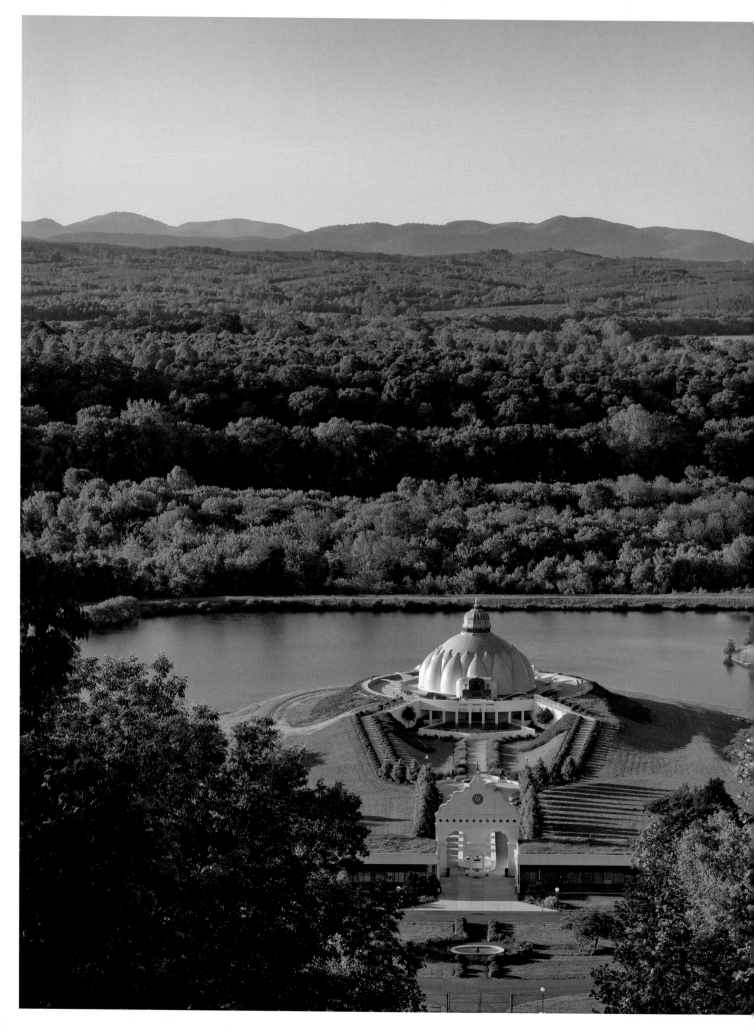

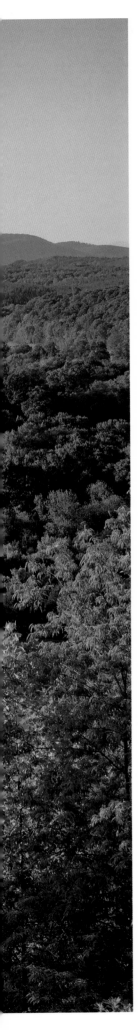

The tried-and-tested mixture of different yoga methods known as Integral Yoga was thought up by one man: Swami Satchidananda. With it, he quickly became a star on the New York hippy scene. In 1969 he was flown by helicopter to Woodstock, so that he could bless the festival. Later, prominent students such as Peter Max, Conrad Rooks, Felix Cavaliere and Alice Coltrane even donated land for his ashram, in the middle of which a rather showy temple in the form of a lotus flower proudly stands. Along with training to become an Integral Yoga teacher, you can also book workshops on the subjects of stress management, yoga and scoliosis, Tantric massage, or freeing the hips; it is also possible simply to visit the daily Hatha Yoga classes or, on Memorial Weekend, sing with Krishna Das.

Books to pack: "Be as You Are" by Ramana Maharshi and "No One Belongs Here More Than You" by Miranda July

Satchidananda Ashram—Yogaville

108 Yogaville Way
Buckingham, VA 23921
USA
Tel. +1 434 969 3121
Fax +1 434 969 1303
ARC@iyiva.org
www.yogaville.org

Directions	53 miles southwest of Charlottesville, 80 miles west of Richmond and 186 miles southwest of Washington, D.C.
Yoga	Hatha, Restorative, meditation, Yoga philosophy
Teachers	Swami Karunananda, Swami Asokananda, David Frawley, Dr. Sandra McLanahan, Nischala Devi
Rooms	207 beds in rooms with two or more beds, as well as dormitories and 12 tents
Food	Predominantly vegan; cheese and yoghurt on request
Treatments	Ayurveda, Panchakarma, Alexander Technique, Thai Yoga massage, myofascial release, shaman healing
Leisure	Swimming, hiking

Die bewährte Mischung verschiedener Yoga-Methoden, *Integral Yoga* genannt, hat sich ein Mann ausgedacht: Swami Satchidananda, der damit in kürzester Zeit ein Star in der New Yorker Hippieszene wurde. 1969 flog man ihn mit einem Helikopter nach Woodstock, damit er das Festival segnete. Später spendierten ihm prominente Schüler wie Peter Max, Conrad Rooks, Felix Cavaliere und Alice Coltrane sogar Land für seinen Ashram, in dessen Mitte ein ziemlicher Angebertempel in Form einer Lotosblüte thront. Neben einer Ausbildung zum Integral-Yogalehrer, kann man hier Workshops zum Thema Stressmanagement, Yoga und Skoliose, Tantrische Massage oder Freie Hüften buchen, einfach nur die täglichen Hatha-Yogaklassen besuchen oder am Memorial Weekend mit Krishna Das singen.

Reisebegleiter: »Sei, was du bist!« von Ramana Maharshi und »Zehn Wahrheiten« von Miranda July

C'est un certain Swami Satchidananda qui a imaginé l'association très probante de différentes méthodes de yoga, portant aussi le nom de yoga intégral, et devint ainsi en peu de temps une star de la scène hippie new-yorkaise. En 1969, on l'envoya par hélicoptère à Woodstock afin qu'il donne sa bénédiction au festival. Plus tard, des étudiants connus comme Peter Max, Conrad Rooks, Felix Cavaliere et Alice Coltrane lui offrirent même un terrain pour son âshram, au centre duquel trône, assez prétentieusement, un temple en forme de fleur de lotus. En plus d'une formation de professeur de yoga intégral, il est possible de s'inscrire à des stages aux thèmes tels que la maîtrise du stress, le yoga et la scoliose, les massages tantriques ou les hanches sans douleurs, de fréquenter simplement chaque jour les classes de Hatha-yoga ou de chanter avec Krishna Das pour célébrer le Memorial Day.

Livres à emporter : « Sois ce que tu es ! » de Ramana Maharshi et « Un bref instant de romantisme » de Miranda July

Anreise	85 km südwestlich von Charlottesville und 300 km südwestlich von Washington, D.C.
Yoga	Hatha, Restorative, Meditation, Yoga-Philosophie
Lehrer	Swami Karunananda, Swami Asokananda, David Frawley, Dr. Sandra McLanahan, Nischala Devi
Zimmer	207 Betten in Doppel- oder Mehrbettzimmern sowie Schlafsäle und 12 Zelte
Küche	Überwiegend vegan, auf Wunsch Käse und Joghurt
Anwendungen	Ayurveda, Panchakarma, Alexander-Technik, Thai-Yoga-Massage, Myofascial Release, Shamanen-Heilung
Aktivitäten	Schwimmen, Wandern

Accès	Situé à 85 km au sud-ouest de Charlottesville et à 300 km au sud-ouest de Washington D.C.
Yoga	Hatha, yoga restauratif, méditation, philosophie du yoga
Professeurs	Swami Karunananda, Swami Asokananda, David Frawley, Dr. Sandra McLanahan, Nischala Devi
Chambres	207 lits dans des chambres doubles et à plusieurs lits, ainsi que des dortoirs et 12 tentes
Restauration	Essentiellement végétalienne, laitages sur demande
Traitements	Ayurveda, panchakarma, technique Alexander, massage de yoga thaïlandais, myofascial release, guérison de chaman
Activités	Natation, randonnées

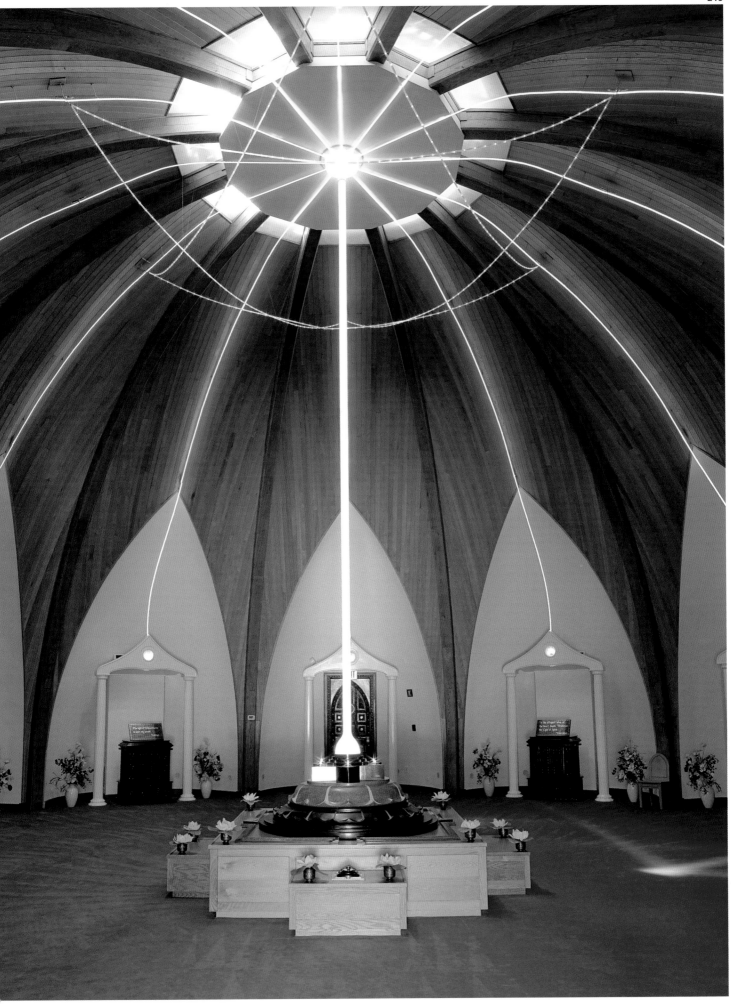

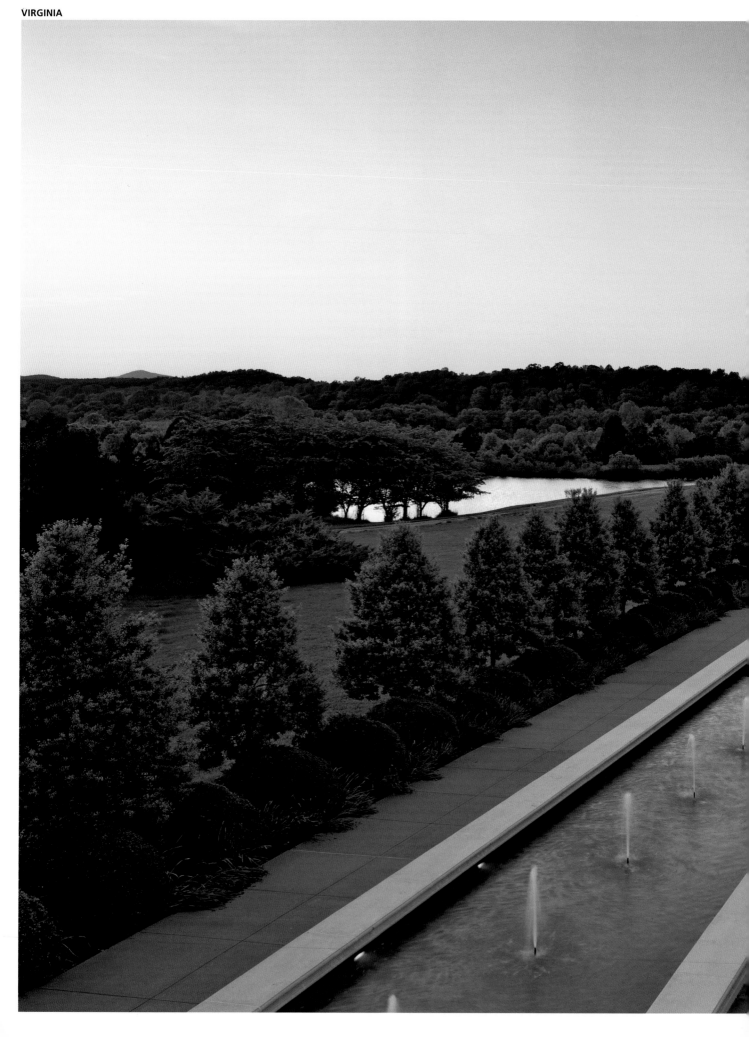

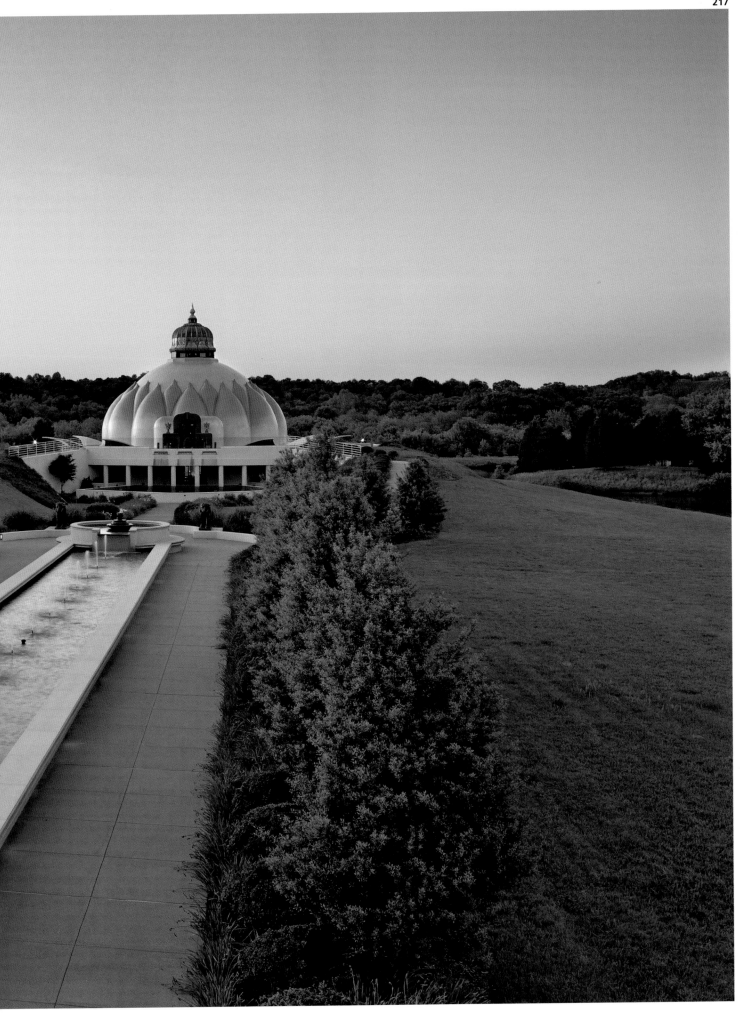

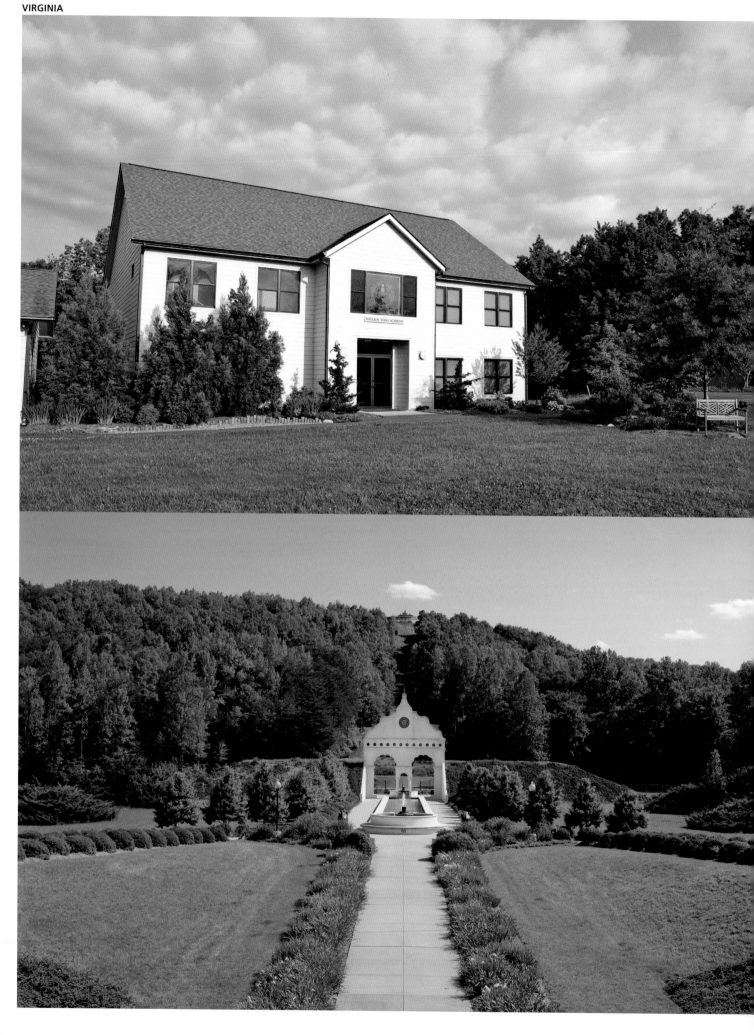

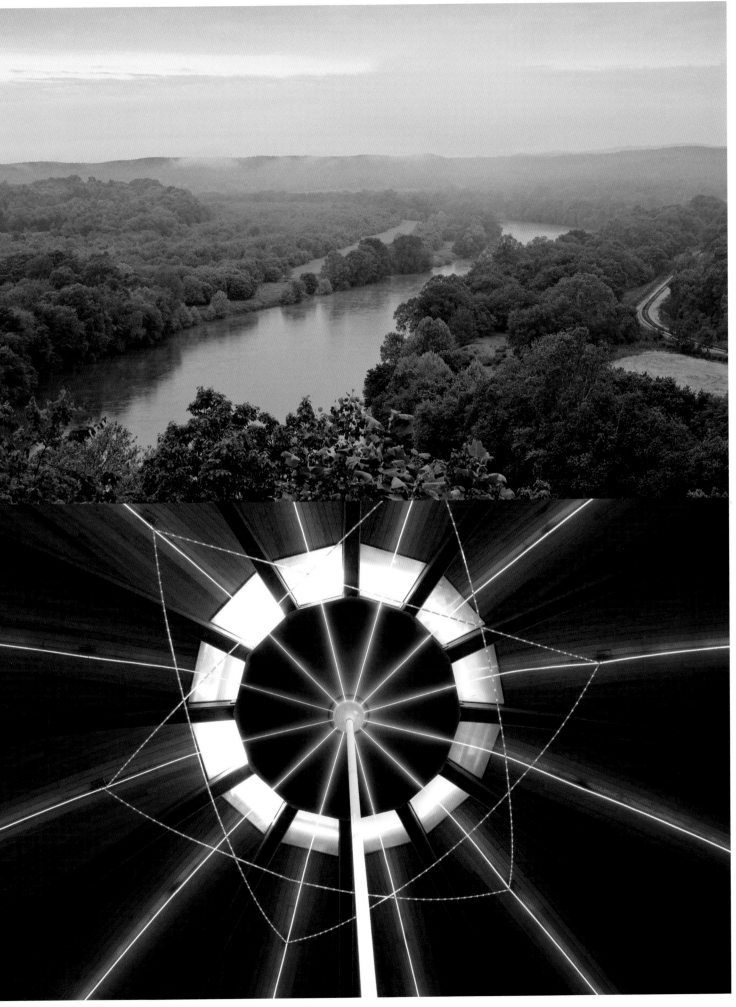

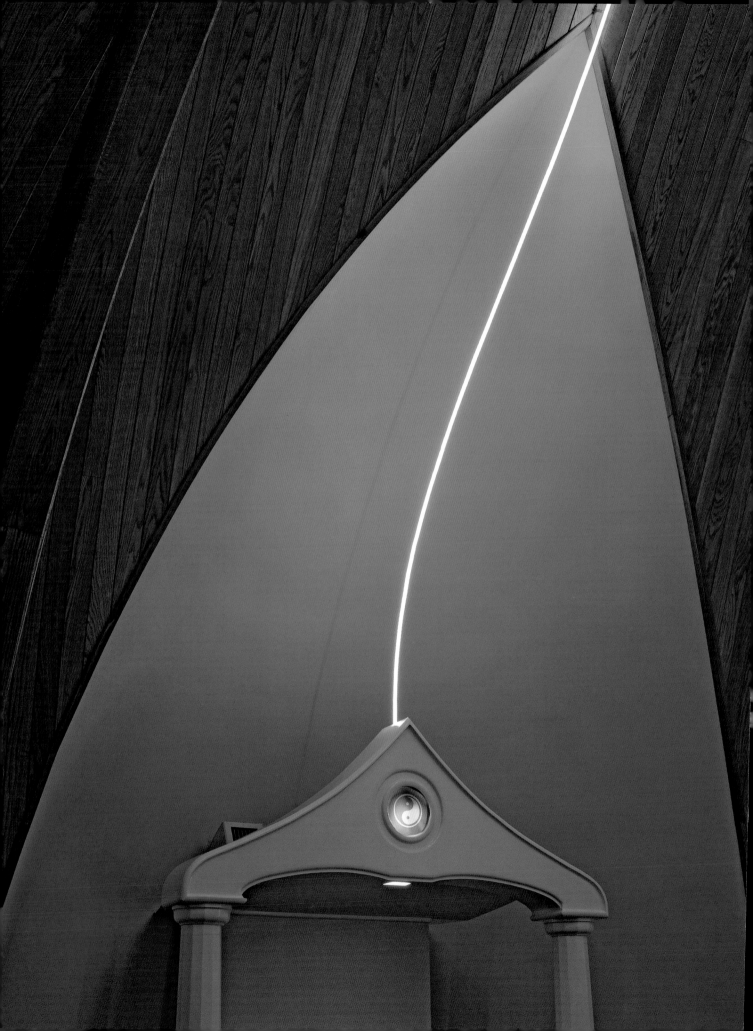

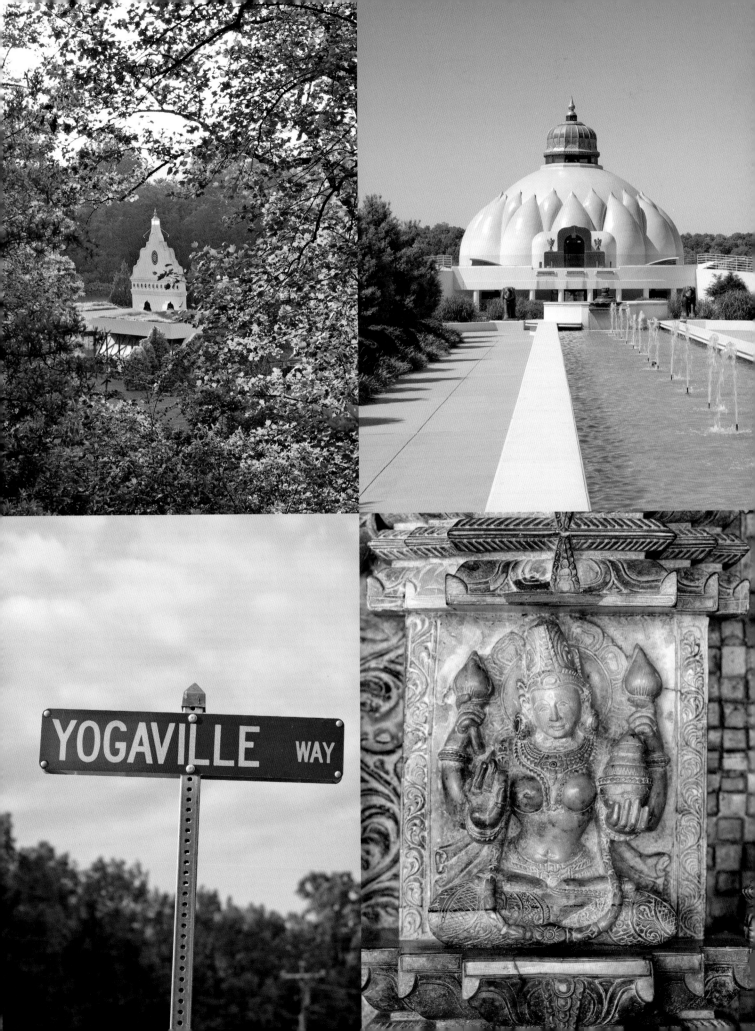

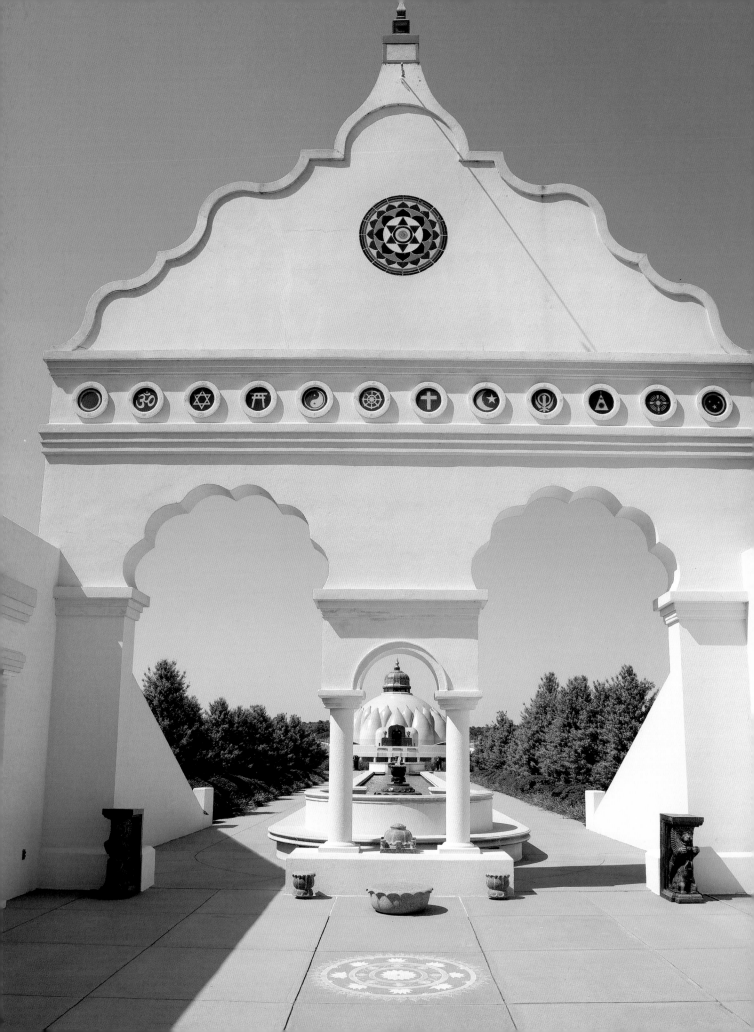

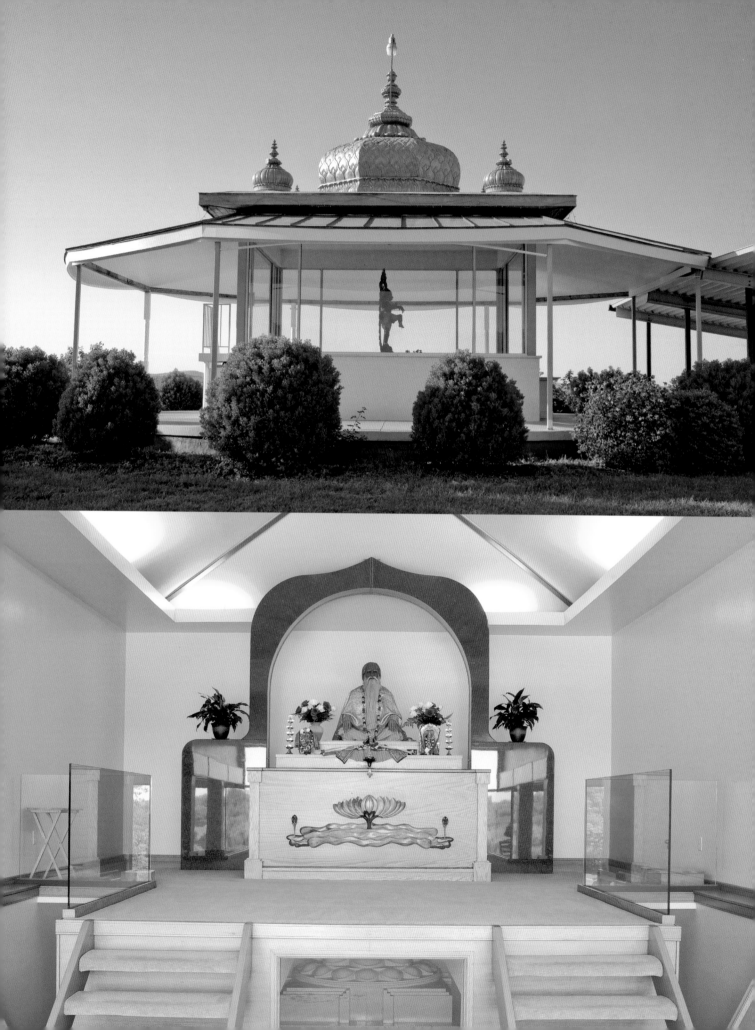

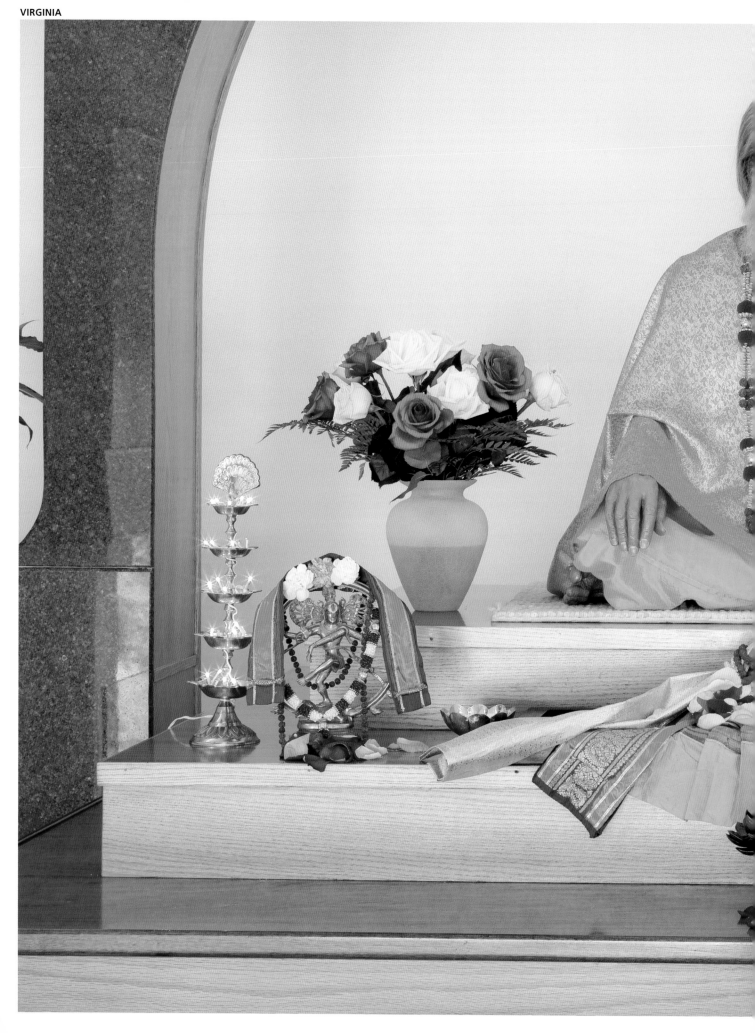

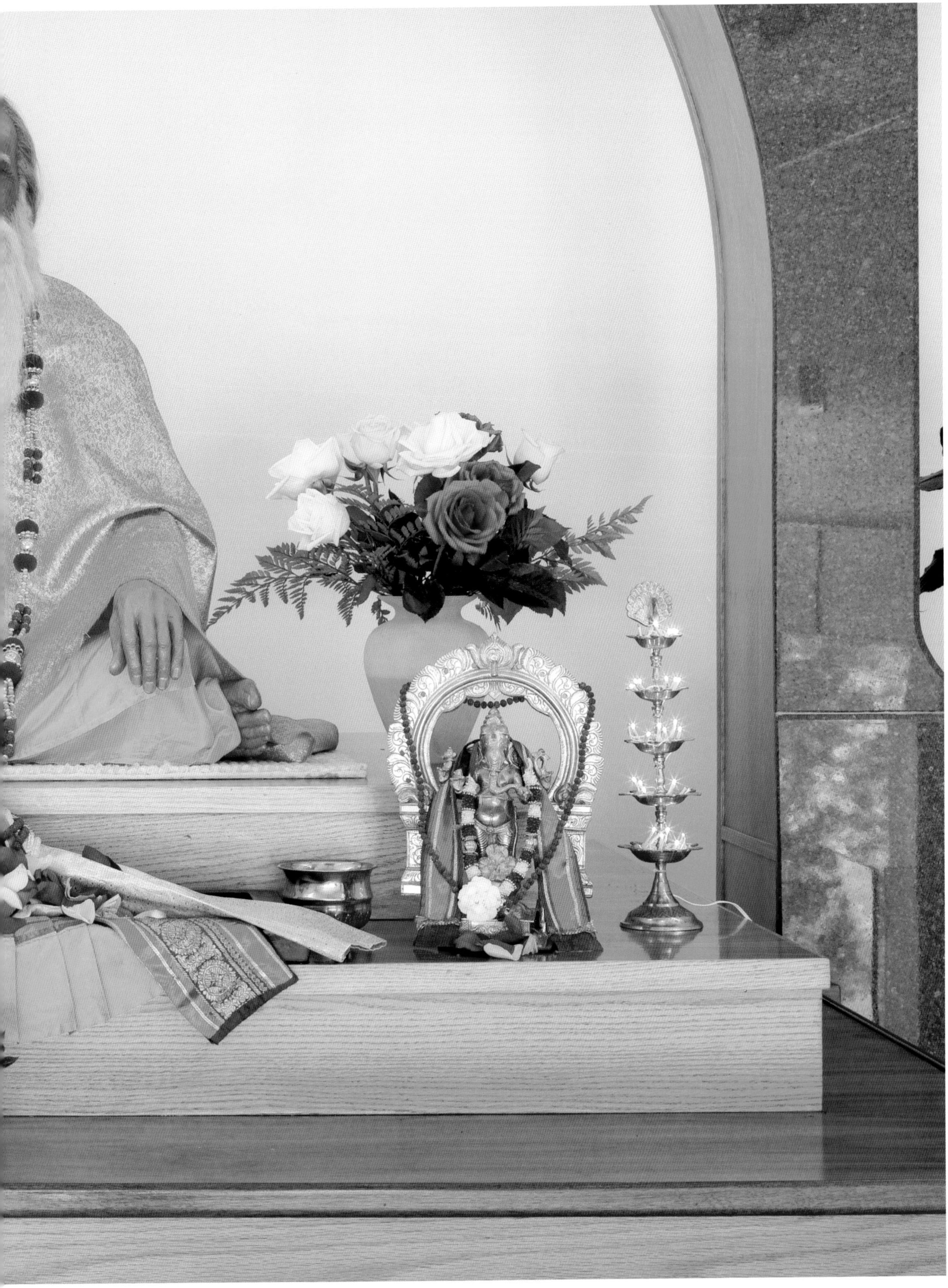

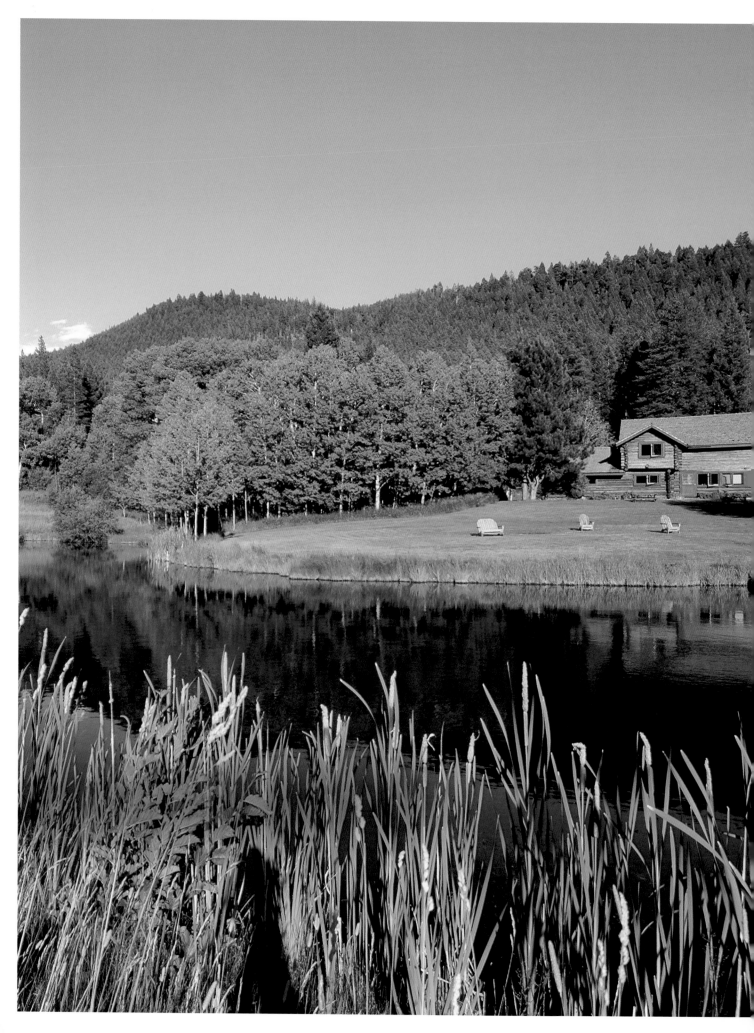

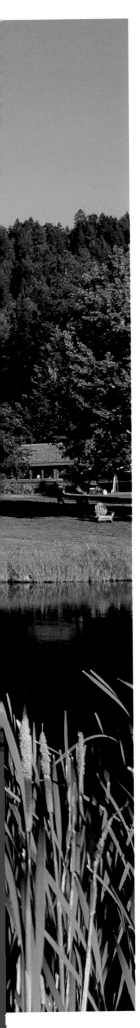

Yoga studios seem to be as ubiquitous and just about as exotic as Starbucks. But establishments like the Feathered Pipe Ranch, where yoga was already being taught before it came into fashion, remind us of what actually matters. You sleep in simple log cabins, comfortably furnished tepees, tents or yurts; as a reward there may be a good, solid massage or a bath in the hot tub. But the intensive yoga classes, taught by the best in the land, for beginners as well as for the more advanced, are the main attraction. When after an hour of sweating in the Chippewa Cree wigwam silence falls on the wild prairies between the Montana Rockies, the sky becomes cloudy and a cool wind blows up, you understand what India Supera saw before her when in 1975 she inherited the old house in the Adirondack style, from which the lawn falls away gently to the lake: a place from which you leave strengthened, peaceful and clear. Added to that, this is probably the world's only yoga studio, with its high walls and chimney, that is decorated by a moose head.

Books to pack: "Touching Peace " by Thich Nhat Hanh and "Fresh Air Fiend" by Paul Theroux

Feathered Pipe Foundation

P.O. Box 1682
Helena, MT 59624
USA
Tel. +1 406 442 8196
Fax +1 406 442 8110
info@featheredpipe.com
www.featheredpipe.com

Directions	Located in the heart of the Montana Rockies, 15 1/2 miles west of the airport in Helena
Yoga	Vinyasa, Iyengar, Anusara, Power Yoga, Restorative, Freedom Style
Teachers	Kira Ryder, Baxter Bell, Richard Miller, Marla Apt, Erich Schiffmann, Lilias Folan
Rooms	Four 4-bed rooms, 9 double rooms, 5 yurts, 5 tepees, and 10 tents, all max. 60 guests altogether
Food	Predominantly organic vegetarian, occasionally chicken and fish
Treatments	Sauna, massage
Leisure	Swimming, hiking, horseback riding, canoeing and rowing

Yogastudios mögen mittlerweile so allgegenwärtig und etwa so exotisch sein wie Starbucks. Aber Adressen wie die Feathered Pipe Ranch, wo Yoga schon unterrichtet wurde, bevor es in Mode kam, erinnern daran, worauf es eigentlich ankommt. Man schläft in einfachen Blockhäusern, in gemütlich eingerichteten Tipis, Zelten oder Jurten, als Belohnung mag es eine tüchtige Massage geben oder ein Bad im Hot Tub. Aber die Hauptattraktion liegt in den intensiven Yogaklassen, die von den Besten des Landes unterrichtet werden, für Anfänger ebenso wie für Fortgeschrittene. Wenn sich nach einer Stunde Schwitzen im Chippewa-Cree-Wigwam gegen Abend Stille senkt auf die Wildwiesen zwischen den Montana Rockies, der Himmel sich bewölkt und ein kühler Wind aufkommt, versteht man, was India Supera vor sich sah, als sie das alte Haus im Adirondack-Stil, von dem die Wiesen sanft zum See abfallen, 1975 von einem Hippiefreund erbte: einen Platz, der einen gestärkt, ruhig und klar wieder entlässt. Außerdem ist das Yogastudio mit seinen hohen Wänden und dem Kamin vermutlich das einzige in der Welt, das ein Elchkopf ziert.

Reisebegleiter: »Das Glück, einen Baum zu umarmen« von Thich Nhat Hanh und »Fresh Air Fiend« von Paul Theroux

Même si les instituts de yoga sont maintenant aussi omni-présents et à peu près aussi exotiques que les cafés Starbucks, des adresses telles que le Feathered Pipe Ranch, où l'on enseignait le yoga bien avant qu'il devienne une mode, rappellent ce qui compte vraiment. On dort dans de simples fustes, dans des tipis, tentes ou yourtes agréablement aménagés et, comme récompense, il peut y avoir un bon massage ou un bain tourbillon. Mais l'attraction majeure, ce sont les cours intensifs de yoga, donnés par les meilleurs professeurs du pays, pour les débutants comme pour les yogis chevronnés. Lorsque, vers le soir, après avoir transpiré une heure durant dans un wigwam Chippewa-Cri, on voit la paix descendre sur les plaines sauvages qui se déploient entre les Rocheuses, le ciel se couvrir de nuages et une brise fraîche se lever, on comprend ce qu'India Supera découvrit quand, en 1975, elle hérita de la vieille maison de style Adirondack, d'où les prairies descendent en pente douce vers le lac : un endroit qui vous rend fort, calme et serein. De plus, l'institut de yoga, avec ses hauts murs et sa cheminée, est sans doute le seul au monde à être décoré d'une tête d'élan.

Livres à emporter : « La plénitude de l'instant » de Thich Nhat Hanh et « Fresh Air Fiend » de Paul Theroux

Anreise	Im Herzen der Montana Rockies, 25 km westlich vom Flughafen in Helena gelegen
Yoga	Vinyasa, Iyengar, Anusara, Power Yoga, Restorative, Freedom style
Lehrer	Kira Ryder, Baxter Bell, Richard Miller, Marla Apt, Erich Schiffmann, Lilias Folan
Zimmer	4 Vierbettzimmer, 9 Doppelzimmer, 5 Jurten, 5 Tipis und 10 Zelte, alle für max. 60 Gäste
Küche	Überwiegend biologisch-vegetarisch, gelegentlich Huhn und Fisch
Anwendungen	Sauna, Massage
Aktivitäten	Schwimmen, Reiten, Wandern, Kanu und Rudern

Accès	Situé au cœur des Rocheuses, à 25 km à l'ouest de l'aéroport de Helena
Yoga	Vinyasa, Iyengar, Anusara, Power Yoga, yoga restauratif, Freedom Style
Professeurs	Kira Ryder, Baxter Bell, Richard Miller, Marla Apt, Erich Schiffmann, Lilias Folan
Chambres	4 chambres à 4 lits, 9 chambres doubles, 5 yourtes, 5 tipis et 10 tentes, en tout pour 60 personnes max.
Restauration	Essentiellement bio et végétarienne, occasionnellement poulet et poisson
Traitements	Sauna, massages
Activités	Natation, randonnées, canoë, aviron et équitation

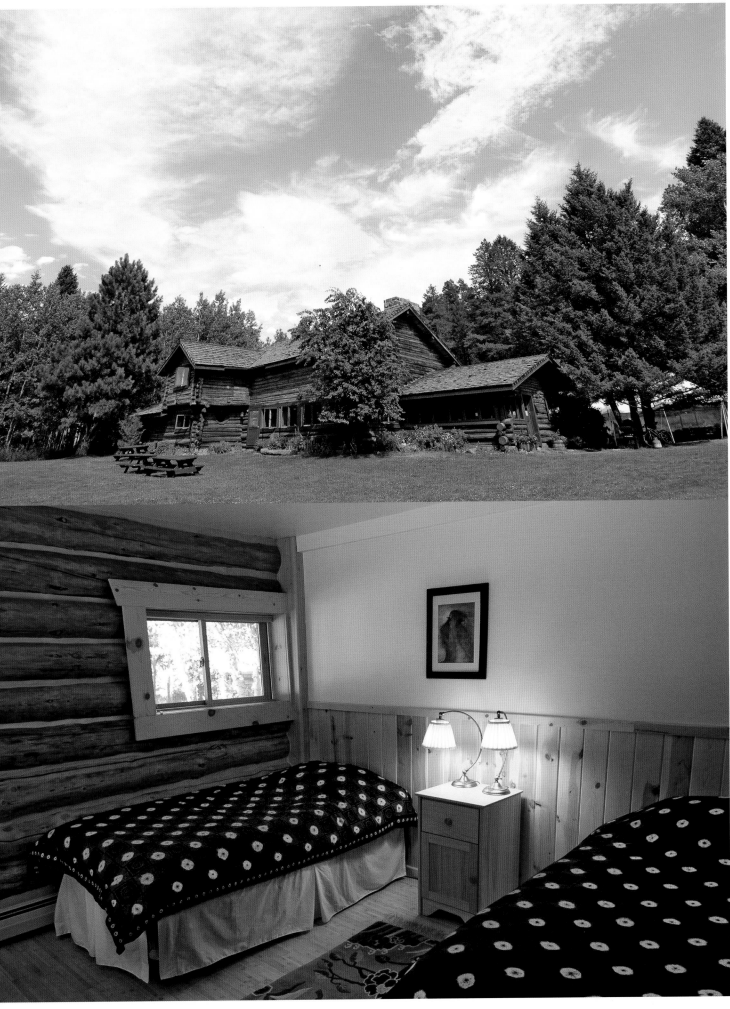

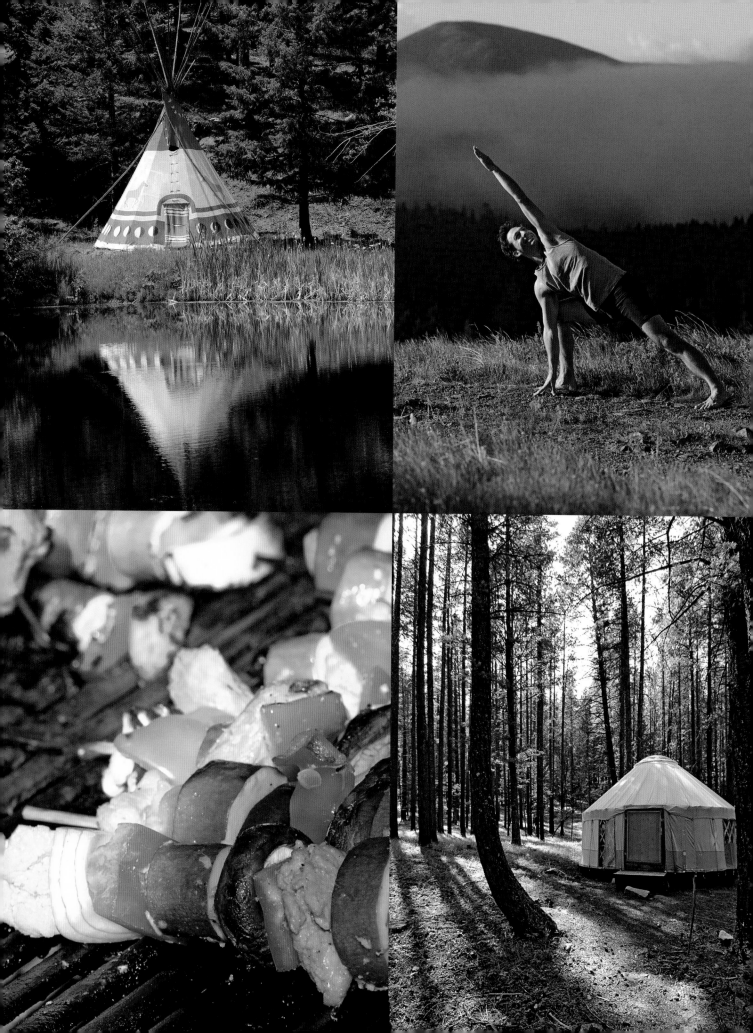

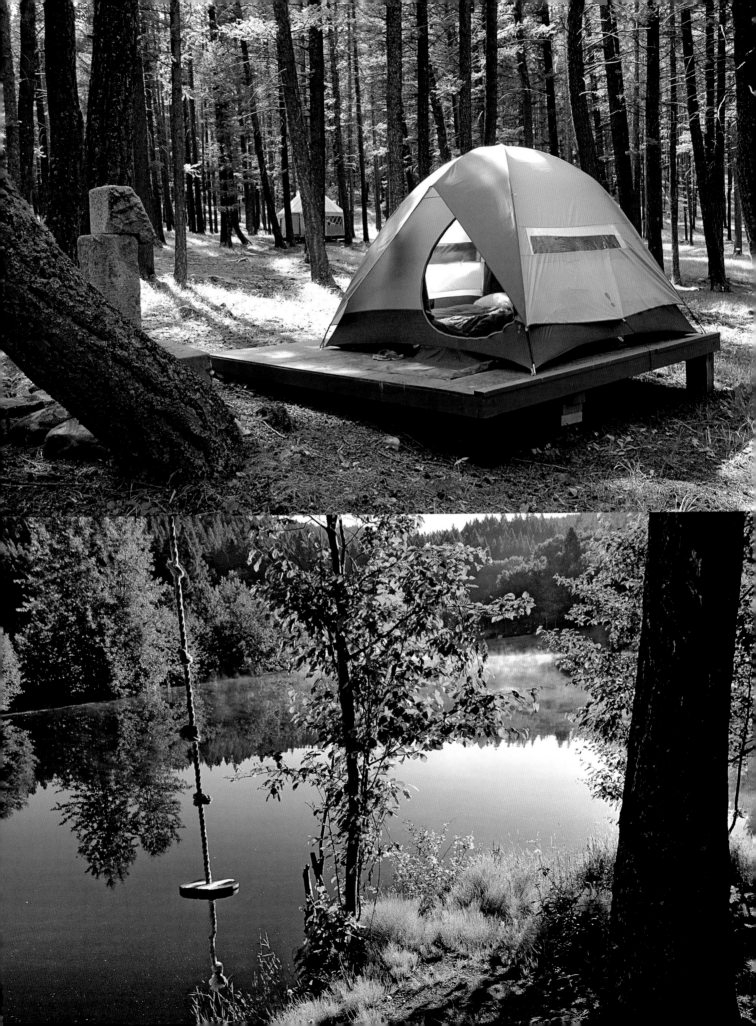

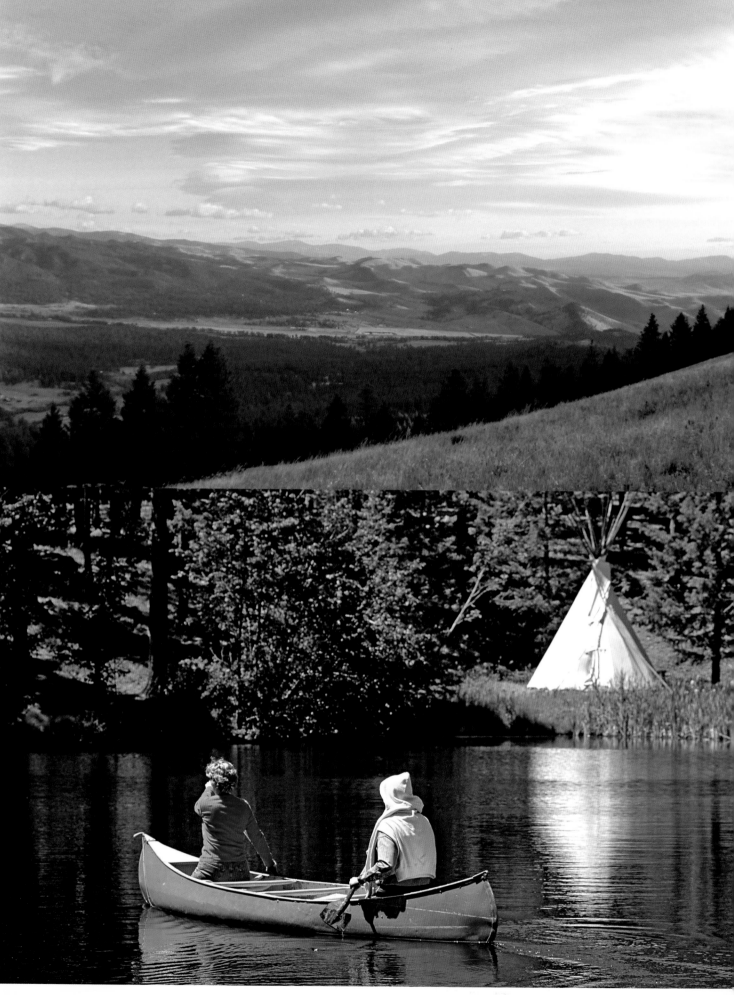

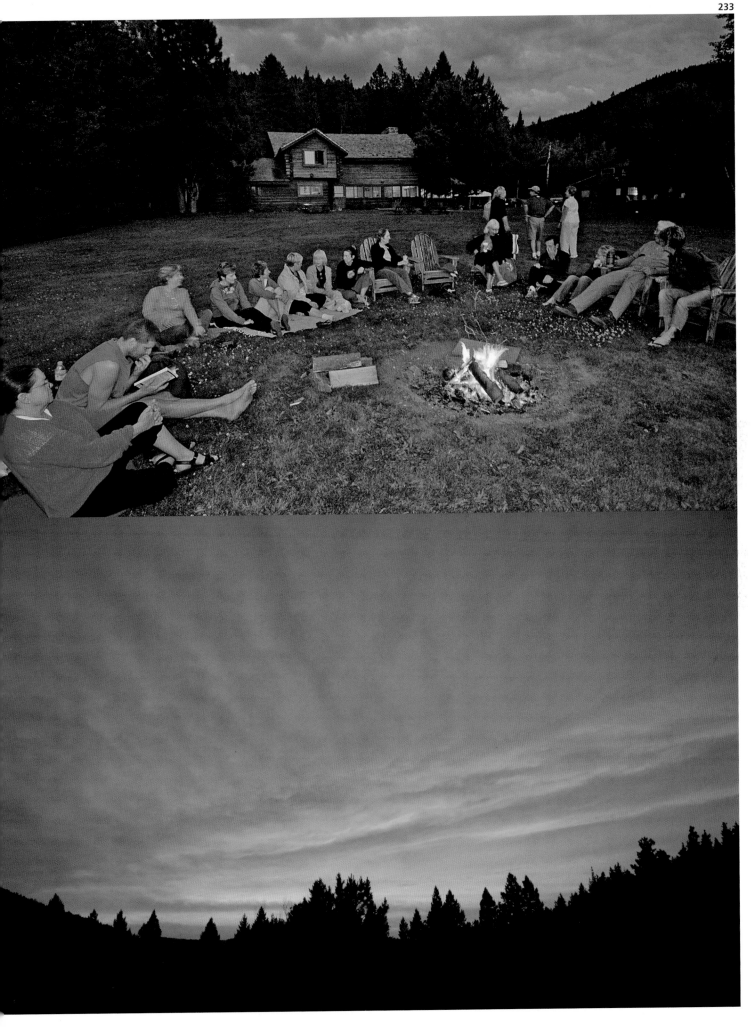

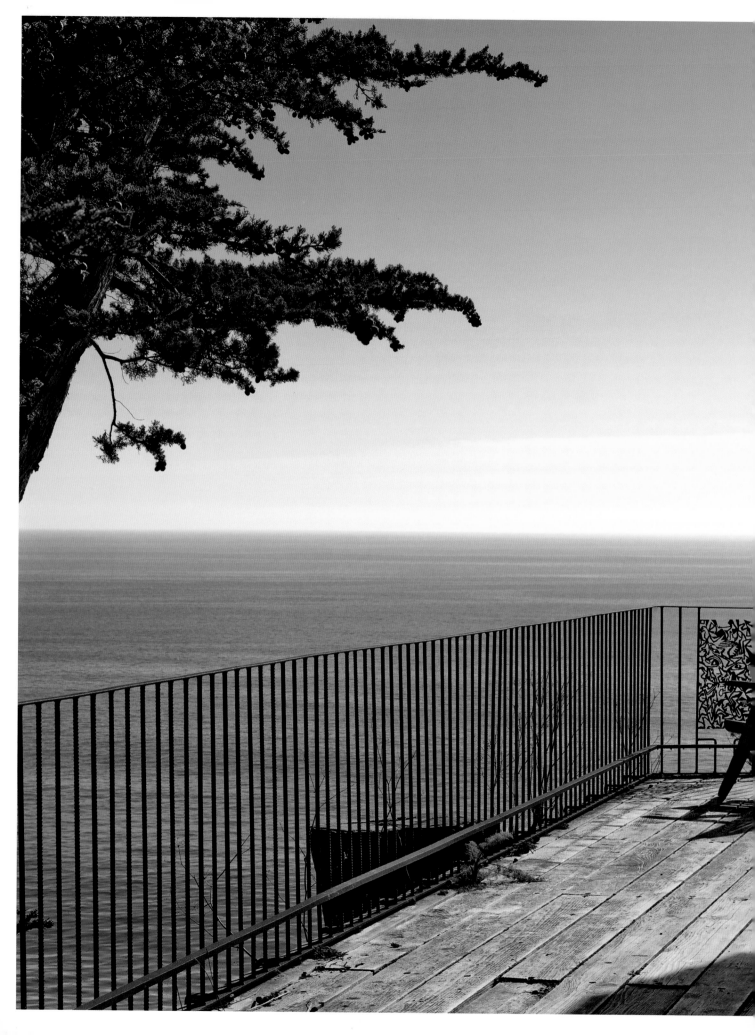

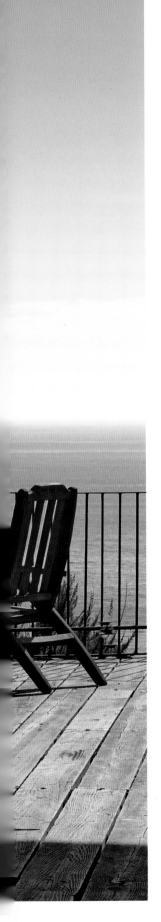

Esalen stands on the edge. In Big Sur, on the legendary Highway 1, it perches on a cliff high above the crashing surf. The institute, part think tank, part refuge, devotes itself to research into "human potential", as Aldous Huxley put it. How a sequence is formed from single Asanas can be learned here from Srivatsa Ramaswami, as well as Chinese Yoga, also known as Qigong, Tantric alchemy from Darren Rhodes or, from the beautiful and intelligent Seane Corn, how you combine yoga and your actions. Even without visiting the excellent workshops you can, if there is room, take part in stimulating yoga and movement sessions with an ensuing dip in the hot springs. The spectacular cliffs, the Santa Lucia Mountains behind, the hot springs and equally heated discussions attracted Joan Baez, Hunter S. Thompson and Henry Miller to Esalen back in the 1960s. The spiritual revolution, which at that time rather shook up the American soul, would have looked meagre without Esalen's thinkers. The thinkers themselves have the hot mineral springs, which bubble powerfully from deep beneath the earth at 119 degrees Fahrenheit, to thank for their cool heads.

Books to pack: "Confessions of an English Opium Eater" by Thomas de Quincey and "Fear and Loathing in Las Vegas" by Hunter S. Thompson

Esalen Institute

55000 Highway 1
Big Sur, CA 93920
USA
Tel. +1 831 667 3000
info@esalen.org
www.esalen.org

Directions	A 3-hr drive south of San Francisco
Yoga	Hatha, Anusara, Raja, Tantra, Chinese Yoga, Tibetan Buddhist meditation, Ashtanga, Sivananda, Iyengar
Teachers	Amy Ipolitti, Thomas Fortel, Saul David Raye, Mark Whitwell, Kia Miller, Janet Stone, Charu Rachlis
Rooms	2–3-bed rooms, single rooms, single-family houses, rooms with bunk beds; places to sleep with sleeping bags
Food	Vegan, vegetarian and meat cuisine, mainly organic, much grown on site
Treatments	Swedish massage, wellness/stress management massage
Leisure	Arts centre, Big Sur National Park, hot springs, night swimming, massage training

Esalen steht am äußersten Rande: In Big Sur, direkt am legendären Highway 1, thront es auf einem Kliff, hoch über der krachenden Brandung. Das Institut ist teils Denkfabrik, teils Refugium für die Erforschung des »menschlichen Potenzials«, wie Aldous Huxley schrieb. Wie man aus einzelnen Asanas eine Sequenz formt, kann man hier von Srivatsa Ramaswami lernen, chinesisches Yoga, auch bekannt als Qigong, oder tantrische Alchemie bei Darren Rhodes, während die schöne wie kluge Seane Corn zeigt, wie man Yoga und Handeln zusammenbringt. Auch ohne die exzellenten Workshops zu besuchen kann man, wenn Platz ist, bei anregenden Kursen mitmachen und anschließend ein Bad in den heißen Quellen nehmen. Die spektakuläre Steilküste, das Santa-Lucia-Gebirge im Rücken, die heißen Quellen und ebenso heißen Diskussionen haben in den 1960ern schon Joan Baez, Hunter S. Thompson und Henry Miller nach Esalen gelockt. Die spirituelle Revolution, die die amerikanische Seele damals ziemlich umkrempelte, hätte ohne Esalens Denker mager ausgesehen. Die Denker selber verdanken bis heute ihre kühlen Köpfe den heißen Mineralquellen, die mit großer Kraft und einer Temperatur von 48 Grad Celcius tief aus der Erde sprudeln.

Reisebegleiter: »Bekenntnisse eines englischen Opiumessers« von Thomas de Quincey und »Angst und Schrecken in Las Vegas« von Hunter S. Thompson

Esalen est situé à l'extrême bord. Il se dresse majestueusement sur une haute falaise de Big Sur, sur la légendaire Highway 1, et surplombe les vagues déferlantes. A la fois fabrique intellectuelle et refuge, cet institut se consacre à la recherche du « potentiel humain », selon l'expression d'Aldous Huxley. On peut y apprendre de Srivatsa Ramaswami comment faire de plusieurs Âsanas une série complète, ou le yoga chinois connu sous le nom de qigong, ou l'alchimie tantrique auprès de Darren Rhodes ou enfin avec la belle et subtile Seane Corn comment associer yoga et action. Même sans assister aux excellents stages, on peut, s'il y a encore des places, suivre des séances inspiratrices de yoga et, ensuite, prendre un bain aux sources chaudes. Déjà dans les années 1960, l'imposante côte escarpée, le massif de Santa-Lucia à l'arrière-plan, les sources chaudes et les discussions également bouillonnantes ont attiré Joan Baez, Hunter S. Thompson et Henry Miller à Esalen. Sans les penseurs d'Esalen, la révolution spirituelle qui, à l'époque, a sensiblement bouleversé l'âme américaine aurait fait piètre figure. Aujourd'hui encore, ces penseurs ont gardé la tête froide grâce aux sources thermales qui, à 48 degrés Celcius, jaillissent puissamment de la terre.

Livres à emporter : « Les Confessions d'un mangeur d'opium anglais » de Thomas de Quincey et « Las Vegas Parano » de Hunter S. Thompson

Anreise	3 Std. Autofahrt südlich von San Francisco
Yoga	Hatha, Anusara, Raja, Tantra, chinesisches Yoga, Tibetan Buddhist Meditation, Ashtanga, Sivananda, Iyengar
Lehrer	Amy Ipolitti, Thomas Fortel, Saul David Raye, Mark Whitwell, Kia Miller, Janet Stone, Charu Rachlis
Zimmer	Zwei- bis Dreibettzimmer, Einzel- und Stockbettzimmer, Einfamilienhäuser, Schlafsackschlafplätze
Küche	Vegan, vegetarisch und Fleischküche
Anwendungen	Schwedische Massage, Wellness-Stressmanagement-Massage
Aktivitäten	Arts Center, Big Sur National Park, heiße Quellen, Nachtbaden, Massagetraining

Accès	Situé à 3 h de voiture au sud de San Francisco
Yoga	Hatha, Anusara, Râja, Tantra, yoga chinois, méditation bouddhiste tibétaine, Ashtânga, Shivananda, Iyengar
Professeurs	Amy Ipolitti, Thomas Fortel, Saul David Raye, Mark Whitwell, Kia Miller, Janet Stone, Charu Rachlis
Chambres	Chambres à 2–3 lits, chambres simples, maisons familiales, chambres avec lits à étages ; places pour dormir avec sacs de couchage
Restauration	Cuisine végétalienne, végétarienne et avec viande
Traitements	Massages suédois, de bien-être et anti-stress
Activités	Centre artistique, Parc national de Big Sur, sources chaudes, bains nocturnes, entraînement au massage

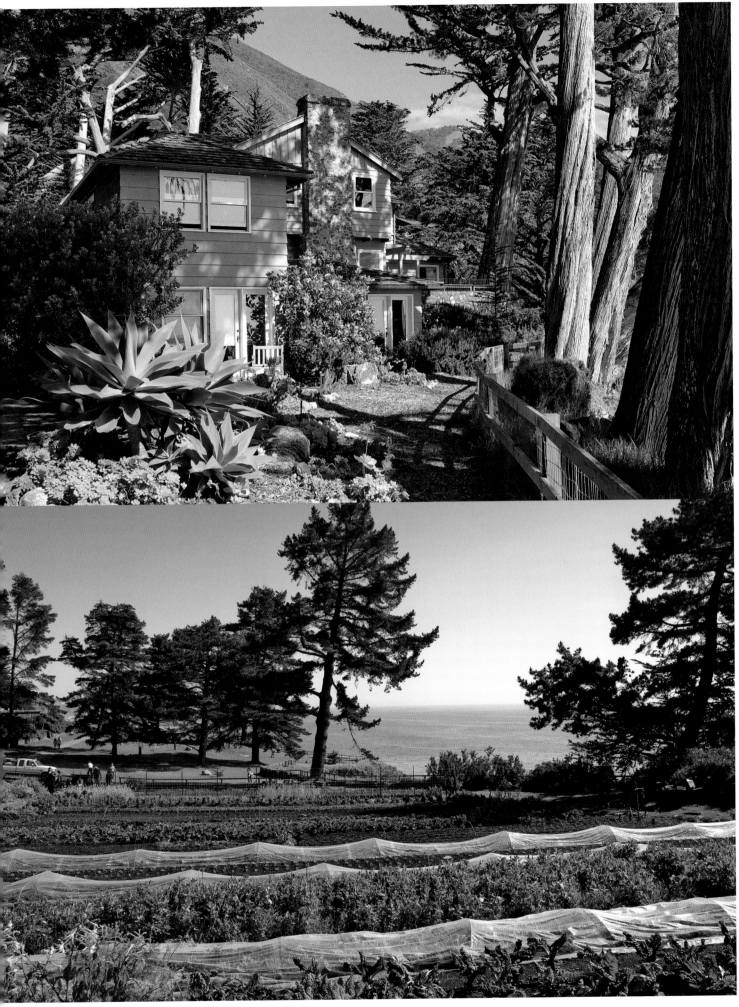

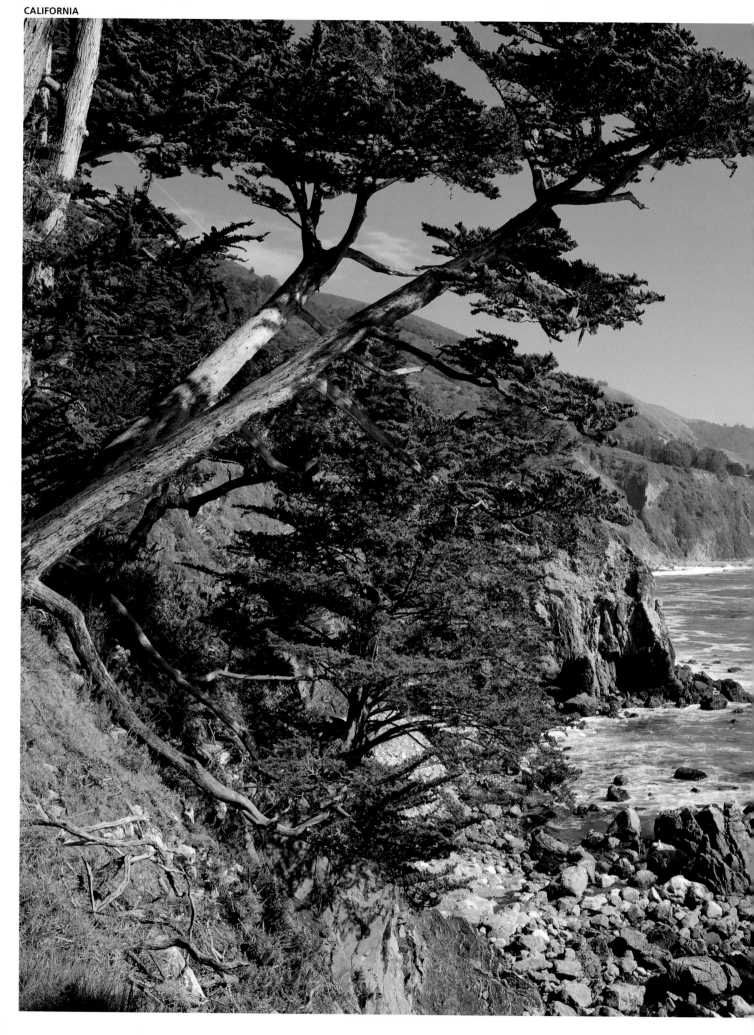

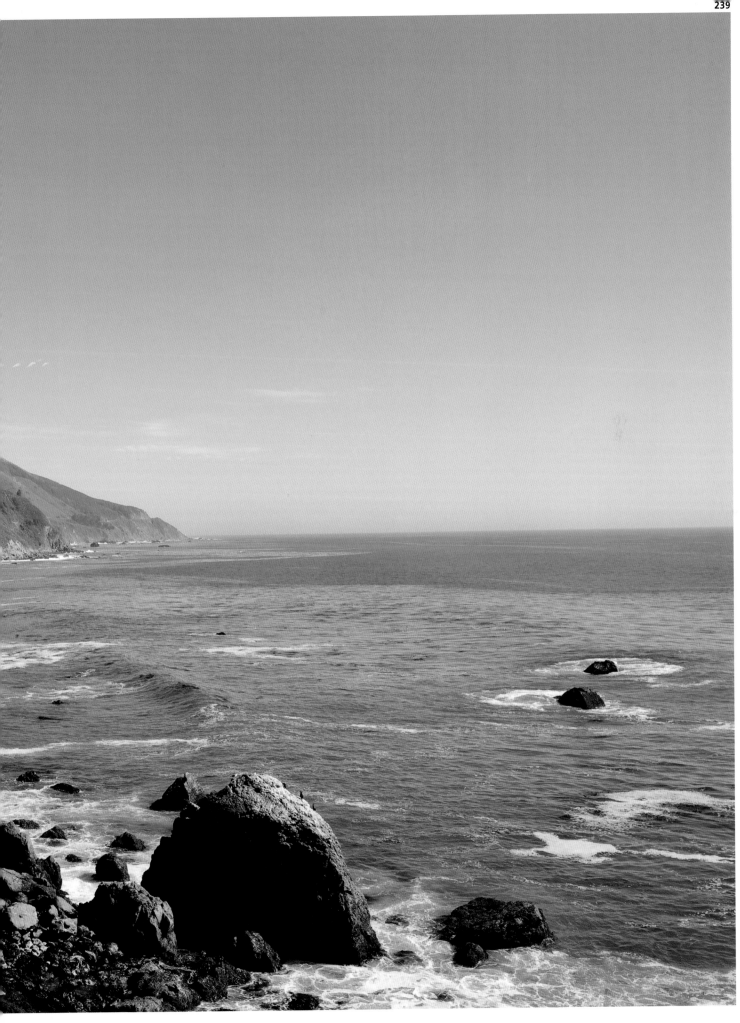

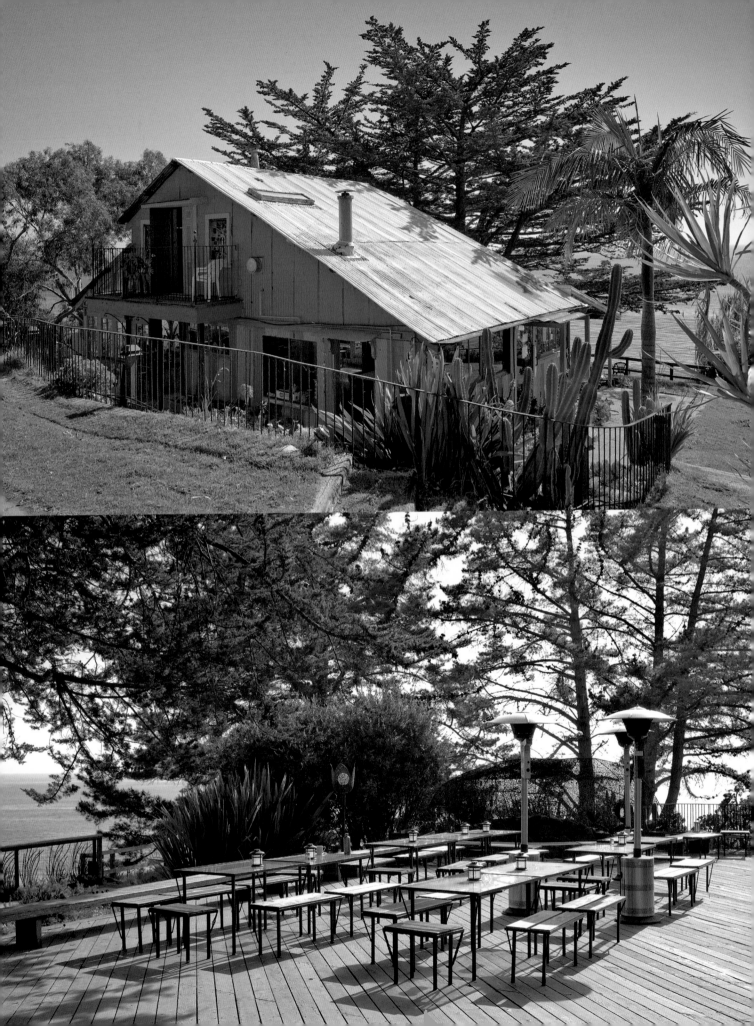

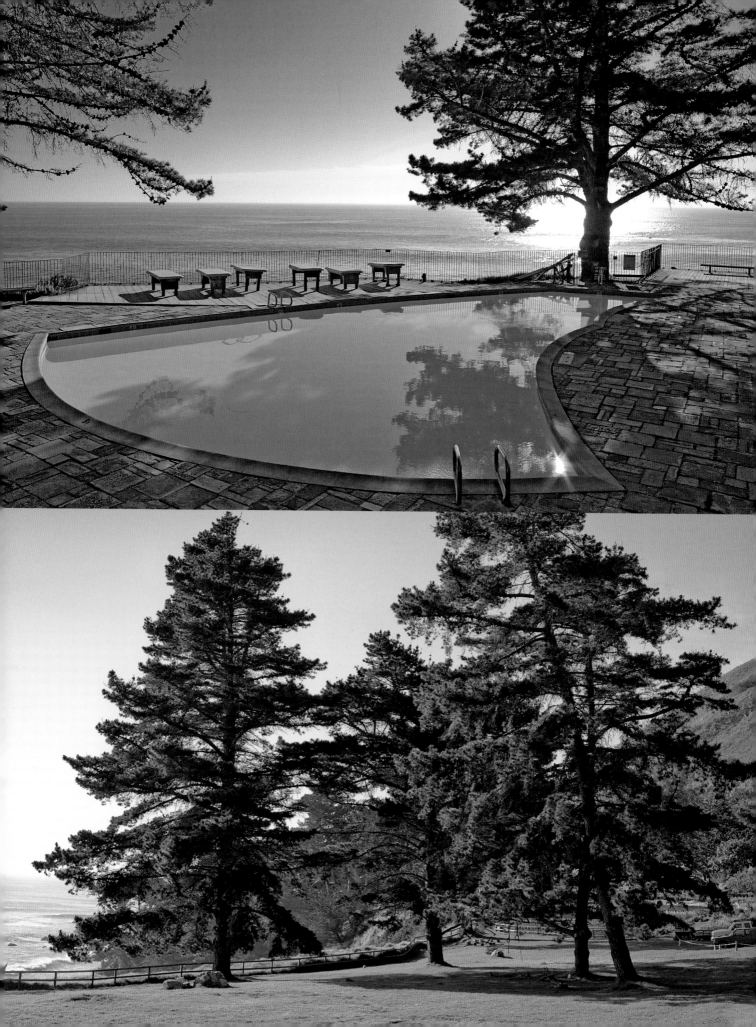

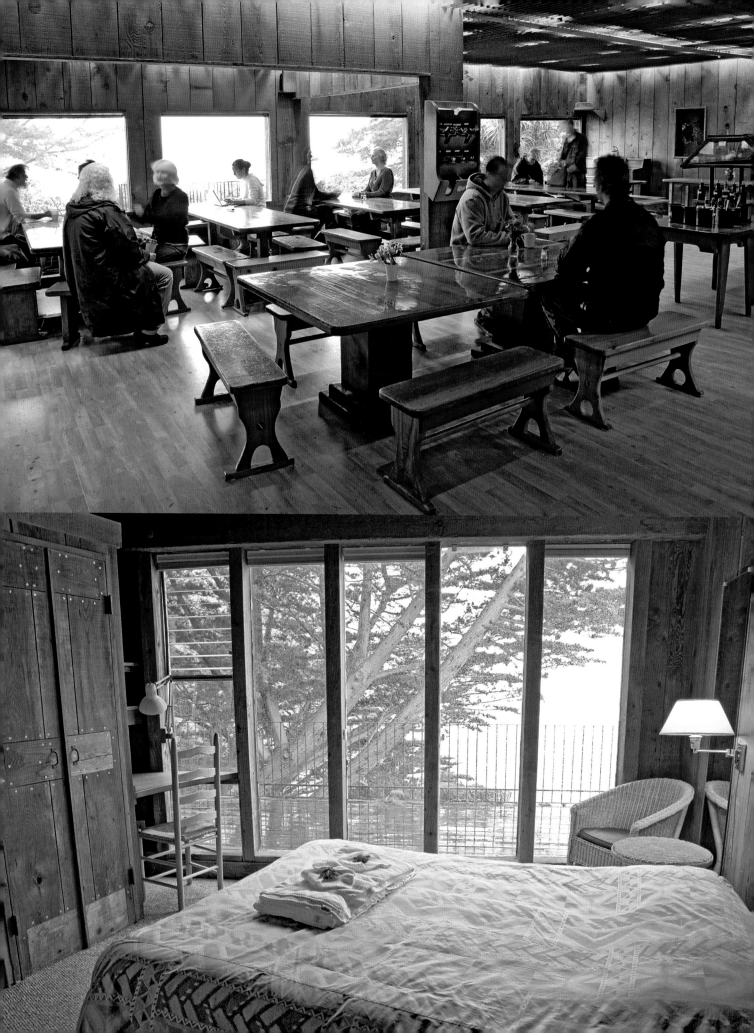

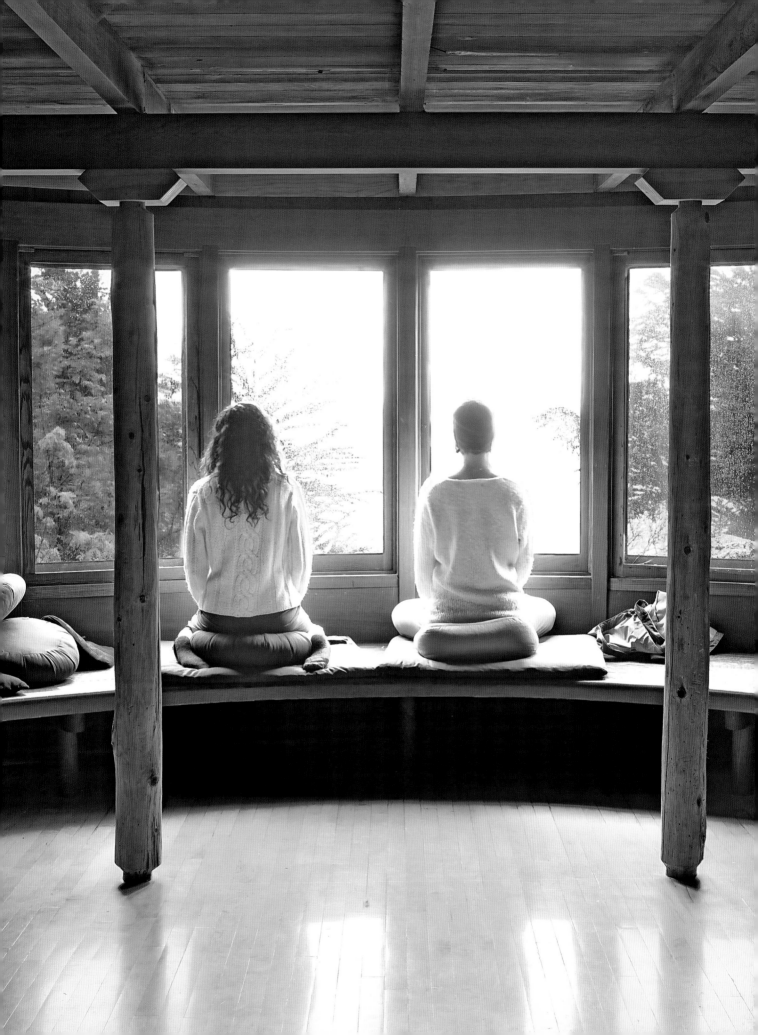

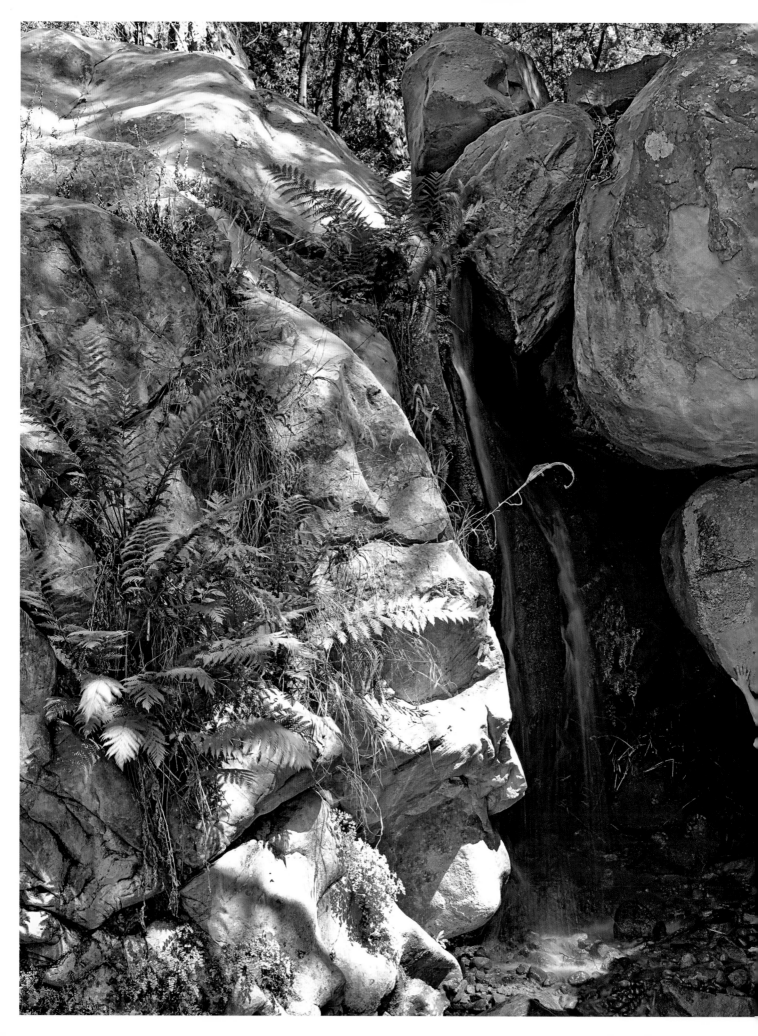

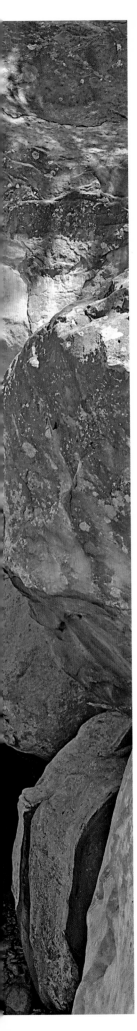

It goes without saying that you would have liked flying over the War Memorial in 1967 during the anti-Vietnam War demonstration in San Francisco with Ganga White in Swami Vishnu's "Peace Plane", throwing flowers and flyers into the air, or watching with curiosity alongside Vietnam War protestor Muhammad Ali as Ganga demonstrated a perfect Dhanurasana (bow pose), but an intensive yoga session with him today is nothing to be sniffed at either. From the tiny beauty salon on Sunset Boulevard in Los Angeles, in which White Lotus began as a yoga school, to the retreat in the mountains above Santa Barbara, the founder has seen a lot of water flow down the San José river. B. K. S Iyengar and Pattabhi Jois were his guests before they became world famous. With its waterfalls, the Indian trails that lead through the steep canyon, the pond full of water lilies, the pretty sandstone bays ideal for bathing, the meditation caves and the enchantingly appointed sleeping tents, the retreat he runs with the impressive Yogini Tracey Rich is a classic like Muhammad Ali's left hook: convincing, clear, a direct hit—with yet the opposite effect of a knock-out.

Books to pack: "Love, Freedom and Aloneness" by Osho and "Budding Prospects" by T. C. Boyle

White Lotus Foundation

2500 San Marcos Pass
Santa Barbara, CA 93105
USA
Tel. +1 805 964 1944
Fax +1 805 964 9617
info@whitelotus.org
www.whitelotus.org

Directions	106 miles north of Los Angeles and 12 miles north of Santa Barbara Airport
Yoga	Undogmatic, Vinyasa Flow, multi-disciplinary
Teachers	Ganga White, Tracey Rich, Sven Holcomb, Cheri Clampett, Kent Bond, James Morrison
Rooms	7 yurts for max. 3 people each, seven 1-2-bed rooms; max. 30 guests
Food	Lacto-ovo-vegetarian, vegan alternatives
Treatments	Hot tub, sauna, bodywork, Thai Yoga therapy
Leisure	Private hiking trails, waterfalls, swimming

Natürlich wäre man mit Ganga White gern in Swami Vishnus »Peace Plane« während der Anti-Vietnam-Demonstration von 1967 über das War Memorial in San Francisco geflogen, um Blumen und Flugblätter abzuwerfen, oder hätte mit Vietnam-Gegner Muhammad Ali neugierig zugesehen, wie Ganga eine perfekte Dhanurasana (Bogen) vorführt. Aber eine intensive Yogasession mit ihm heutzutage ist auch nicht übel. Von dem winzigen Schönheitssalon auf dem Sunset Boulevard in Los Angeles, in dem White mit seiner Yogaschule anfing, bis zum Retreat in den Bergen oberhalb Santa Barbaras hat der Gründer eine Menge Wasser den San-José-Fluss hinunterfließen sehen. B. K. S Iyengar und Pattabhi Jois waren seine Gäste, noch bevor sie weltberühmt wurden. Mit seinen Wasserfällen, den indianischen Wanderwegen, die durch den steilen Canyon führen, dem Teich voller Seerosen, hübschen Schwimmbuchten aus Sandstein, den Meditationshöhlen und den bezaubernd eingerichteten Schlafzelten ist das Retreat, das er zusammen mit der beeindruckenden Yogini Tracey Rich führt, ein Klassiker wie die Linke von Muhammad Ali: überzeugend, klar, ein Volltreffer. Nur eben ohne K. o.

Reisebegleiter: »Liebe, Freiheit, Alleinsein« von Osho und »Grün ist die Hoffnung« von T. C. Boyle

Bien sûr, on aurait aimé accompagner Ganga White dans le « Peace Plane » de Swami Vishnu, en 1967, pendant la manifestation contre la guerre du Vietnam et survoler le War Memorial de San Francisco pour lancer des fleurs et des tracts ou encore avec Muhammad Ali, opposant à la guerre du Vietnam, observer avec intérêt Ganga en train d'effectuer une parfaite Dhanurasana (posture d'extension), mais une séance intensive de yoga avec lui, de nos jours, n'est pas mal non plus. Du petit institut de beauté sur le Sunset Boulevard de Los Angeles, où White Lotus fut d'abord une école de yoga, au domaine retiré dans les montagnes au-dessus de Santa Barbara, le fondateur a vu beaucoup d'eau couler sous les ponts du fleuve San José. B. K. S Iyengar et Pattabhi Jois comptaient déjà parmi ses hôtes avant de devenir mondialement célèbres. Avec ses cascades, ses sentiers de randonnée indiens qui sillonnent le canyon escarpé, l'étang aux nénuphars, les jolies criques aux roches de grès, les cavernes de méditation et les tentes-dortoirs délicieusement aménagées, le domaine qu'il codirige avec l'extraordinaire yogini Tracey Rich est un classique, au même titre que le gauche de Muhammad Ali : convaincant, clair, droit au but. Mais sans K.O.

Livres à emporter : « Amour, liberté et solitude » d'Osho et « La belle affaire » de T. C. Boyle

Anreise	170 km nördlich von Los Angeles und 20 km nördlich vom Flughafen Santa Barbara gelegen
Yoga	Undogmatisch und interdisziplinär, Vinyasa Flow
Lehrer	Ganga White, Tracey Rich, Sven Holcomb, Cheri Clampett, Kent Bond, James Morrison
Zimmer	7 Jurten (für jeweils max. 3 Personen), 7 Ein- bis Zweibettzimmer; max. 30 Gäste
Küche	Lacto-ovo-vegetarisch, vegane Alternativen
Anwendungen	Hot Tub, Sauna, Bodywork, Thai-Yoga-Therapie
Aktivitäten	Private Wanderwege, Wasserfälle, Schwimmen

Accès	Situé à 170 km au nord de Los Angeles et à 20 km au nord de l'aéroport de Santa Barbara
Yoga	Hors dogme, Vinyasa Flow, pluridisciplinaire
Professeurs	Ganga White, Tracey Rich, Sven Holcomb, Cheri Clampett, Kent Bond, James Morrison
Chambres	7 yourtes pour 3 personnes max., 7 chambres à 1 et 2 lits ; 30 personnes max.
Restauration	Cuisine lacto-ovo-végétarienne, alternatives végétaliennes
Traitements	Bain tourbillon, sauna, bodywork, thérapie de yoga thailandais
Activités	Chemins de randonnée privés, cascades, natation

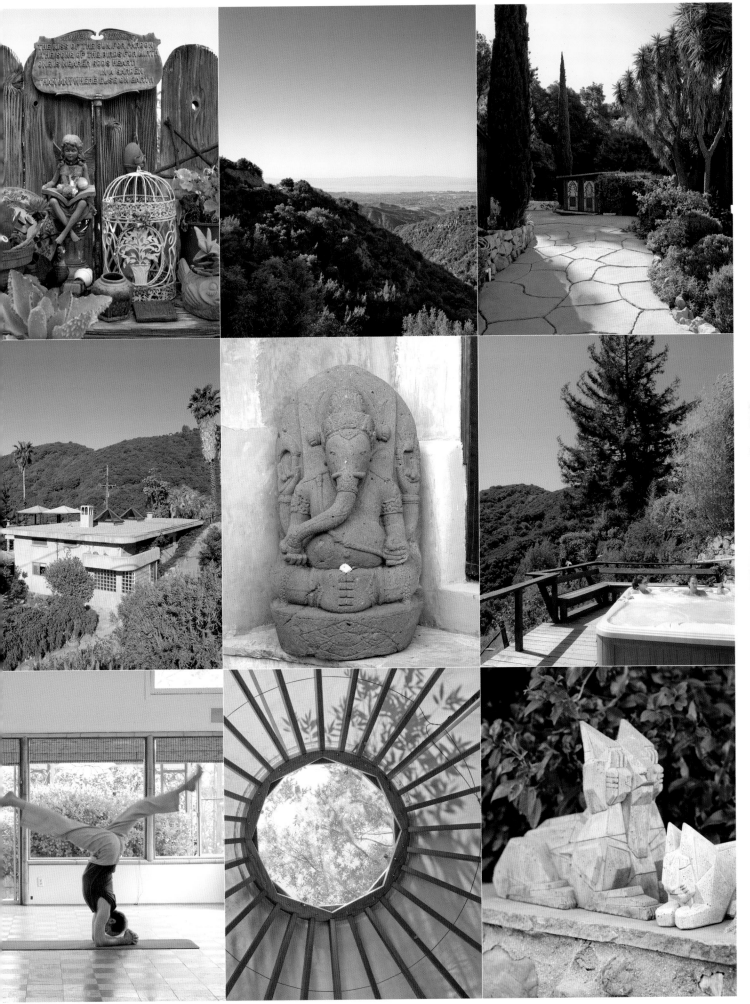

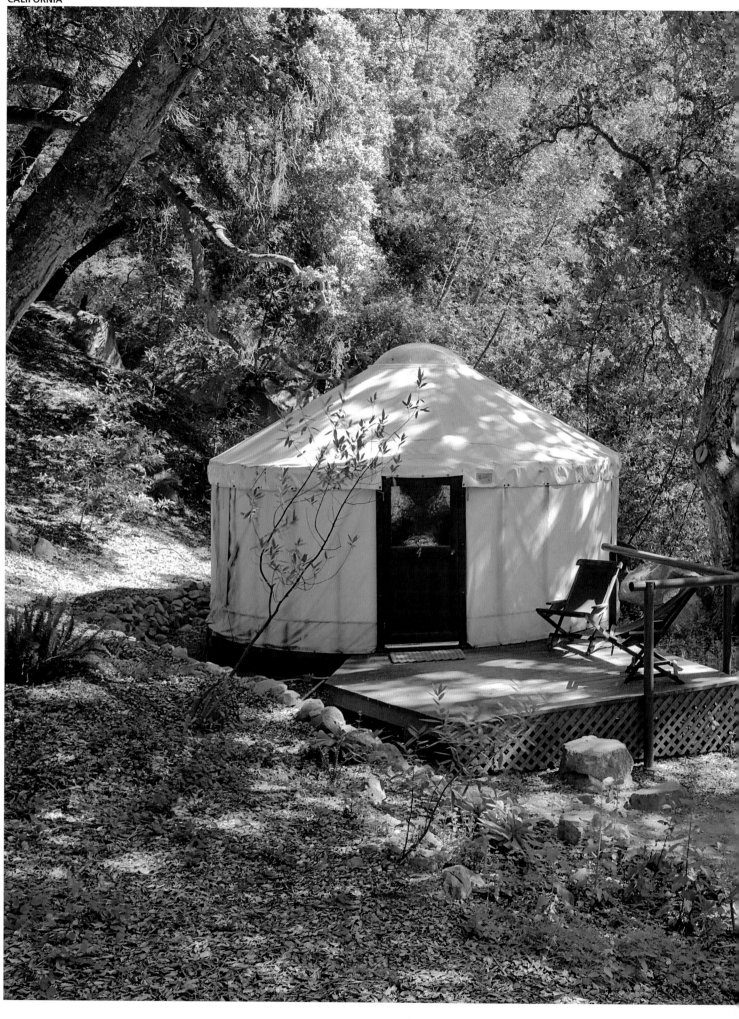

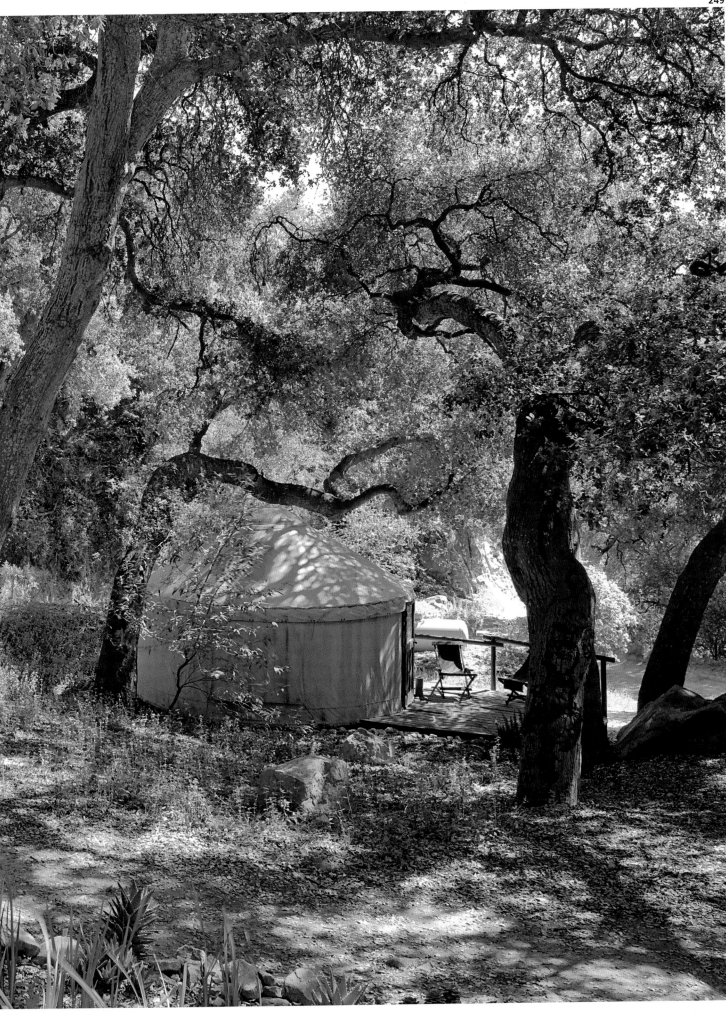

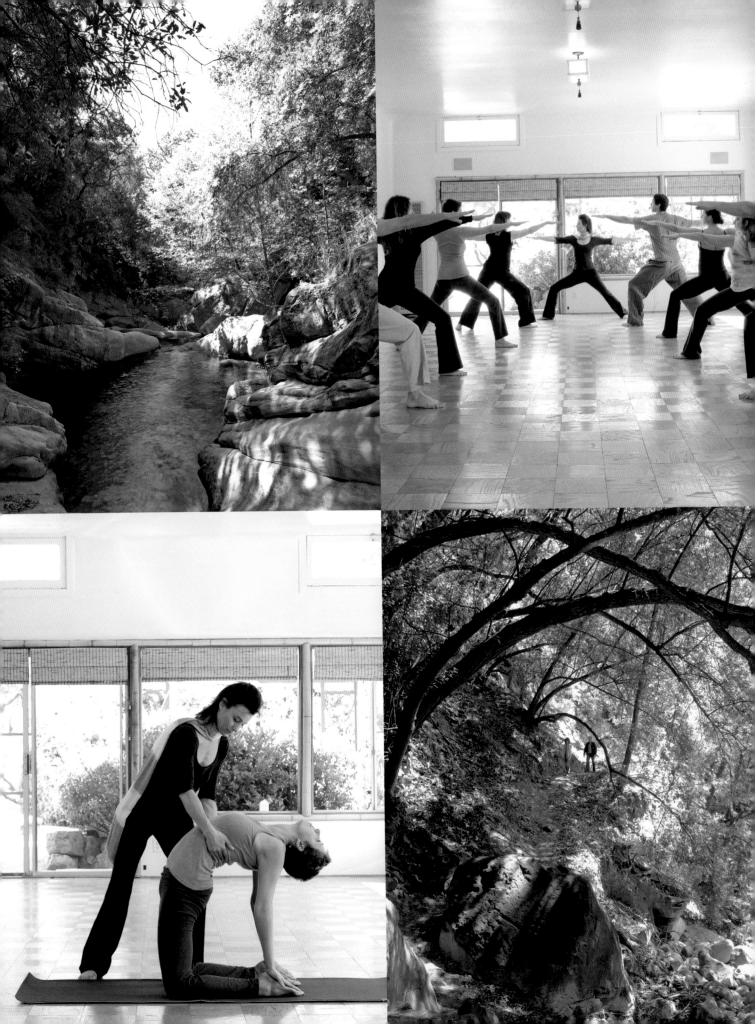

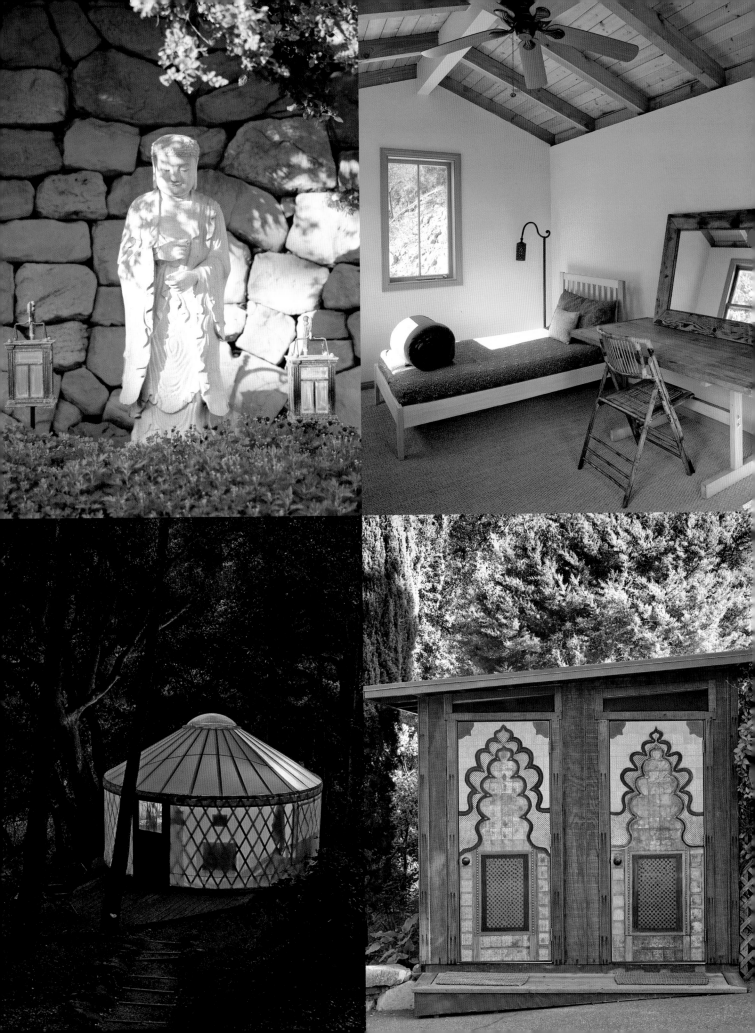

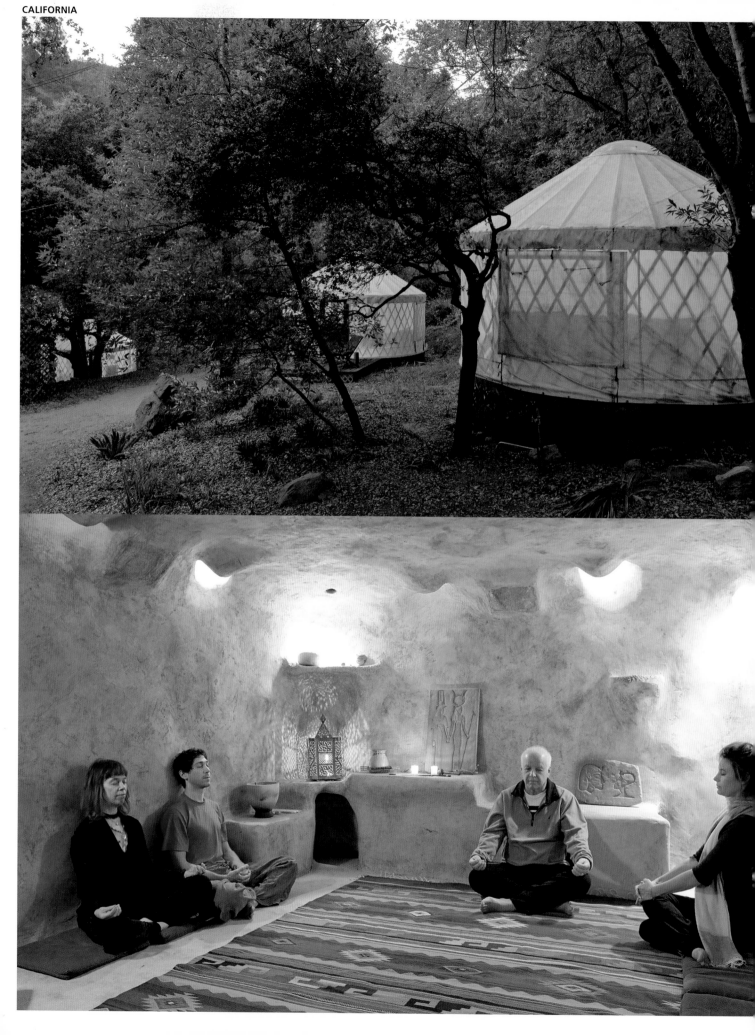

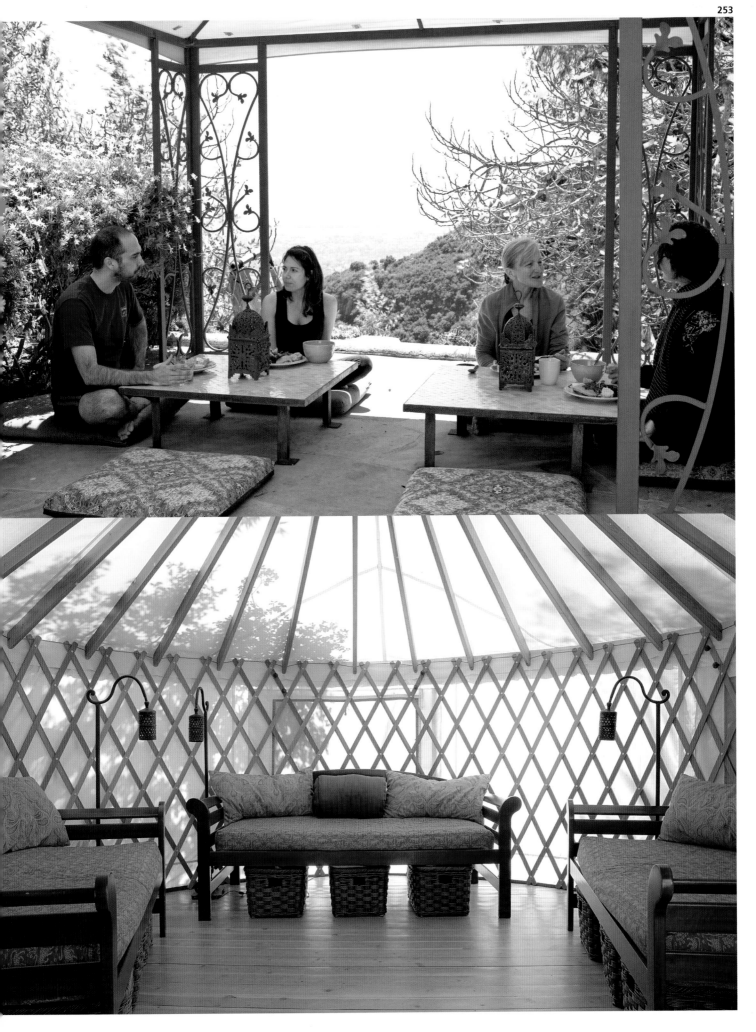

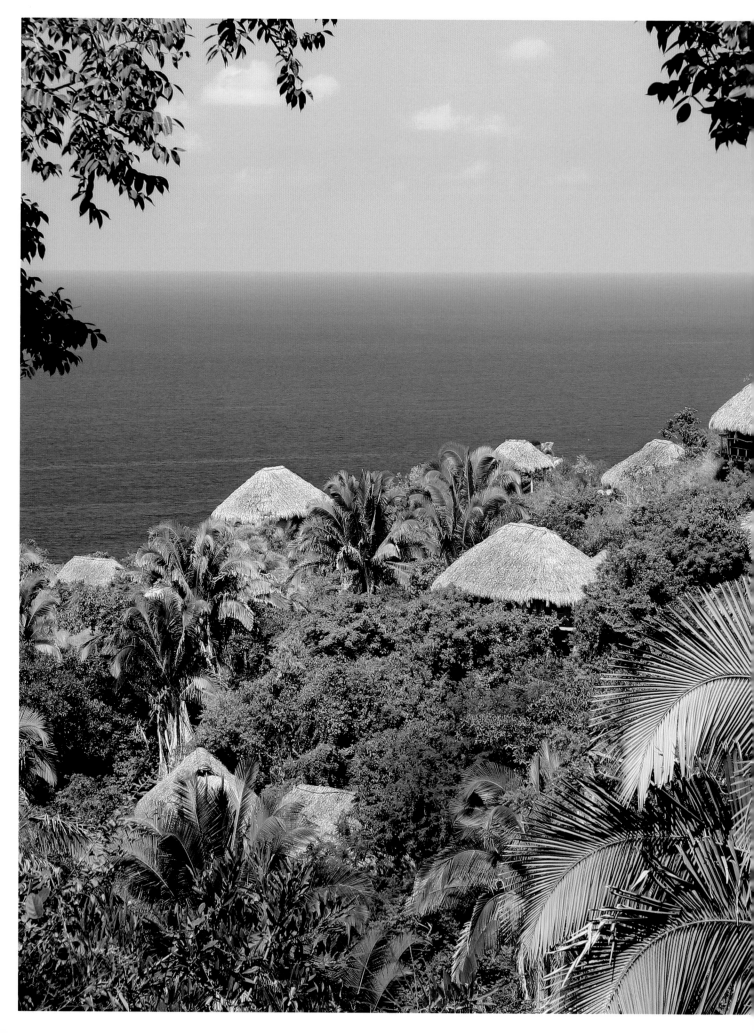

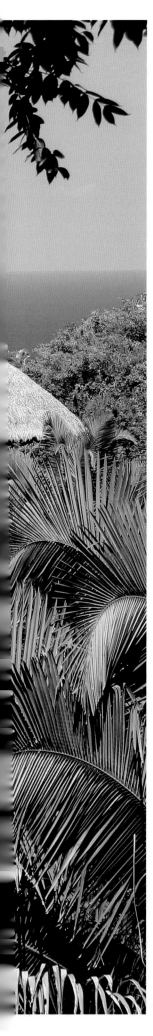

How many shades of green are there? How does the green of the grasses, bushes, ferns and the pine forests on the mountain crests on the horizon disappear into the white-blue of the sky, merging from there into the turquoise-blue of the sea, and transform itself from the grey-brown of the forgotten rocks on the beach into the golden yellow of the sand? Wherever you look at the Haramara Retreat, colors explode. The yoga sessions in the yoga pavilion that is open 360 degrees and stands high on the hill are an adventure in themselves. A fabulous view onto the entangled jungle all about you comes as the reward after intense practice. If the thicket in your own head has not been wonderfully cleared after that, Vipassana meditation is a possibility. Or simply the luxury of a good old-fashioned midday nap. When the sky hovers hot over Haramara, time stands still for a couple of hours. And the spirit finds peace. If you hadn't booked one of the world-class massages, wild horses couldn't drag you from the hand-woven linen of the romantic and charmingly furnished bungalows. Only the whales—also in evidence here, by the way—might just manage it.

Books to pack: "The Maya End Times" by Patricia Mercier and "Living Yoga" by Christy Turlington

Haramara Retreat

Tamarindos 13
Sayulita, Nayarit
Mexico
Tel. +52 29 329 291 3038
haramara@comcast.net
www.haramararetreat.com

Directions	40 min north of Puerto Vallarta Airport, airport transfer by arrangement
Yoga	Hatha, Ashtanga, Sivananda, Iyengar, Anusara, Kundalini, Istha, SUP Yoga
Teachers	Rodney Yee, Janet Stone, Desiree Rumbaugh, Sherri Baptiste, Anne Dyer, Peggy Orr, Darren Rhodes
Rooms	16 rooms with one, two or more beds for max. 44 guests; additional dormitory for 8 guests; exclusive use of property available
Food	Vegan, vegetarian, with fish and seafood
Treatments	Full spa service including massages and facials
Leisure	Snorkelling, whale watching, surfing and jungle hikes

Wie viele Schattierungen von Grün gibt es? Wie taucht das Grün der Gräser, Sträucher, Farne, der Kiefernwälder auf den Bergkämmen am Horizont ins weißlich Blaue des Himmels, von dort ins Türkisblau des Meers – und verwandelt sich vom Graubraun der am Strand vergessenen Felsbrocken ins Goldgelbe des Sands? Wohin auch immer man blickt im Haramara Retreat, es explodieren Farben. Ein Abenteuer für sich sind die Yogastunden in dem rundum offenen Yoga-Pavillon, der einen Hügel bekrönt. Ein sagenhafter Ausblick auf den verknoteten Dschungel ringsum ist die Belohnung nach intensivem Üben. Wenn sich danach das Dickicht im eigenen Kopf nicht auf wundersame Weise löst, gibt es die Möglichkeit zur Vipassana-Meditation – oder einfach den Luxus einer altmodischen Mittagsruhe. Spätestens dann, wenn der Himmel heiß über Haramara schwebt, bleibt für ein paar Stunden die Zeit stehen, und der Geist findet Ruhe. Hätte man nicht eine der Weltklasse-Massagen gebucht, würden einen keine zehn Pferde von den handgewebten Laken der romantisch-charmant eingerichteten Bungalows trennen können. Höchstens Wale. Die gibt es hier nämlich auch.

Reisebegleiter: »Der Ruf der Mayas« von Wiek Lenssen und »Living Yoga« von Christy Turlington

Combien de tons de vert existe-t-il ? Comment exactement le vert des herbes, buissons, fougères et forêts de pins sur les cimes montagneuses à l'horizon se fond-il au bleu pâle du ciel, puis dans le bleu turquoise de la mer, avant de passer du gris brun des rochers oubliés sur la plage au jaune doré du sable ? Au Hamarara Retreat, où que le regard se pose, les couleurs explosent. Les séances de yoga, véritables événements, ont lieu dans le pavillon de yoga ouvert à 360 degrés qui trône tout en haut de la colline. Une splendide vue panoramique sur la forêt vierge enchevêtrée tout autour est la récompense après un entraînement intensif. Si, après cela, la jungle de l'esprit n'est toujours pas défrichée, une méditation Vipassana est possible. Ou tout simplement le luxe d'une sieste classique. Au plus tard à cet instant-là, tandis que le ciel brûlant plane au-dessus de Hamarara, le temps s'arrête pour quelques heures. Et l'esprit trouve la paix. Si l'on n'était pas inscrit à l'un des massages haut de gamme, dix chevaux ne pourraient pas vous tirer des toiles de lin tissées main des charmants bungalows romantiques. Tout au plus des baleines. Parce qu'il y en a ici aussi.

Livres à emporter: : « Le code Maya » de Barbara Hand Clow et « Living Yoga » de Christy Turlington

Anreise	40 min vom Flughafen Puerto Vallarta entfernt; Flughafentransfer nach Absprache
Yoga	Hatha, Ashtanga, Sivananda, Iyengar, Anusara, Kundalini, Istha, SUP Yoga
Lehrer	Rodney Yee, Janet Stone, Desiree Rumbaugh, Sherri Baptiste, Anne Dyer, Peggy Orr, Darren Rhodes
Zimmer	16 Einzel-, Doppel und Mehrbettzimmer für max. 44 Gäste; zusätzlicher Schlafsaal für 8 Gäste; exklusive Anmietung des gesamten Retreats möglich
Küche	Vegan, vegetarisch, Fisch und Meeresfrüchte
Anwendungen	Komplettes Spa-Angebot, u. a. Massagen und Facials
Aktivitäten	Schnorcheln, Whale Watching, Surfen und Dschungelwanderungen

Accès	Situé à 40 min de l'aéroport de Puerto Vallarta ; transfert de l'aéroport après accord
Yoga	Hatha, Ashtânga, Shivananda, Iyengar, Anusara, Kundalinî, Ishta, SUP Yoga
Professeurs	Rodney Yee, Janet Stone, Desiree Rumbaugh, Sherri Baptiste, Anne Dyer, Peggy Orr, Darren Rhodes
Chambres	16 chambres simples, doubles et à plusieurs lits pour 44 personnes max. ; dortoir supplémentaire pour 8 personnes ; privatisations possibles
Restauration	Végétalienne, végétarienne, poisson et fruits de mer
Traitements	Service spa complet comprenant massages et soins du visage
Activités	Plongée, observation des baleines, randonnées

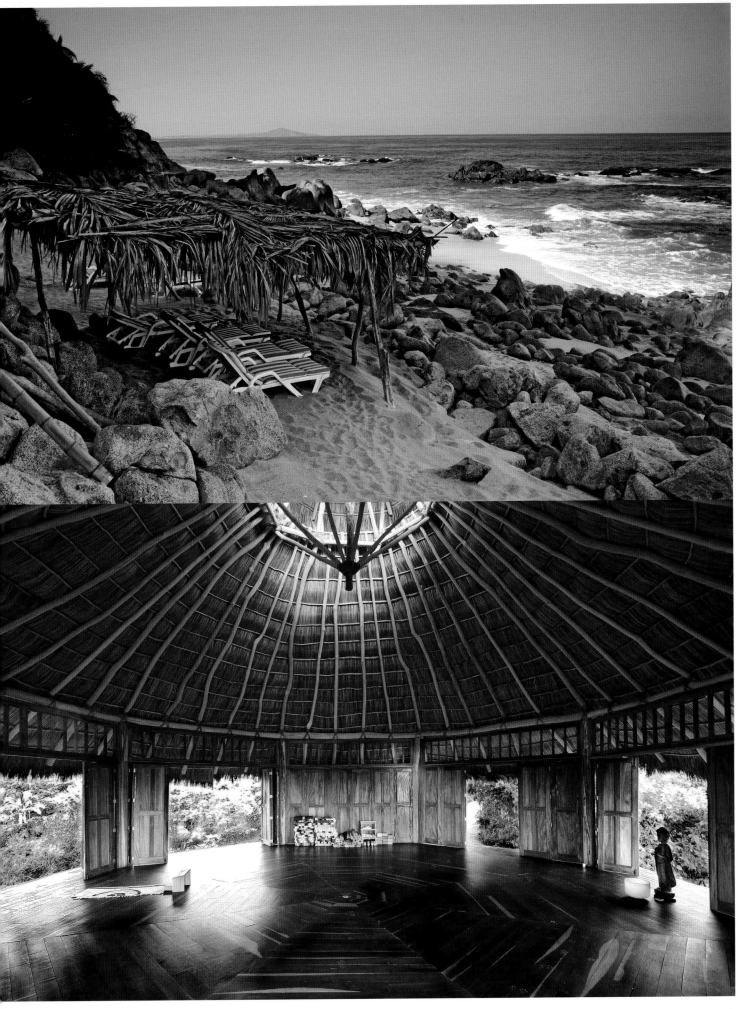

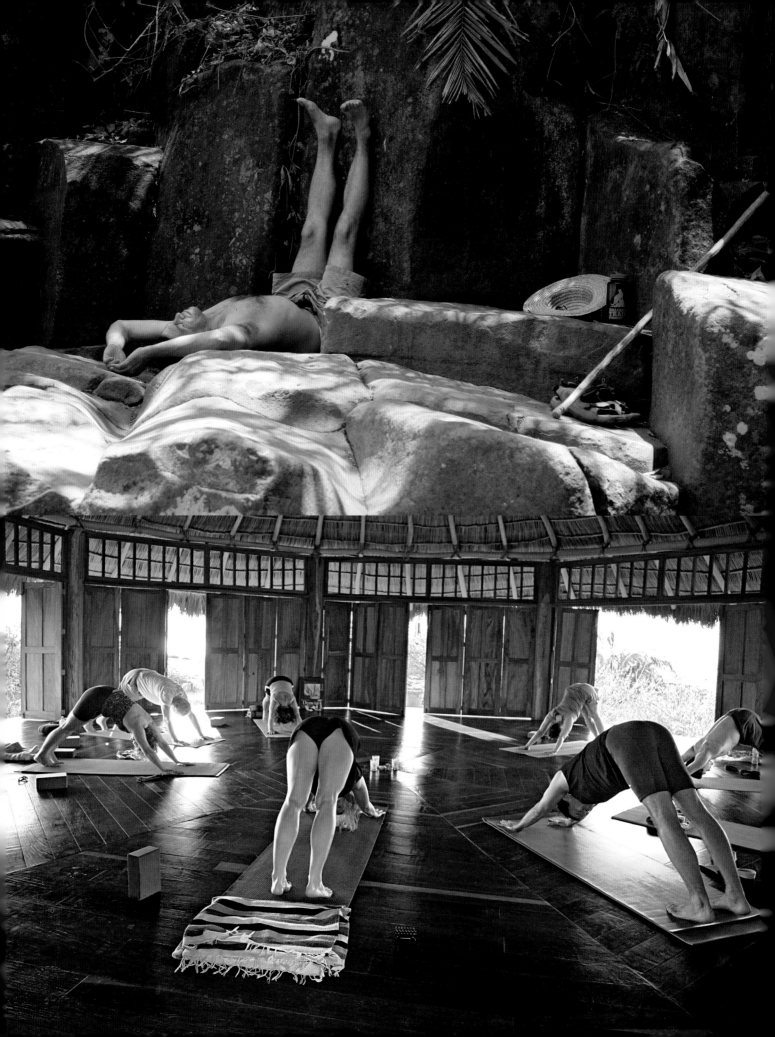

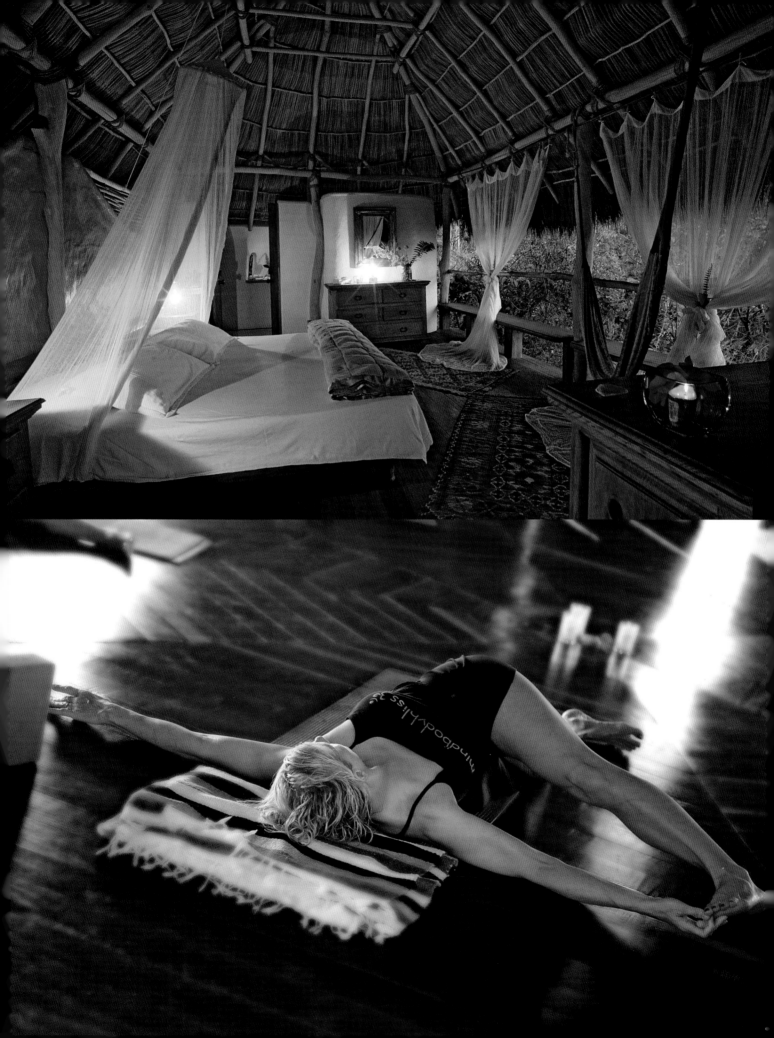

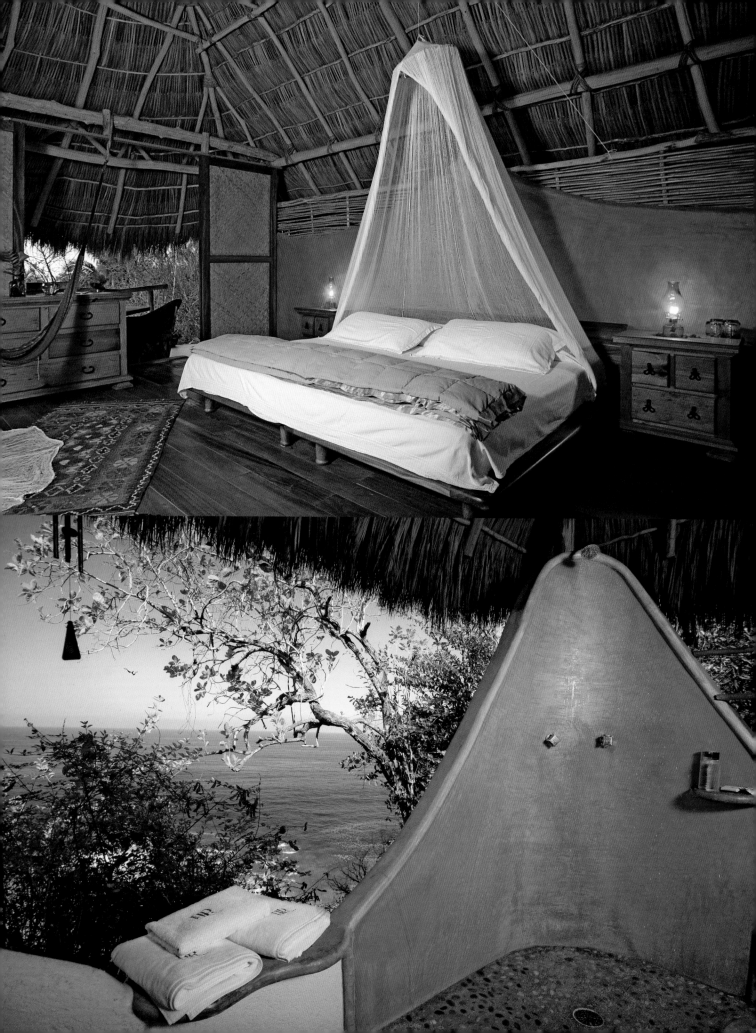

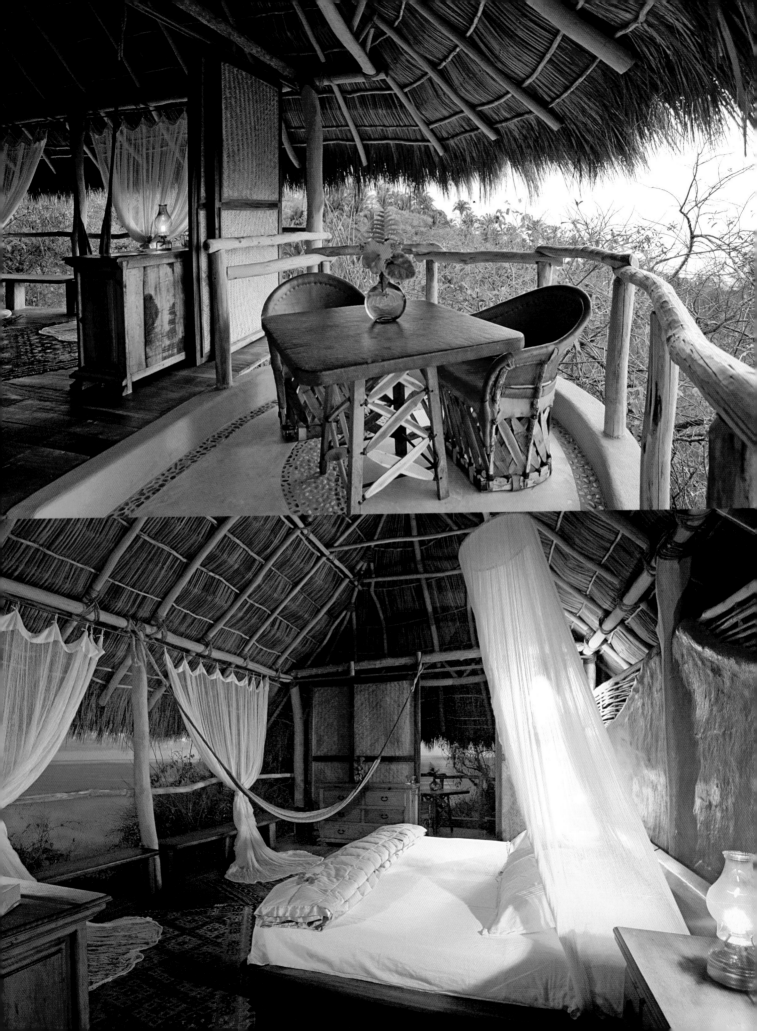

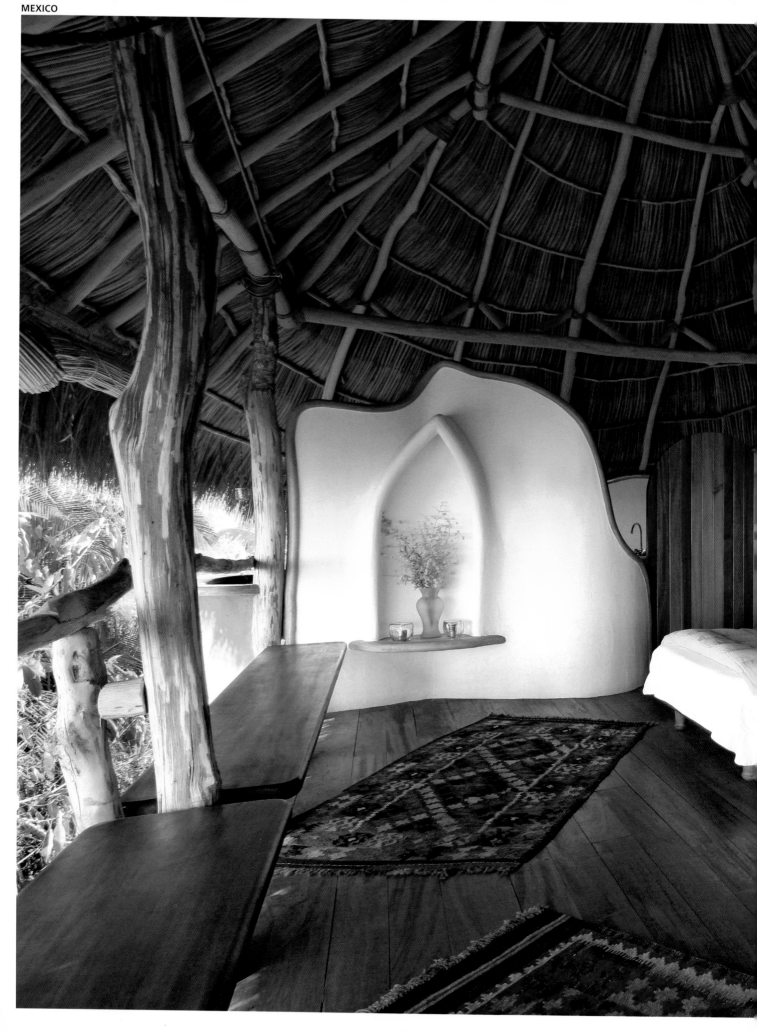

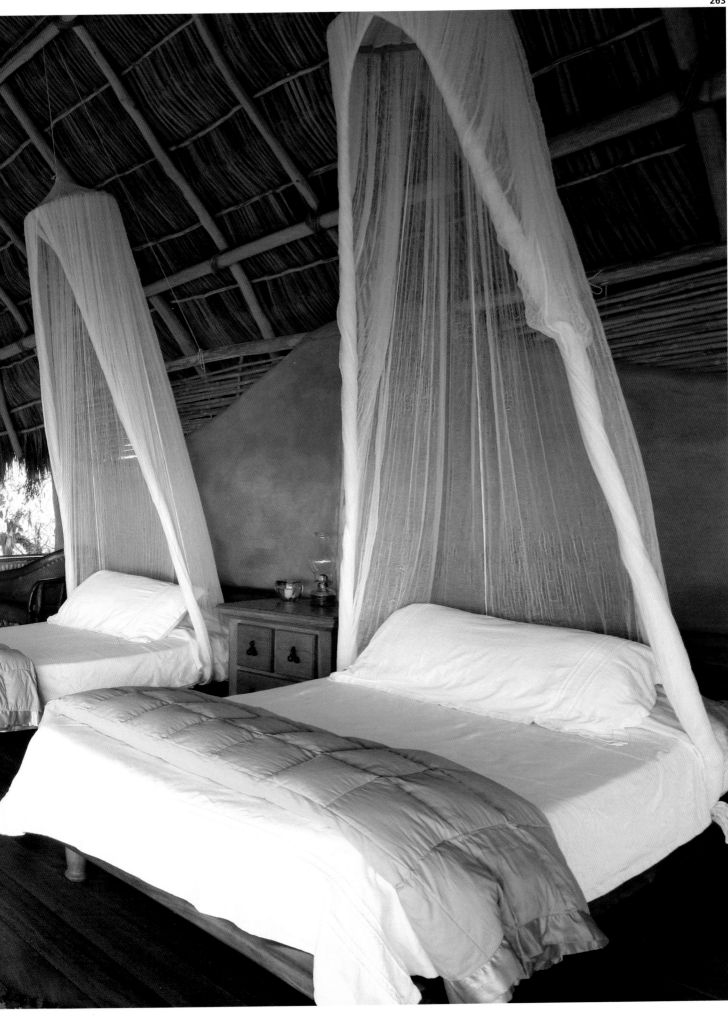

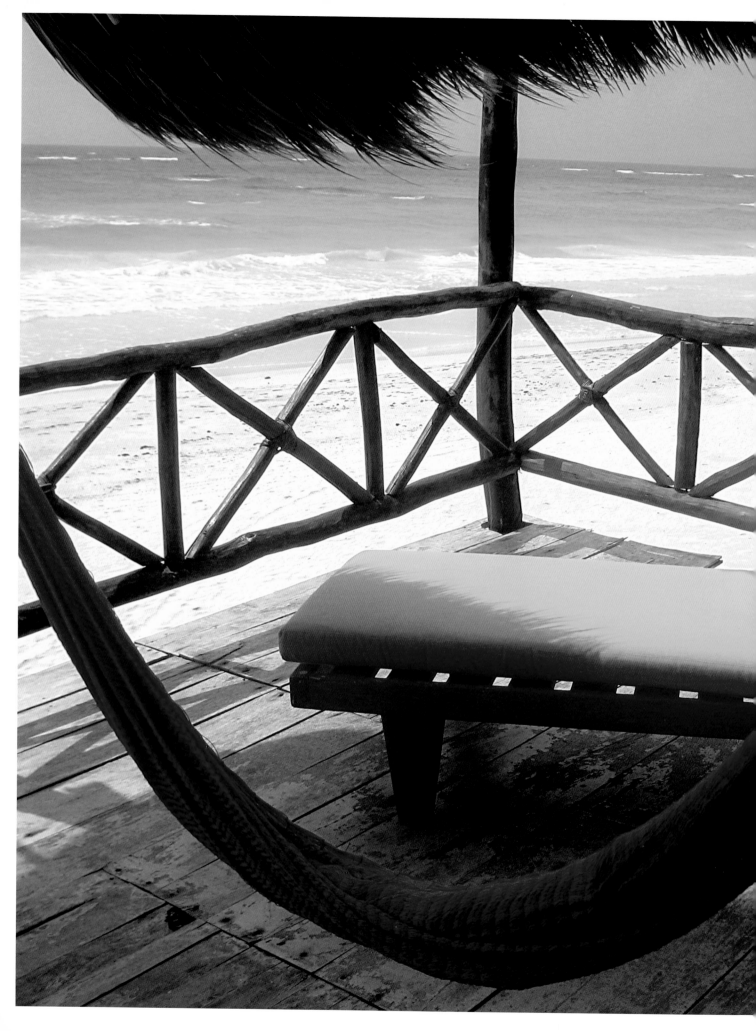

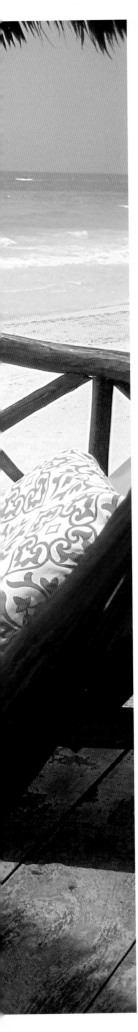

An instructor in Wellington boots who makes a row of shivering girls do sit-ups in the wet sand before sunrise? And in bikinis? All wrong. Amansala means "peaceful water" and in this solar-powered resort right beside the sea the guest is permitted to calmly select from the numerous activities on offer. Power Yoga perhaps, or maybe you'd prefer relaxing Restorative Yoga, a day trip on a bike, a sightseeing tour of the Mayan ruins, a kayak tour or a treatment with Mayan clay. If the bikini is a little too tight, why not sign up for the boot camp? You'll begin the day with a brisk power walk, and then after yoga, swimming, massages and another march, after tasty grilled fish and a fresh pineapple juice, sink into the distinctly non-rustic Frette linen under the mosquito net in your little hut. If need be you can still drink one of the best margaritas in the world on the veranda of the hippy-chic little wooden houses. In the candlelight, no one will see you.

Books to pack: "The Girls' Guide to Hunting and Fishing" by Melissa Bank and "The Tortilla Curtain" by T. C. Boyle

Amansala Eco Chic Resort

Km 5.5 Boca Paila
Tulum
Mexico
Tel. +52 998 185 7428
www.amansalaresort.com

Directions	2 hrs south of Cancun Airport
Yoga	Hatha, Ashtanga, Sivananda, Iyengar, Anusara, Vinyasa Flow
Teachers	Jessica Belafonte, Cole Williston, Ian Lopatin
Rooms	25 cabanas
Food	According to the needs of the group vegetarian-vegan with fish, Mexican specialities like ceviche, tacos, mango, papaya, jicama, jalapeño
Treatments	Massage, treatments with Mayan clay
Leisure	Swimming, hiking, snorkelling, kayaking, day trips to Mayan ruins

Ein Ausbilder in Gummistiefeln, der eine Reihe zitternder Mädchen im nassen Sand vor Sonnenaufgang Sit-ups machen lässt – im Bikini? Falsch. Amansala bedeutet »friedliches Wasser«, und in diesem solarbetriebenen Resort direkt am Meer darf der Gast in aller Ruhe entscheiden, welches der vielen Angebote er wahrnehmen möchte. Power-Yoga oder lieber Yoga zur Entspannung (Restorative), Ausflüge mit dem Fahrrad, eine Besichtigung der Maya-Ruinen, eine Kajaktour oder eine Behandlung mit Maya-Tonerde? Sollte der Bikini zu sehr zwicken, warum sich nicht doch dem *boot camp* anschließen? Beginnen wird man den Tag zum Beispiel mit einem strammen Power-Walk, um dann nach Yoga, Schwimmen, Massagen, erneutem Marsch, nach würzig gegrilltem Fisch und einem frischen Ananassaft in seiner kleinen Hütte unter das Moskitonetz in die völlig unbäuerlichen Frette-Laken zu sinken. Wenn's sein muss, kann man davor noch auf der Veranda der hippieschicken Holzhäuschen einen der besten Margaritas der Welt trinken. Bei Kerzenlicht sieht das keiner so genau.

Reisebegleiter: »Wie Frauen fischen und jagen« von Melissa Bank und »América« von T. C. Boyle

Un instructeur en bottes de caoutchouc qui, avant l'aube, fait faire dans le sable mouillé des abdominaux à une rangée de filles grelottantes ? En bikini ? Erreur. Amansala signifie « eau paisible », et dans ce site en bordure de mer, alimenté à l'énergie solaire, le client peut choisir en toute quiétude ce qu'il aimerait faire parmi les nombreux programmes qui lui sont proposés. Yoga dynamique ou plutôt yoga de relaxation (restauratif), des randonnées à vélo, une visite des sites mayas, un tour en kayak ou un traitement à base d'argile maya ? Si le bikini vous serre un peu trop, pourquoi ne pas aller rejoindre le camp d'entraînement ? Et commencer la journée par une marche soutenue, et après le yoga, la nage, les massages, une nouvelle marche, après avoir dégusté un poisson grillé aux épices et un jus d'ananas frais, se laisser tomber dans des draps de lin griffés Frette sous la moustiquaire de sa petite hutte. Au besoin, on peut toujours boire une des meilleures Margaritas du monde sur la véranda des jolies maisonnettes de bois de style hippie. A la lueur des bougies personne n'y regarde de si près.

Livres à emporter : « Manuel de chasse et de pêche à l'usage des filles » de Melissa Bank et « América » de T. C. Boyle

Anreise	2 Std. südlich vom Flughafen Cancun
Yoga	Hatha, Ashtanga, Sivananda, Iyengar, Anusara, Vinyasa Flow
Lehrer	Jessica Belafonte, Cole Williston, Ian Lopatin
Zimmer	25 Hütten
Küche	Je nach Gruppe vegetarisch-vegan, mit Fisch, mexikanische Spezialitäten wie Ceviche, Tacos, Mango, Papaya, Jicama, Jalapeño
Anwendungen	Massage, Behandlung mit Maya-Tonerde
Aktivitäten	Schwimmen, Wandern, Schnorcheln, Kajak, Ausflüge zu Maya-Ruinen

Accès	Situé à 2 h au sud de l'aéroport de Cancun
Yoga	Hatha, Ashtânga, Shivananda, Iyengar, Anusara, Vinyasa Flow
Professeurs	Jessica Belafonte, Cole Williston, Ian Lopatin
Chambres	25 cabanes
Restauration	Selon le groupe, cuisine végétarienne-végétalienne avec poisson, spécialités mexicaines comme le ceviche, les tacos, la mangue, la papaye, le jicama, le piment japaleño
Traitements	Massage, traitement à base d'argile maya
Activités	Natation, randonnées, plongée libre, kayak, visites des sites mayas

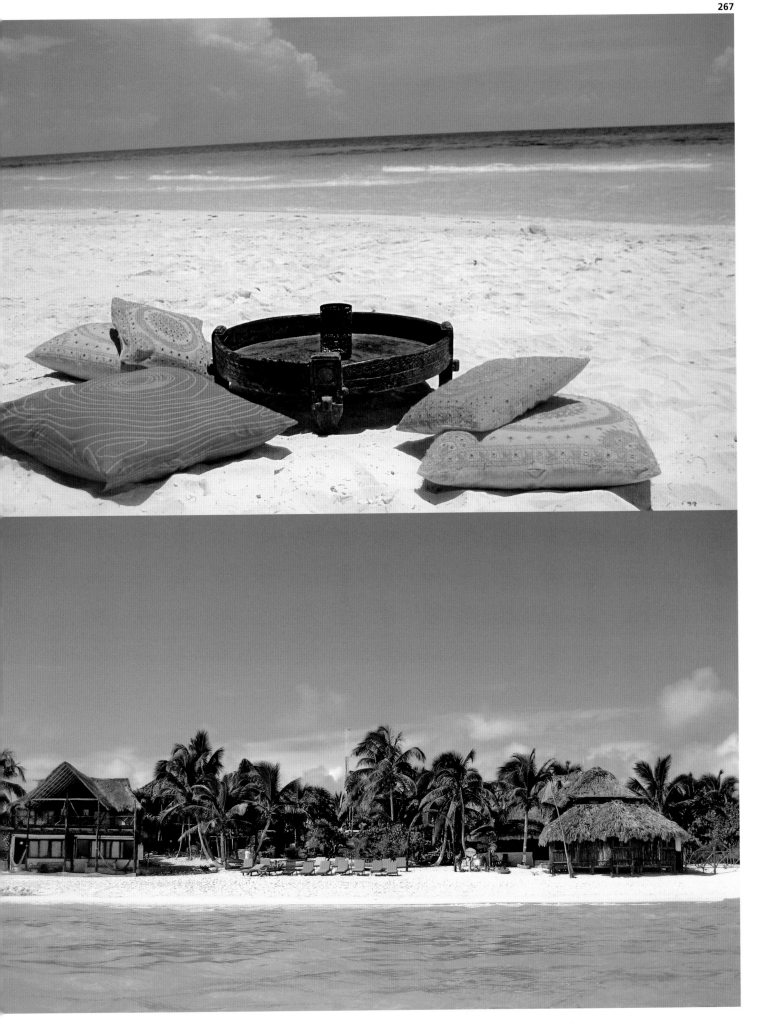

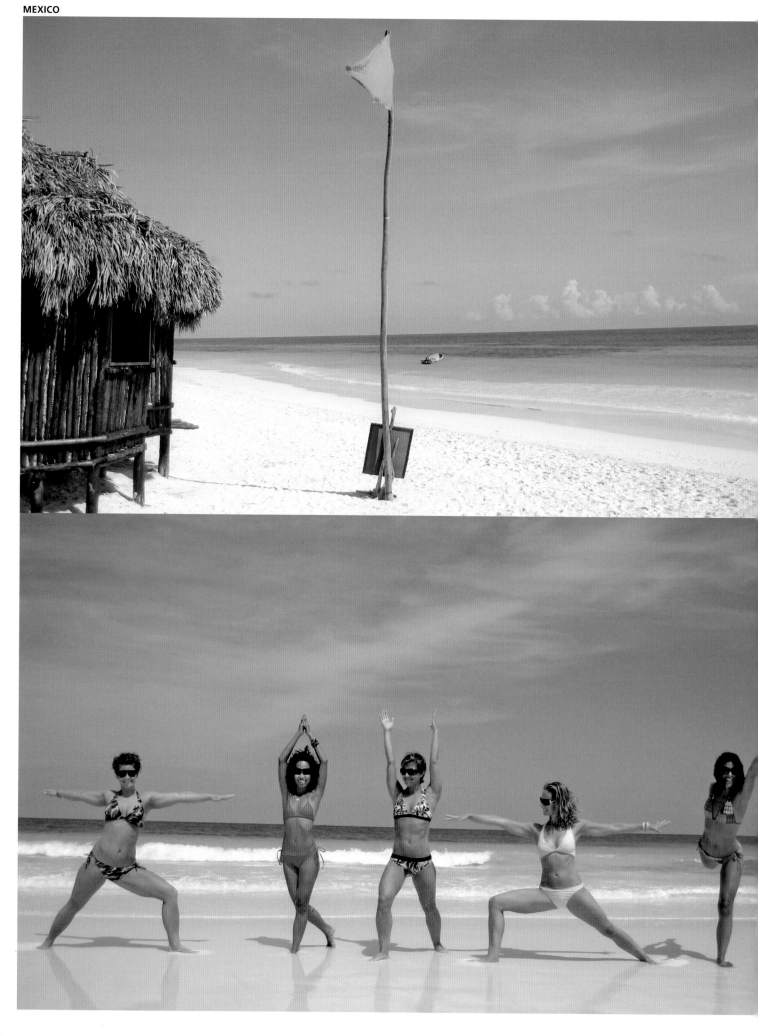

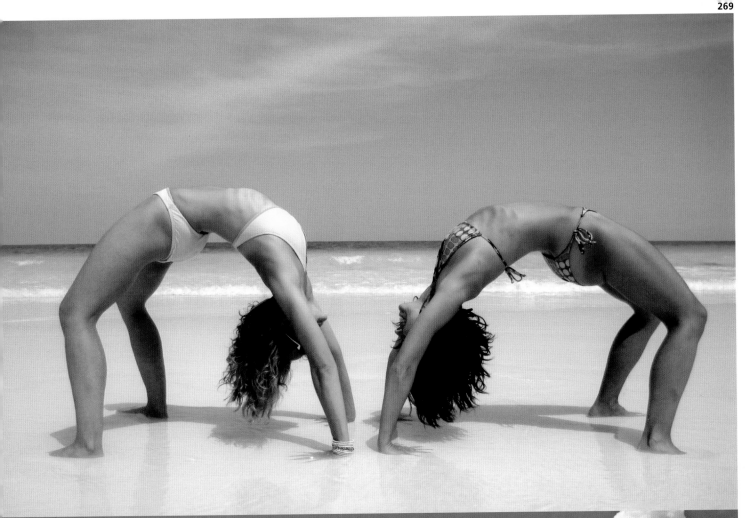

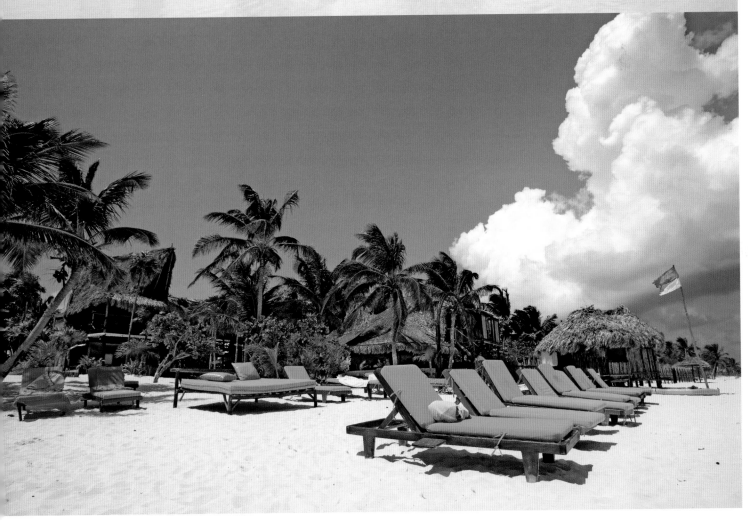

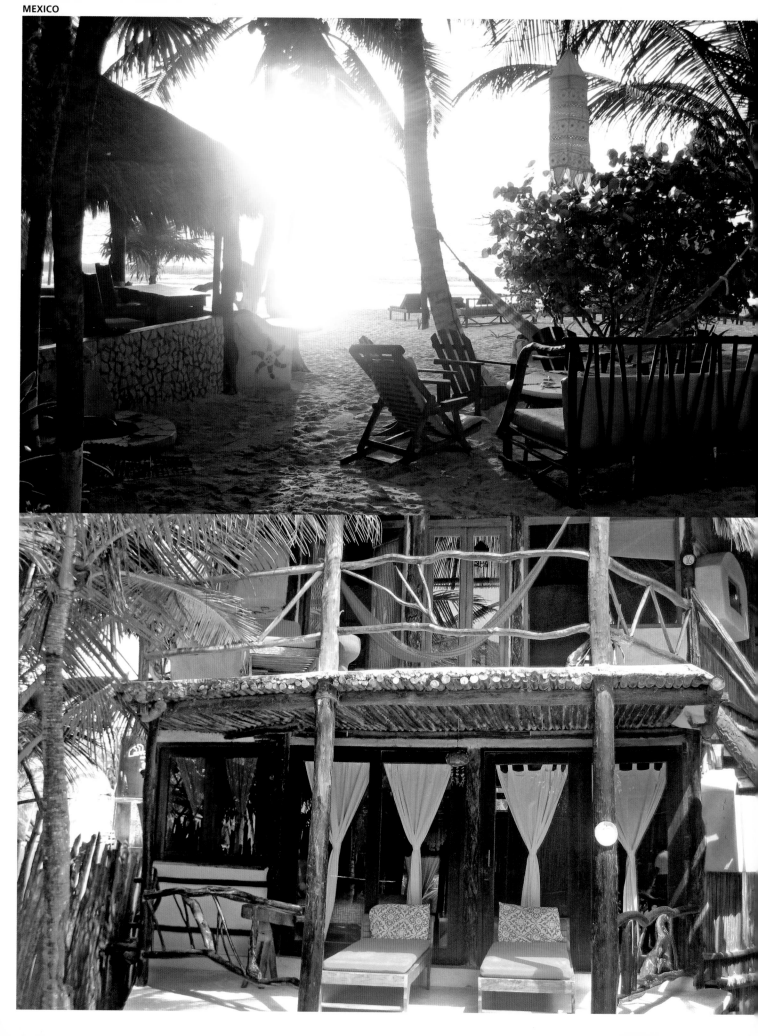

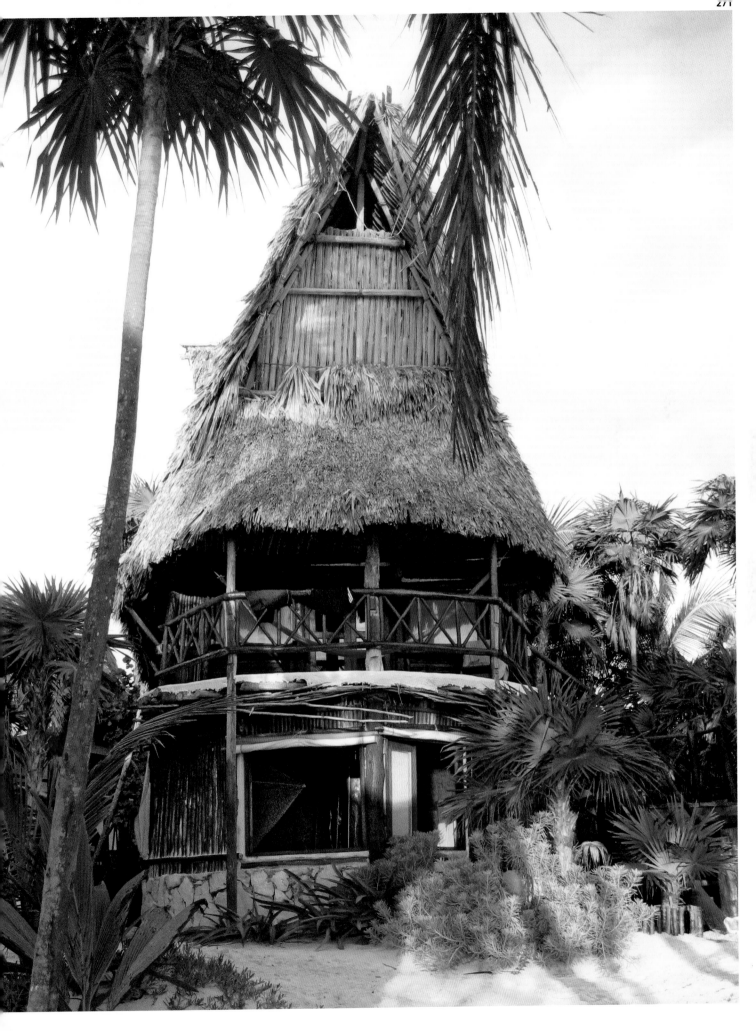

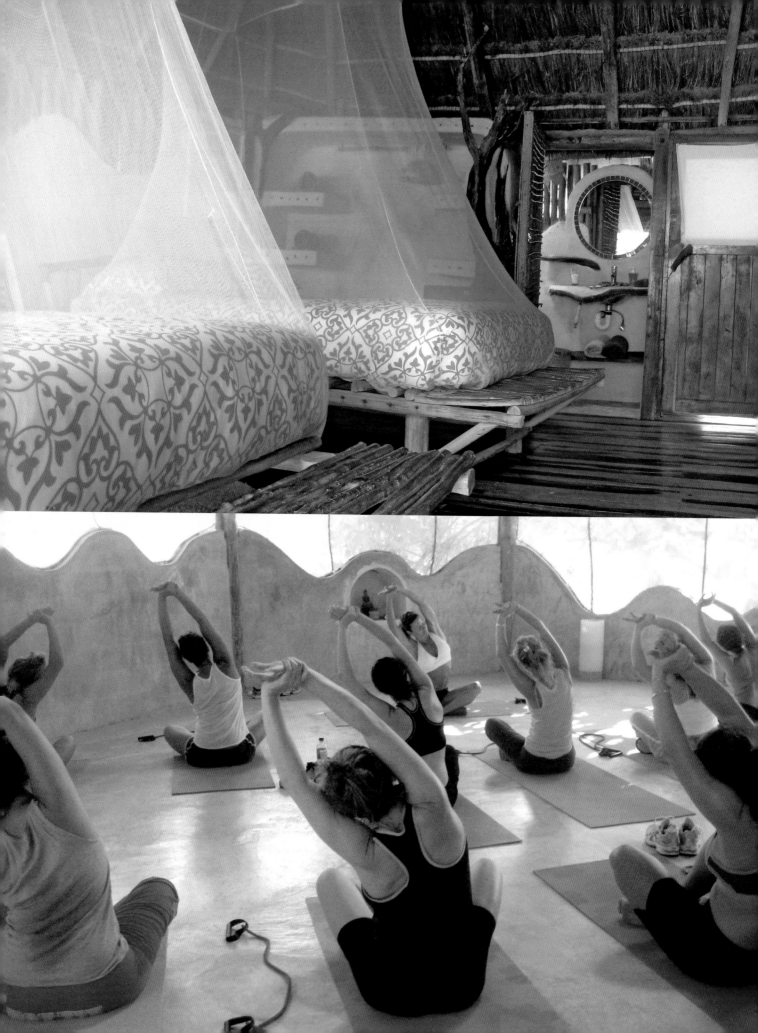

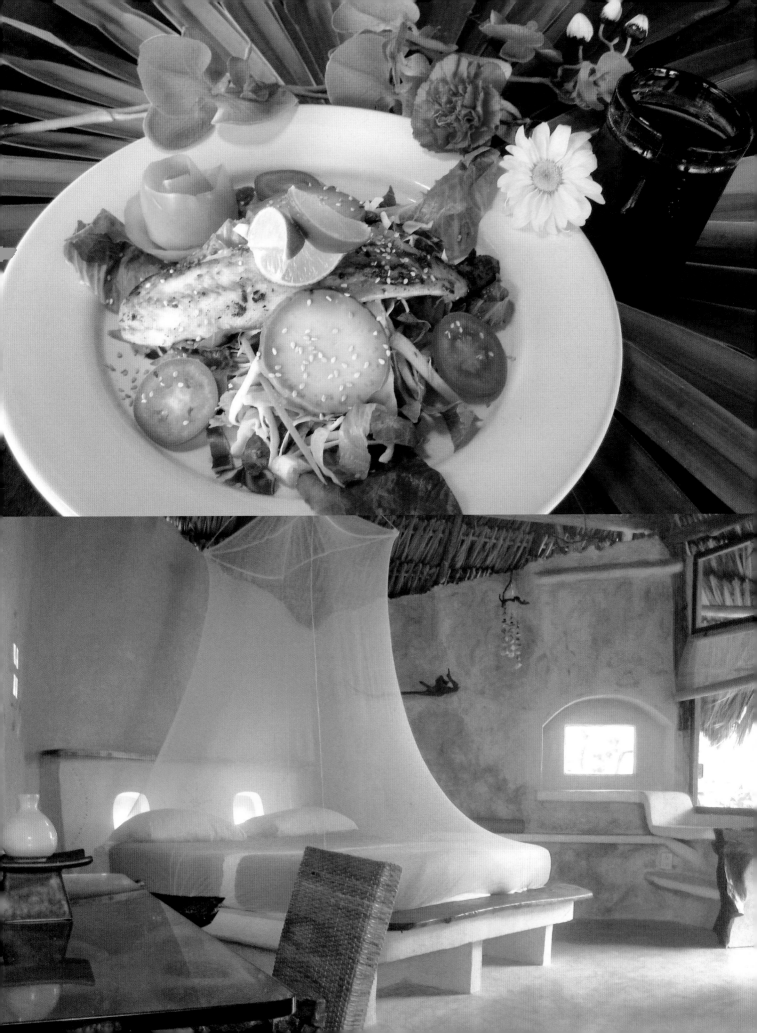

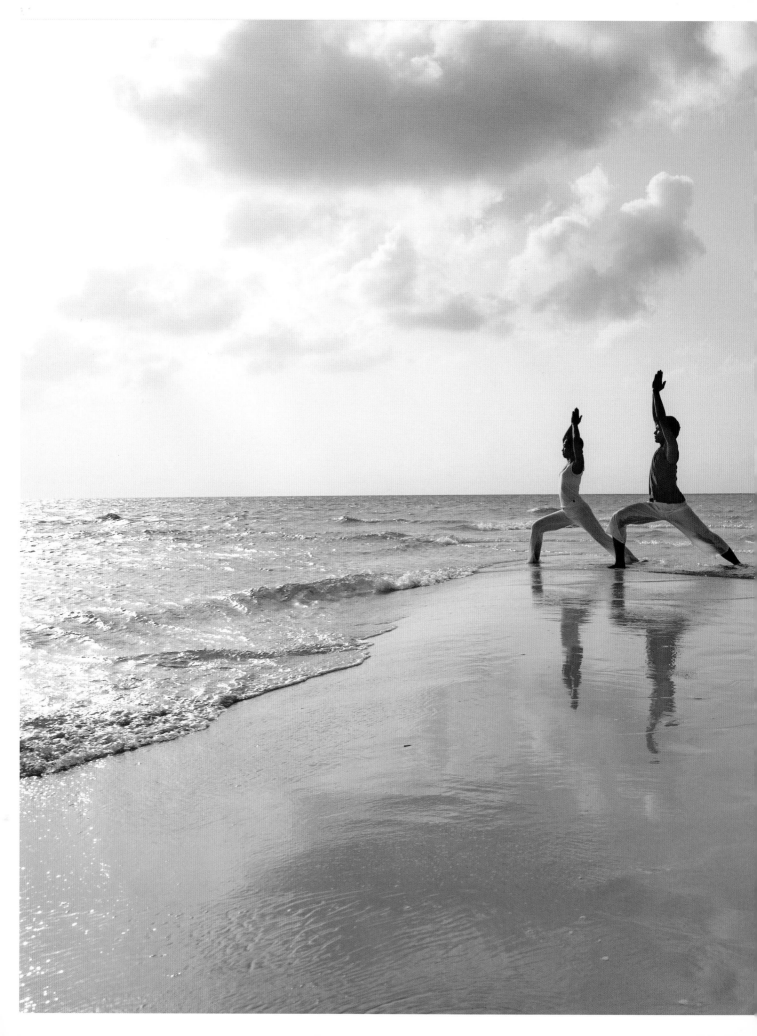

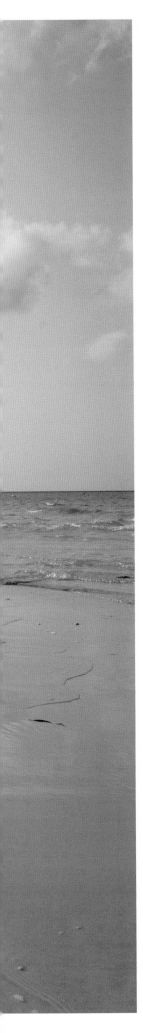

Outside it is well over 86 degrees Fahrenheit; inside the ventilator whirrs, and the sweating guests hold Downward Facing Dog. Was that more than five breaths? The cheek of it. But the almost unnatural blue of the Caribbean, which reminds one of a drink for the ladies, or a visit to the world's most elegant spa, quickly calms the temper. What's the use anyway? There is no escape from this small private island, which lies in the Caribbean as though James Bond had taken up residence there as a pensioner. And why would you want to leave? Private butlers fulfil every wish, and the scent of hibiscus flowers hangs heavy in the air above the tennis courts and the infinity pool. Supermodels, world-famous Yogis and their followers escape here to enjoy, to a sound-track of silver herons and the quietly hissing spray of the sea, what Shambhala means in Sanskrit: peace and harmony. Maybe indulge in a facial, too, and the best "organic" piña colada in the world.

Book to pack: "The Power of Now" by Eckhart Tolle

Parrot Cay by COMO

P.O. Box 164
Providenciales, Turks & Caicos Islands
British West Indies
Tel. +1 649 946 7788
Fax +1 649 946 7789
res@parrotcay.como.bz
www.parrotcay.como.bz

Directions	One of the 40 small Turks & Caicos Islands, about 70 min flying time southwest of Miami; airport transfer from the main island of Providenciales by boat included in the price
Yoga	Iyengar, Vinyasa, Hatha, Anusara
Teachers	Erich Schiffmann, Elena Brower, Rodney Yee, Colleen Saidman
Rooms	A total of 60 rooms, including beach houses and villas
Food	Caribbean, Southeast Asian, Continental, Italian
Treatments	Holistic therapies, Ayurveda, massage, facial treatments, Abhyanga package
Leisure	Pilates, catamaran sailing, water-skiing, diving, tennis, swimming

Draußen sind es weit über 30 Grad, drinnen surrt der Ventilator, schwitzend harrt man im »Herabschauenden Hund« aus. Waren das nicht mehr als fünf Atemzüge? Frechheit. Doch das fast schon unnatürliche Blau der Karibik, das an einen Drink für Ladys erinnert, oder ein Besuch im elegantesten Spa der Welt besänftigt schnell die Gemüter. Was würde es auch nützen? Es gibt kein Entkommen von dieser kleinen Privatinsel, die in der Karibik liegt, als warte sie darauf, dass sich James Bond dort als Rentner niederlässt. Und warum auch? Private Butler erfüllen einem jeden Wunsch, schwer hängt der Duft nach Hibiskusblüten über den von Flutlicht erhellten Tennisplätzen und dem Infinity-Pool. Supermodels, weltberühmte Yogis und ihre Anhänger flüchten hierher, um beim Soundtrack von Silberreihern und leise zischender Meeresgischt zu genießen, was Shambhala auf Sanskrit bedeutet: Frieden und Harmonie. Vielleicht sollte man noch ein Facial buchen, und dann wartet schon die beste »organic« Piña Colada der Welt.

Buchtipp: »Jetzt! Die Kraft der Gegenwart« von Eckhart Tolle

A l'extérieur, le thermomètre grimpe bien au-dessus de 30 degrés, à l'intérieur le ventilateur bourdonne, les hôtes en sueur gardent stoïquement la posture du « chien tête en bas ». Mais c'était plus que cinq inspirations, non ? Quel toupet. Cependant, le bleu presque irréel des Caraïbes, couleur d'un drink pour dames, ou un passage dans le spa le plus élégant du monde, calme vite les esprits. D'ailleurs, à quoi bon ? On ne s'évade pas de cette petite île privée, posée là dans la mer des Caraïbes, comme si James Bond s'y était installé à l'âge de la retraite. Et puis, pourquoi s'enfuir ? Un maître d'hôtel à votre service satisfait tous vos désirs, le parfum lourd des fleurs d'hibiscus plane au-dessus des courts de tennis baignés par la lumière des projecteurs et de la piscine à débordement. Top modèles, yogis mondialement connus et leurs adeptes viennent se réfugier ici et, avec en fond sonore les cris des grandes aigrettes et le bruit de l'écume frémissante, goûtent le shambhala, qui signifie en sanskrit : paix et harmonie. Peut-être encore un traitement facial et le meilleur drink bio au monde, une Piña Colada.

**Livre à emporter : « Le Pouvoir du moment présent »
d'Eckhart Tolle**

Anreise	Eine der 40 kleinen Turks- und Caicosinseln, etwa 70 min Flugzeit südöstlich von Miami gelegen; Flughafentransfer von der Hauptinsel Providenciales per Boot
Yoga	Iyengar, Vinyasa, Hatha, Anusara
Lehrer	Erich Schiffmann, Elena Brower, Rodney Yee, Colleen Saidman
Zimmer	60 Zimmer inklusive Beach-Häuser und Villen
Küche	Karibisch, südostasiatisch, kontinental, italienisch
Anwendungen	Ganzheitliche Therapien, Ayurveda, Massage, Gesichtsbehandlungen, Abhyanga-Package
Aktivitäten	Pilates, Katamaransegeln, Wasserski, Tauchen, Tennis, Schwimmen

Accès	Une des 40 petites îles Turques-et-Caïques, située à environ 70 min de vol au sud-est de Miami ; transfert par bateau inclus, de l'aéroport de l'île principale
Yoga	Iyengar, Vinyasa, Hatha, Anusara
Professeurs	Erich Schiffmann, Elena Brower, Rodney Yee, Colleen Saidman
Chambres	60 chambres, y compris maisons de plage et villas
Restauration	Cuisine des Caraïbes, du Sud-Est asiatique, italienne
Traitements	Thérapies intégrales, Ayurveda, massage, soins du visage, Abhyanga-Package
Activités	Pilates, nautisme (catamaran), ski nautique, plongée, tennis, natation

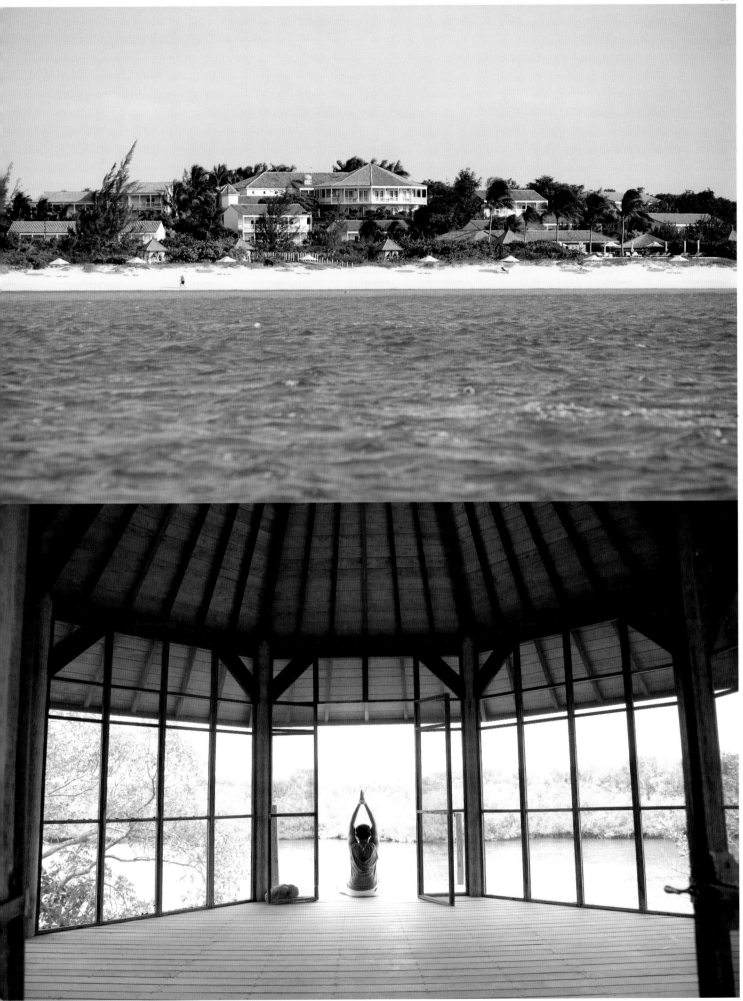

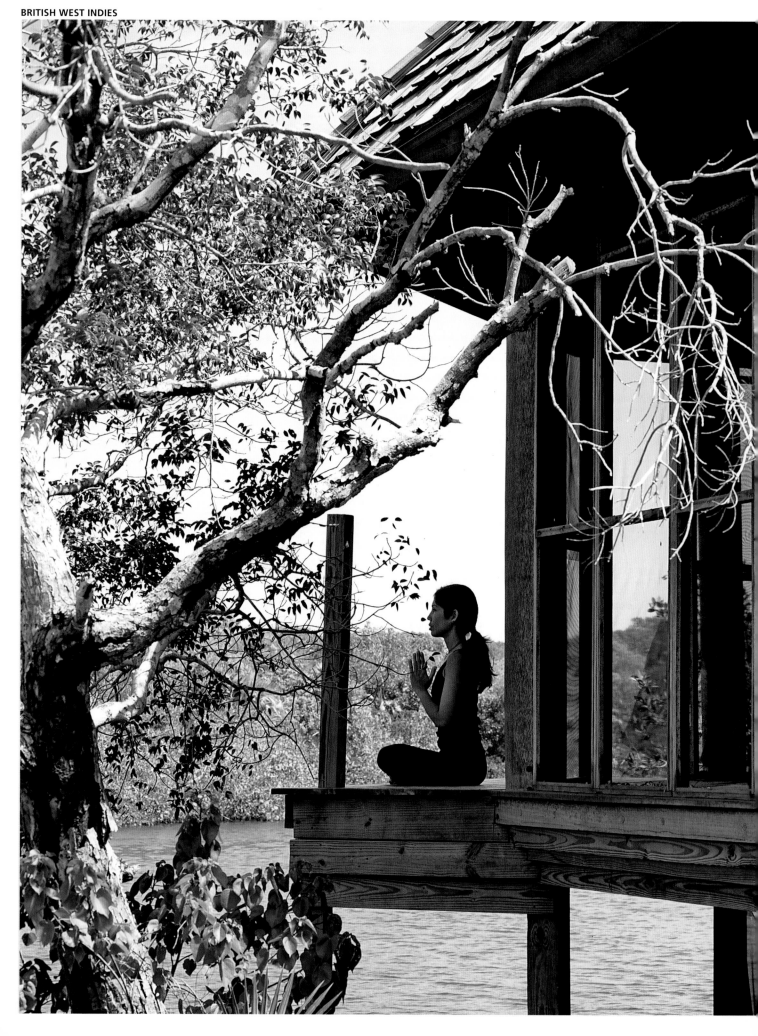

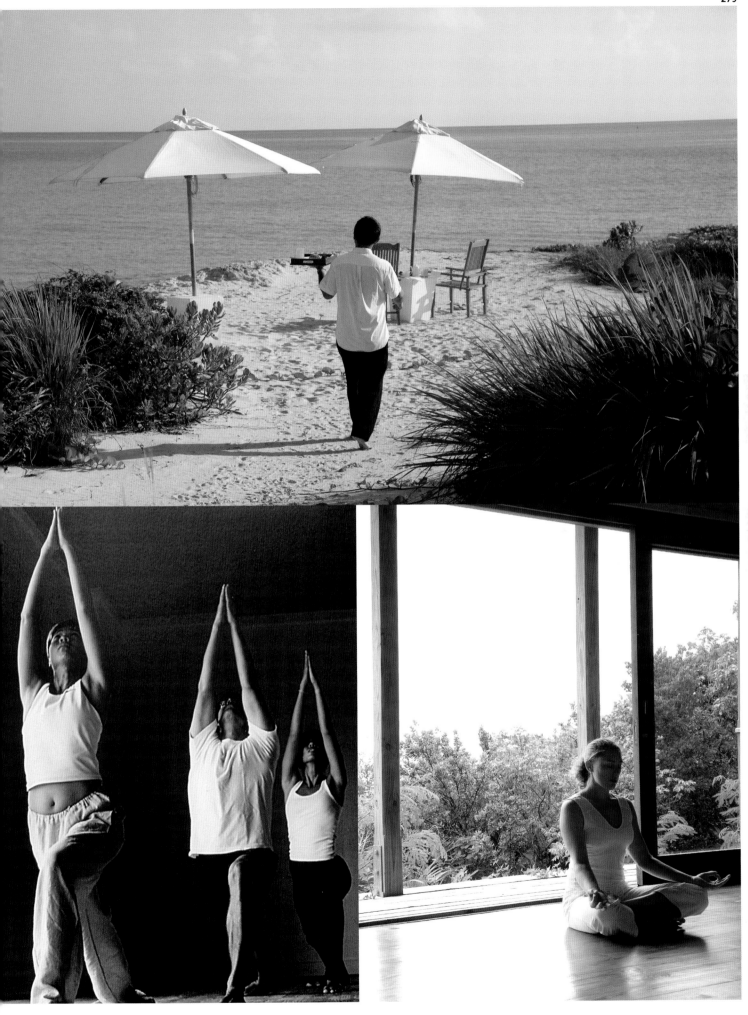

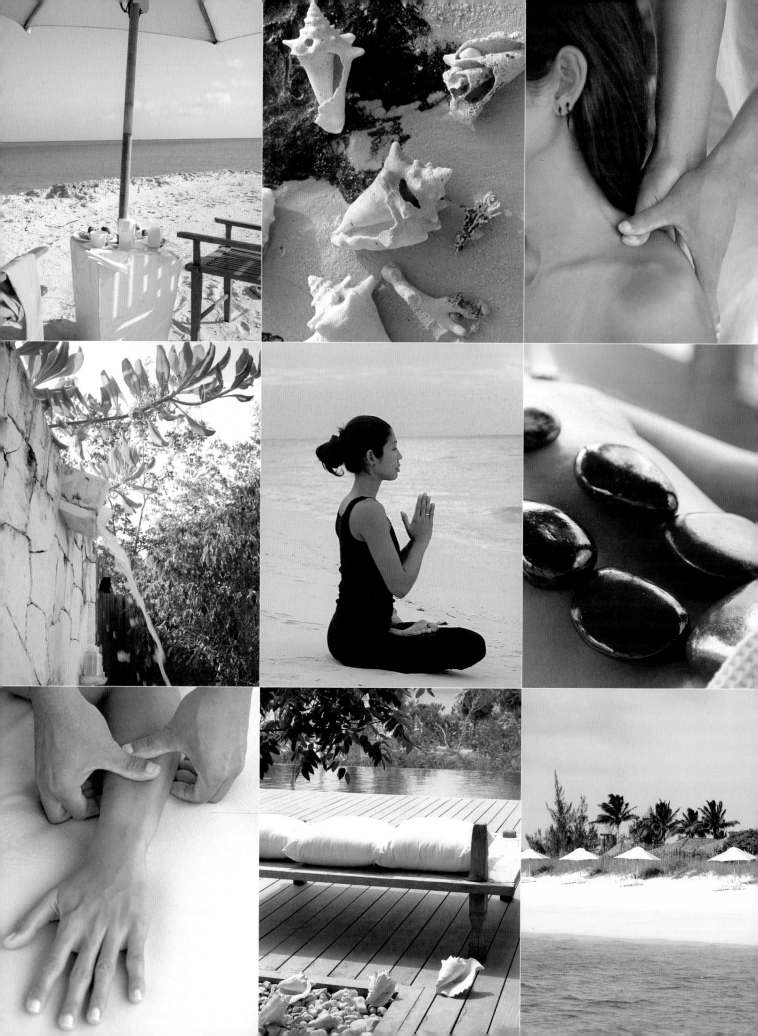

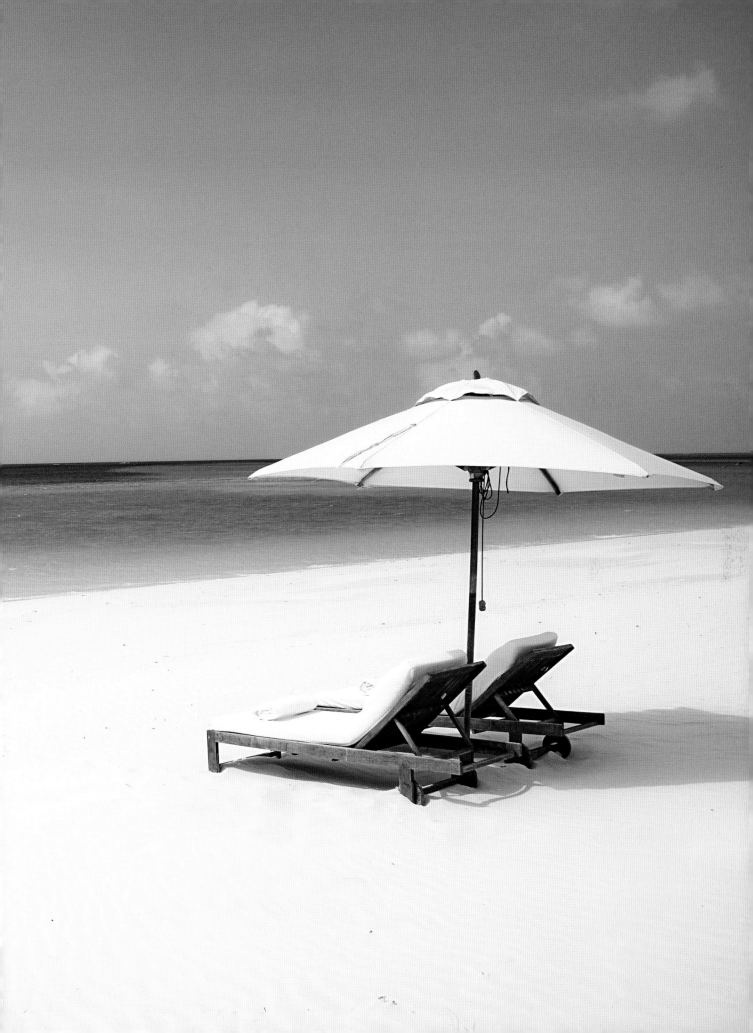

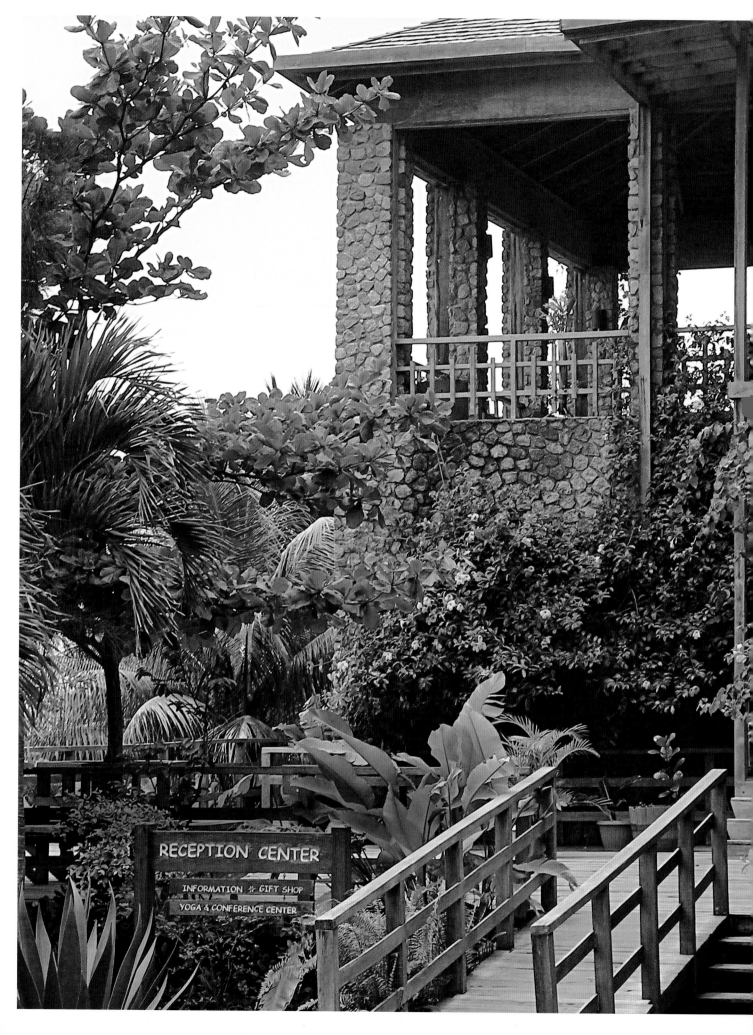

RECEPTION CENTER

INFORMATION & GIFT SHOP

YOGA & CONFERENCE CENTER

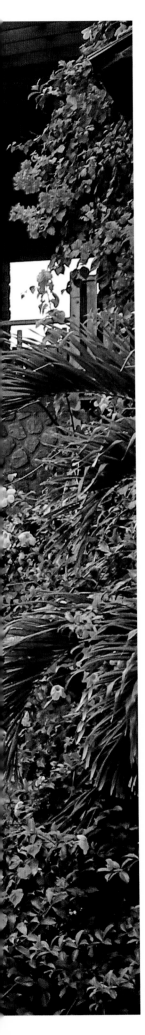

If the Dominican Republic is the Pamela Anderson of the Caribbean—shiny surface, instant fun, occasionally chaotic—then Dominica is the Julia Roberts of the Lesser Antilles: intense, idiosyncratic, unpolished, but really quite sexy. With its black sandy beaches, primeval rain forest, huge ferns, orchids, banana trees and red-throated parrots, the Morne Trois Pitons National Park is on Unesco's World Heritage list. At daybreak in the Jungle Bay eco lodge, opened in 2005, you can face east for a sun salutation on the veranda; in case you oversleep, you can also have a good stretch later in the large hall of volcanic stone. Sometimes the view over the Atlantic is enough to make you feel somewhat closer to heaven. Those who survive the ten-hour trek through mud and over steep cliffs to the 4747-foot-high Mount Diablotin will need a deep-tissue massage in the spa pavilion, built on the slope as if hovering above the surf. Curse of the Caribbean? On the contrary—the place is a blessing.

Book to pack: "The Green Pope" by Miguel Angel Asturias

Jungle Bay Resort & Spa

Point Mulatre
Commonwealth of Dominica
British West Indies
Tel. +1 767 446 1789
Fax +1 767 446 1090
info@junglebaydominica.com
www.junglebaydominica.com

Directions	Dominica lies in the eastern Caribbean between Guadeloupe and Martinique and has two small airports: Melville Hall Airport and Canefield Airport
Yoga	Hatha, Anusara, Vinyasa Flow, Iyengar
Teachers	Sheree Mullen, Chrissy Carter, Nikki Vilella, Jillian Turecki, Joanne Silver, Ashleigh Beyer, Laureen Rueckner
Rooms	35 huts with a king-size bed or 2 double beds
Food	Caribbean—freshly caught fish, breadfruit salad, beetroot salad, baked bananas, fresh tamarind juice
Treatments	Massage, facial, pedicure, manicure, aromatherapy, detoxifying body rub, honeymoon massage
Leisure	Hiking, day trips, snorkelling, kayaking, diving, hot springs

Wenn die Dominikanische Republik die Pamela Anderson der Karibik ist – glänzende Oberfläche, schneller Spaß, gelegentlich chaotisch – ist Dominica die Julia Roberts der Kleinen Antillen: intensiv, eigen, unaffektiert, dabei durchaus sexy. Mit seinem urzeitlichen Regenwald, den schwarzen Sandstränden, dicken Farnen, Orchideen, Bananenbäumen und rothalsigen Papageien gehört der Morne Trois Pitons National Park zum UNESCO-Welterbe. In der 2005 eröffneten Jungle-Bay-Öko-Lodge kann man bereits in der Morgendämmerung auf der Veranda seine Sonnengrüße Richtung Osten richten, oder aber, sollte man verschlafen, sich später in der großen Halle aus Vulkanstein stretchen. Manchmal genügt schon der Blick über den Atlantik, um sich dem Himmel etwas näher zu fühlen. Wer die zehnstündige Wanderung durch Matsch und über steile Felsen zum 1447 Meter hohen Mount Diablotin übersteht, wird eine Deep-Tissue-Massage im Spa-Pavillon brauchen, der oberhalb der Brandung gleichsam schwebend in den Hang gebaut ist. Fluch der Karibik? Im Gegenteil – der Platz ist ein Segen.

Buchtipp: »Der grüne Papst« von Miguel Angel Asturias

Si la République dominicaine est la Pamela Anderson des Caraïbes – look éblouissant, plaisir facile, quelquefois chaotique –, la Dominique est la Julia Roberts des Petites Antilles : intense, capricieuse, naturelle mais ô combien sexy. Avec ses plages de sable noir, sa forêt pluviale, ses fougères touffues, ses orchidées, ses bananiers et ses perroquets à cou rouge, le Parc national de Morne Trois Pitons est classé au patrimoine mondial de l'UNESCO. Dans les pavillons écologiques de Jungle Bay, inaugurés en 2005, on peut adresser sur la véranda, dès l'aurore, un salut au soleil en se tournant vers l'est, ou plus tard, si l'on a dormi trop longtemps, faire des exercices d'assouplissement dans la grande salle en pierre volcanique. Parfois, un regard posé sur l'Atlantique suffit pour se sentir plus près du ciel. Pour qui vient de marcher dix heures dans la boue au-dessus des roches escarpées du Mont Diablotin (1447 mètres), un massage en profondeur dans le pavillon Spa, suspendu à même le coteau au-dessus du ressac, s'impose. Pas de pirates ni de malédiction ici, au contraire, cet endroit est béni des dieux.

Livre à emporter : « Le Pape Vert » de Miguel Angel Asturias

Anreise	Dominica liegt in der Ostkaribik zwischen Guadeloupe und Martinique und hat zwei kleine Flughäfen: Melvill Hall Airport oder Canefield Airport
Yoga	Hatha, Anusara, Vinyasa Flow, Iyengar
Lehrer	Sheree Mullen, Chrissy Carter, Nikki Vilella, Jillian Turecki, Joanne Silver, Ashleigh Beyer, Laureen Rueckner
Zimmer	35 Hütten mit einem Kingsize-Bett oder 2 Doppelbetten
Küche	Karibisch – frischer Fisch, Brotfruchtsalat, Rote-Bete-Salat, geröstete Bananen, frischer Tamarindensaft
Anwendungen	Massage, Facial, Pediküre, Maniküre, Aromatherapie, Detox-Body-Rub, Honeymoon-Massage
Aktivitäten	Wandern, Ausflüge, Schnorcheln, Kajak, Tauchen, Thermalbäder

Accès	La Dominique se trouve entre la Guadeloupe et la Martinique et dispose de deux petits aéroports: Melvill Hall Airport et Canefield Airport
Yoga	Hatha, Anusara, Vinyasa Flow, Iyengar
Professeurs	Sheree Mullen, Chrissy Carter, Nikki Vilella, Jillian Turecki, Joanne Silver, Ashleigh Beyer, Laureen Rueckner
Chambres	35 bungalows avec un lit extra-large ou deux lits
Restauration	Caraïbe – poisson pêché sur place, salade d'uru, salade de betteraves rouges, bananes grillées, jus de tamarin
Traitements	Massage, soins du visage, pédicurie, manucurie, aromathérapie, massage de détox, massage « lune de miel »
Activités	Randonnées, excursions, sources chaudes, plongée libre, kayak, plongée sous-marine

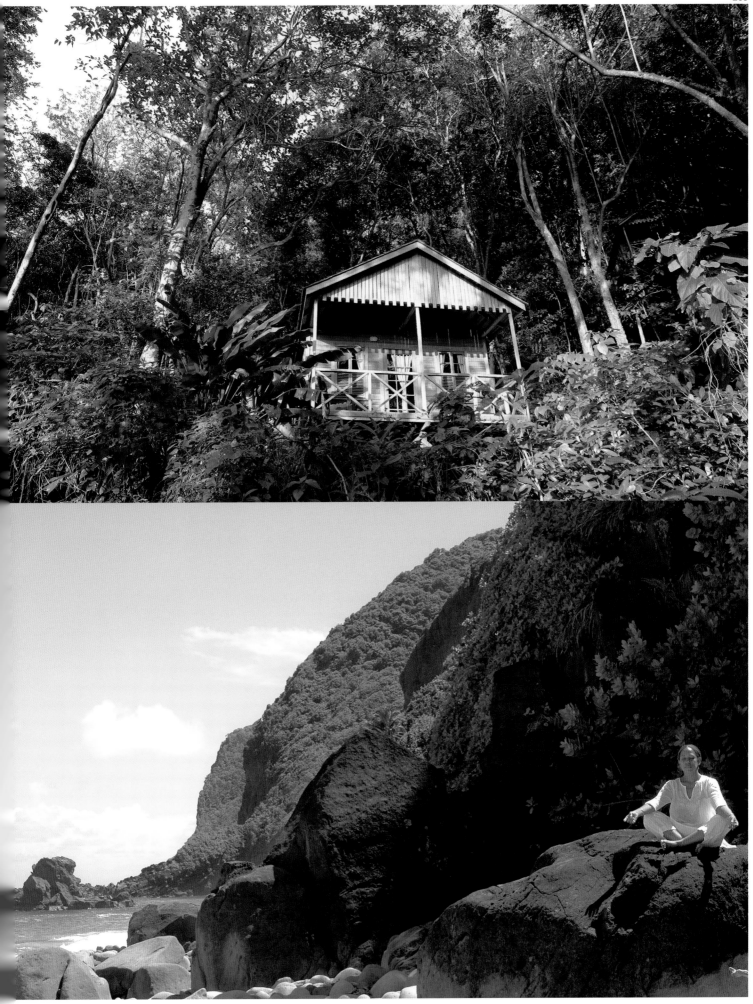

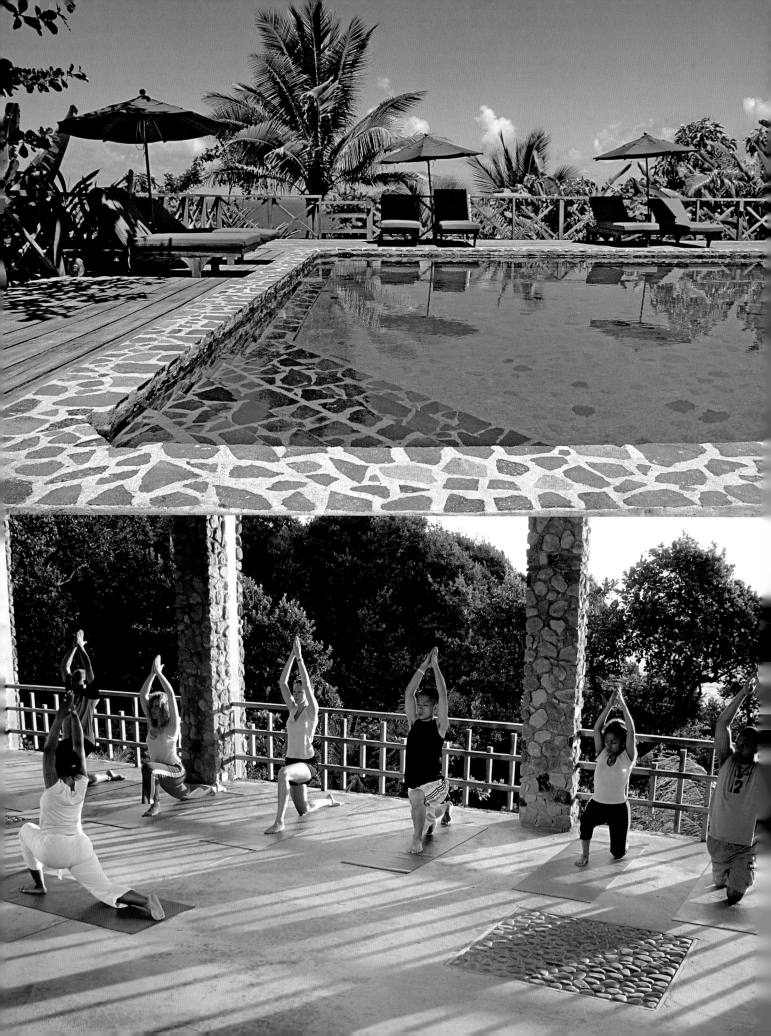

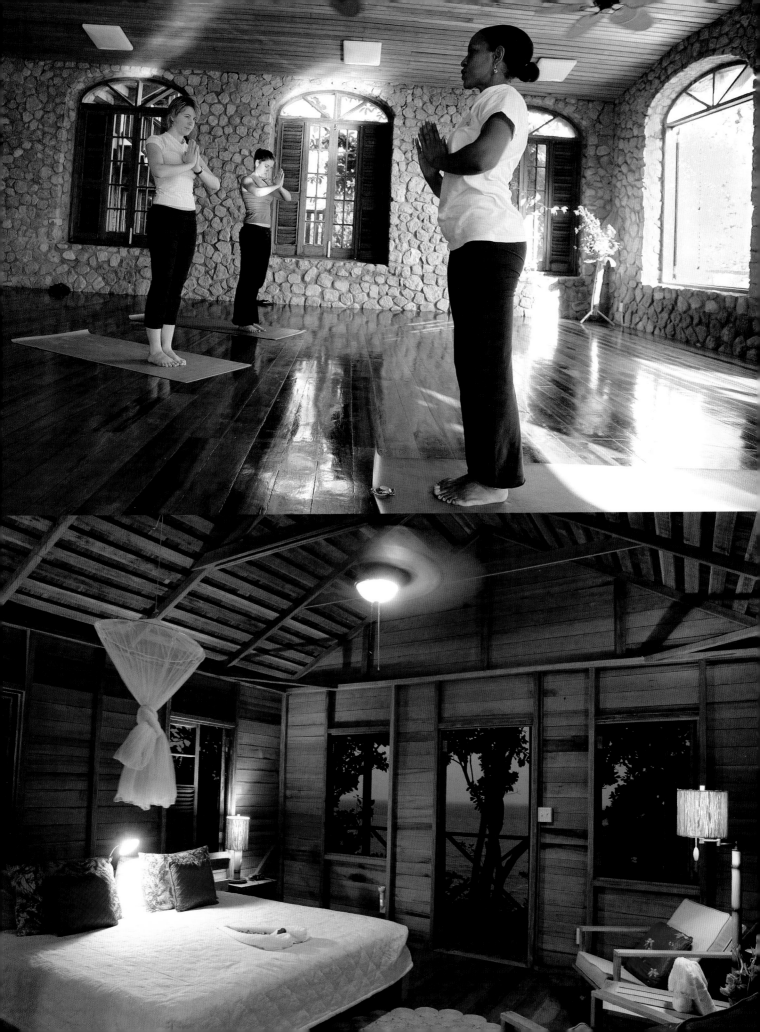

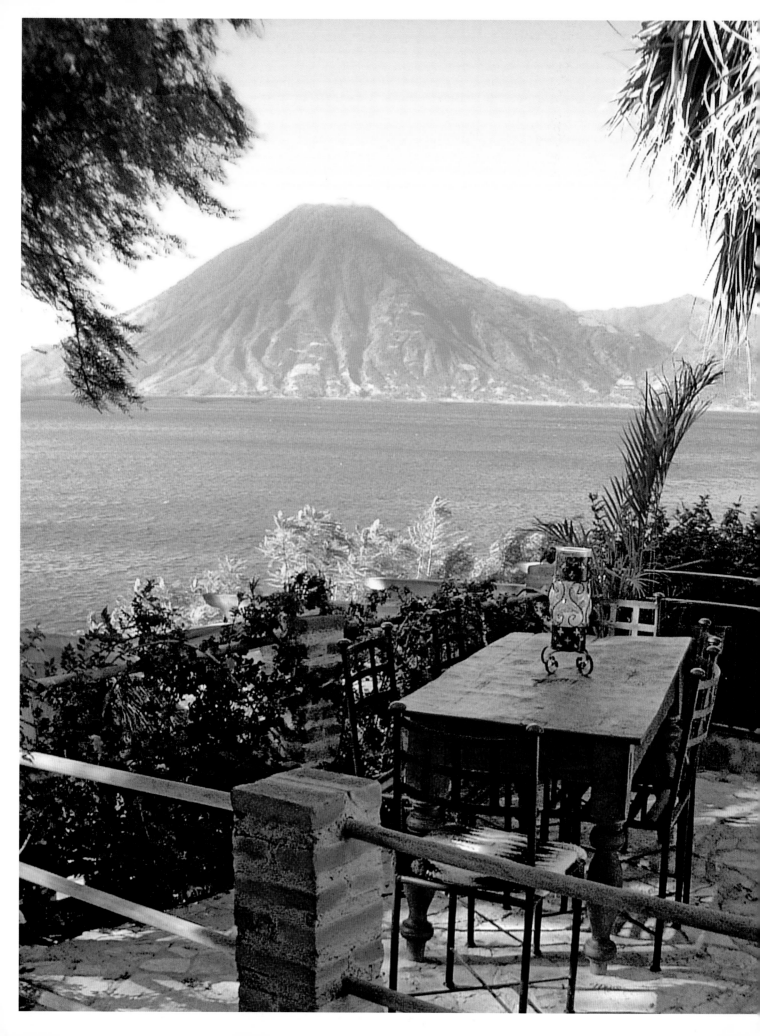

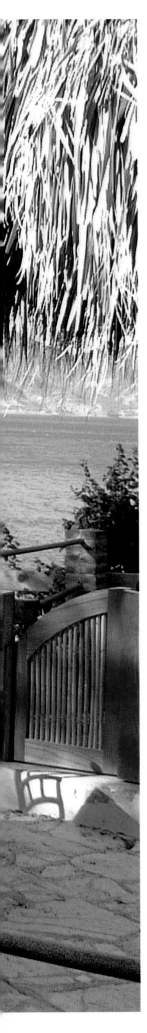

The morning fog banks rise, clearing the view onto the mighty volcanoes on the opposite shore of the unique deep blue lake, and from the kitchen comes the aroma of freshly baked bread and coffee. Even if the advanced civilisation of the Mayas met its mysterious end more than a thousand years ago, the fertile soil of the mountain ridge, the lakes and the avocado and coffee forests became home to the Cack'chiquel, Quek'chi, Mam and Tzutujil—ethnic Mayan groups whose traditional culture still exists today. How did they pass the time back then? In Villa Sumaya, at any rate, there is no reason for cultural pessimism. Under the huge dome of the straw roof, not only is yoga practised on the parquet floor, but also, mindful of the ruins of a unique civilisation, an insight is gained into the transitoriness of one's own culture. But as long as there is the solar-heated pool and fresh enchiladas, home-made sauces with chili peppers and organic fruit, no problem. The rest is taken care of by the sweet Guatemalan worry dolls, which are on sale in the hotel's delightful shop, Spirit Dog.

Book to pack: "Under the Volcano" by Malcolm Lowry

Villa Sumaya

Santa Cruz La Laguna,
Lake Atitlan
Guatemala
Tel. +502 402 61390 and +502 402 61455
info@villasumaya.com
www.villasumaya.com

Directions	Located on the shores of Lake Atitlan at a height of of 5,000 feet, about 3 hrs drive from the airport in Guatemala City
Yoga	All 8 arms of Yoga, Hatha, Iyengar
Teachers	Paula Tursi, Will Duprey, Laurie Ellis Young, Ernesto Ortiz
Rooms	15 rooms, max. 35 guests
Food	Slow Food, fish, local specialities
Treatments	Massage
Leisure	Maya seminar, Spanish course, dance, creative arts, pool, hot tub, sauna, kayaking, diving, water-skiing, hiking, horseback riding, birdwatching, boat trips

Die morgendlichen Nebelbänke heben sich, der Blick wird frei auf die mächtigen Vulkane am anderen Ufer des einzigartigen tiefblauen Sees, und aus der Küche dringt der Geruch von frisch gebackenem Brot und Kaffee. Auch wenn die Hochkultur der Mayas vor mehr als 1000 Jahren ihr mysteriöses Ende fand, wurden die fruchtbare Erde der Bergzüge, die Seen, Avocado- und Kaffeewälder zur Heimat der Cack'chiquel, Quek'chi, Mam und Tzutujil – der ethnischen Maya-Gruppen, deren traditionelle Kultur noch heute besteht. Wie sie sich damals wohl die Zeit vertrieben haben? In der Villa Sumaya besteht jedenfalls kein Grund zum Kulturpessimismus. Unter der riesigen Kuppel des Strohdachs wird auf Holzparkett nicht nur Yoga geübt, sondern eingedenk der Ruinen einer einzigartigen Zivilisation auch die Einsicht in die Vergänglichkeit der eigenen Kultur. Solange es den solargeheizten Pool und frische Enchiladas, selbst gemachte Soßen aus Chillies und naturbelassenes Obst gibt, ist das kein Problem. Den Rest erledigen die niedlichen guatemaltekischen Sorgenpüppchen, die es in dem entzückenden Laden »Spirit Dog« im Hotel zu kaufen gibt.

Buchtipp: »Unter dem Vulkan« von Malcolm Lowry

Les nappes de brumes matinales s'évaporent, libérant la vue sur les puissants volcans dressés sur l'autre rive du fantastique lac d'un bleu profond, tandis que de la cuisine monte l'odeur de pain frais et de café. Si la civilisation maya s'éteignit mystérieusement il y a plus de mille ans, la terre fertile des flancs de montagne, les lacs, les forêts d'avocatiers et de caféiers sont devenus la patrie des Cack'chiquel, Quek'chi, Mam et Tzutujil, groupes ethniques mayas dont la culture traditionnelle subsiste de nos jours. Comment ont-ils tué le temps autrefois ? Dans la Villa Sumaya, en tout cas, il n'y a aucune raison de s'adonner à une vision pessimiste de la civilisation. Sous l'immense voûte du toit de paille ont lieu des séances de yoga sur le parquet en bois mais aussi, face aux ruines d'une civilisation extraordinaire, on prend conscience de la fragilité de notre propre culture. Pas de souci, tant qu'il y aura la piscine chauffée au soleil et des enchiladas, les sauces maison à base de piment fort et les fruits bio. Les ravissantes poupées anti-soucis guatémaliennes que l'on peut acheter à l'hôtel dans le joli magasin Spirit Dog se chargent du reste.

Livre à emporter : « Au-dessous du volcan » de Malcolm Lowry

Anreise	Am Ufer des Lake Atitlan auf 1.500 Höhenmetern gelegen, etwa 3 Std. Autofahrt vom Flughafen in Guatemala City entfernt
Yoga	Die 8 Glieder des Yoga, Hatha, Iyengar
Lehrer	Paula Tursi, Will Duprey, Laurie Ellis Young, Ernesto Ortiz
Zimmer	15 Zimmer, max. 35 Gäste
Küche	Slow Food, Fisch, lokale Spezialitäten
Anwendungen	Massagen
Aktivitäten	Maya-Seminar, Spanischkurs, Tanz und kreative Künste, Pool, Hot Tub, Sauna, Kajak, Tauchen, Wasserski, Wandern, Reiten, Vogelschau, Bootsfahrten

Accès	Au bord du lac Atitlán situé à 1500 m d'altitude, env. à 3 h de voiture de l'aéroport de Guatemala ville
Yoga	Les huit membres, Hatha, Iyengar
Professeurs	Paula Tursi, Will Duprey, Laurie Ellis Young, Ernesto Ortiz
Chambres	15 chambres pour 35 personnes max.
Restauration	Slow Food, poisson, spécialités locales
Traitements	Massages
Activités	Séminaire maya, cours d'espagnol, écriture créative, piscine, jacuzzi, sauna, kayak, plongée sous-marine, ski nautique, randonnées, équitation, observation d'oiseaux, promenades en bateau

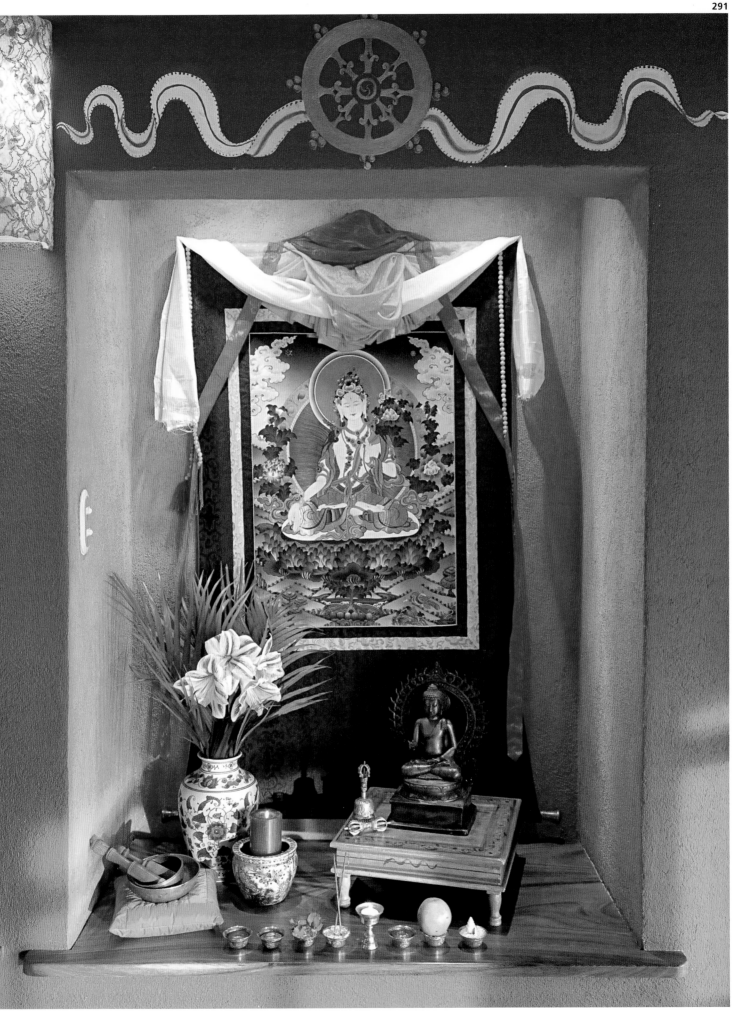

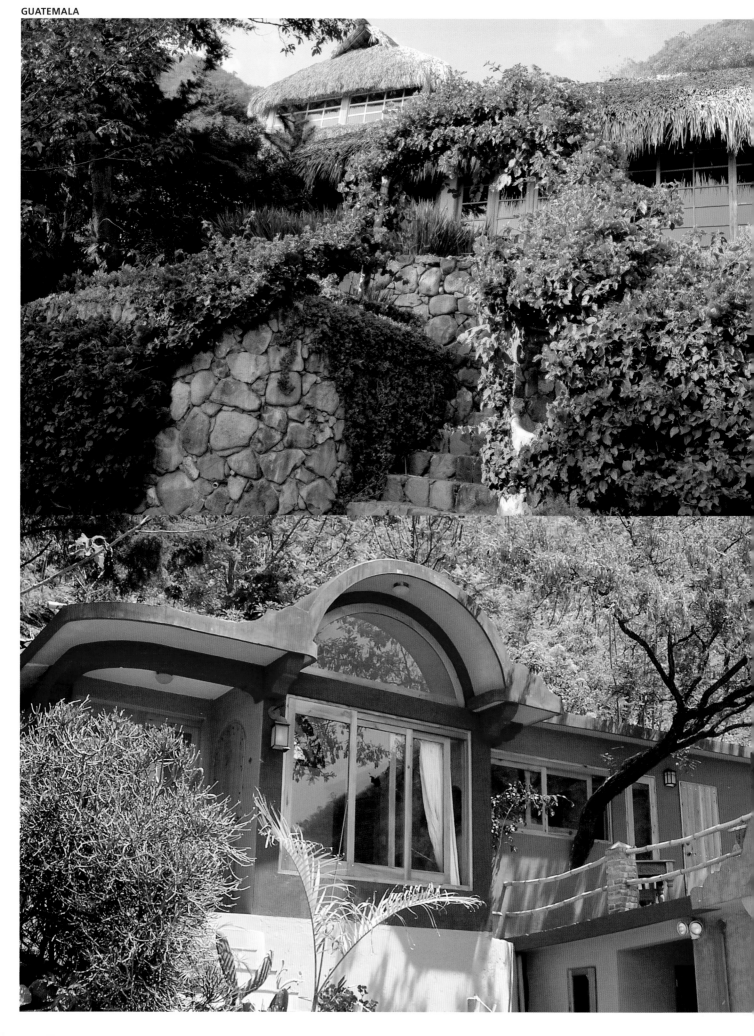

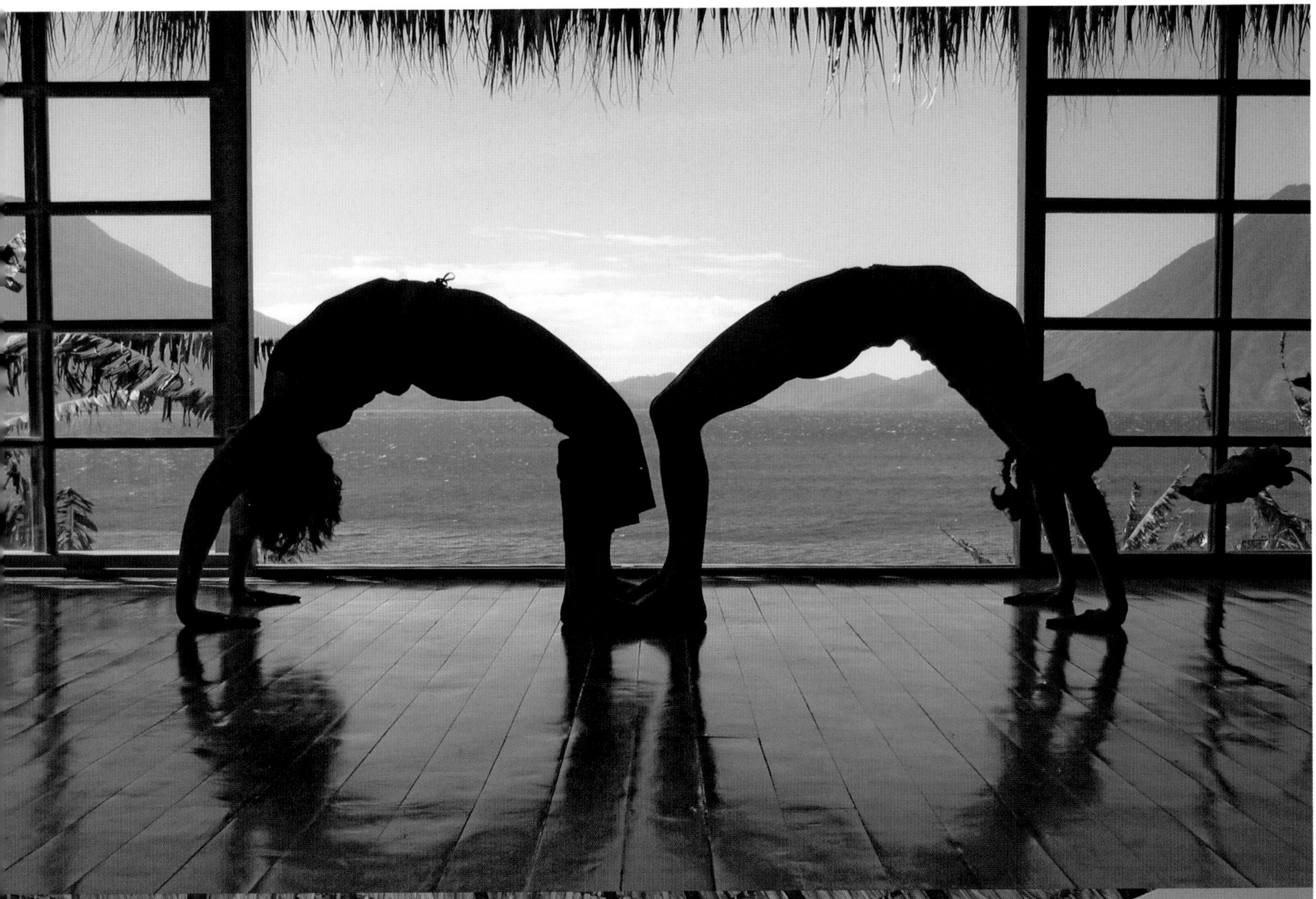

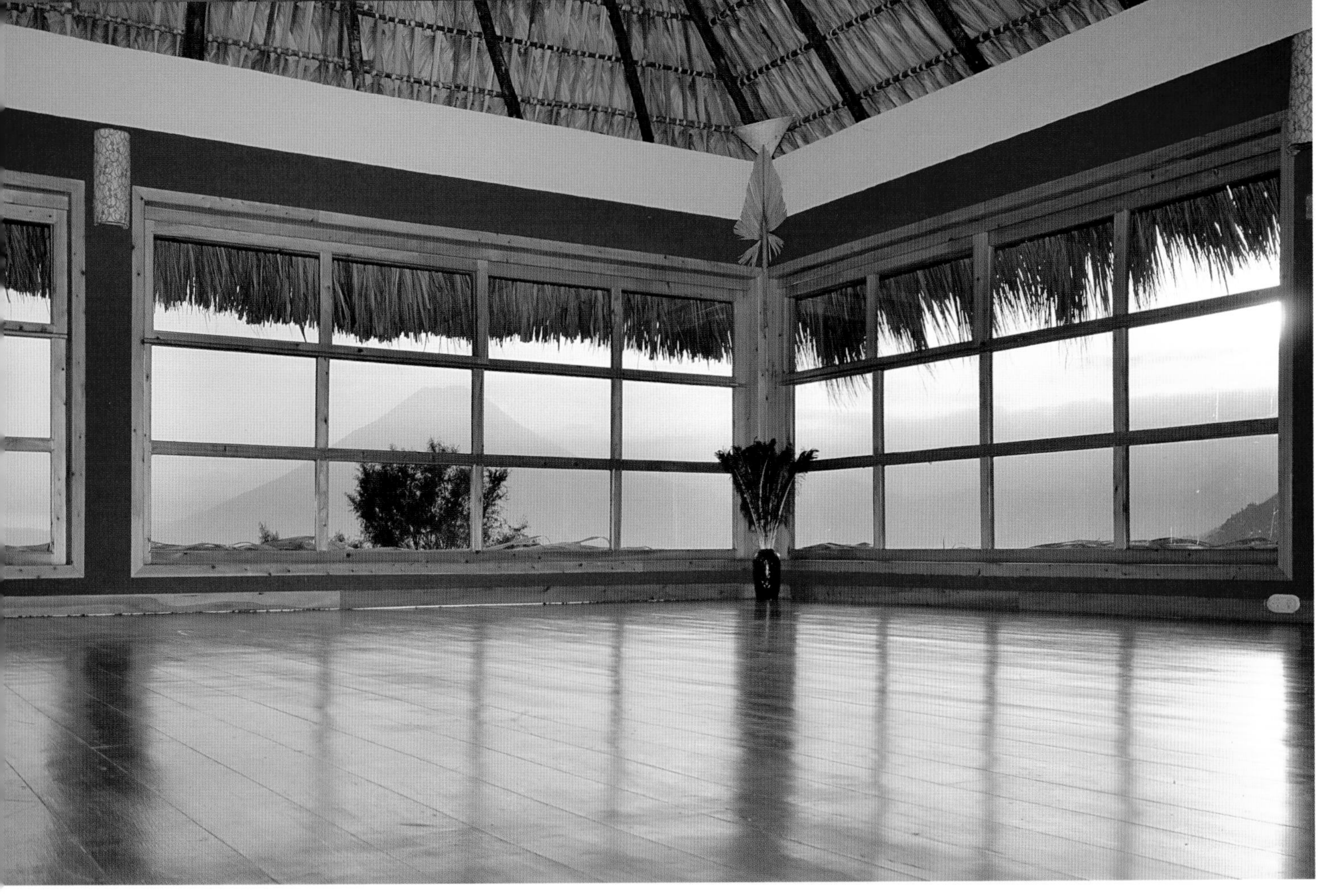

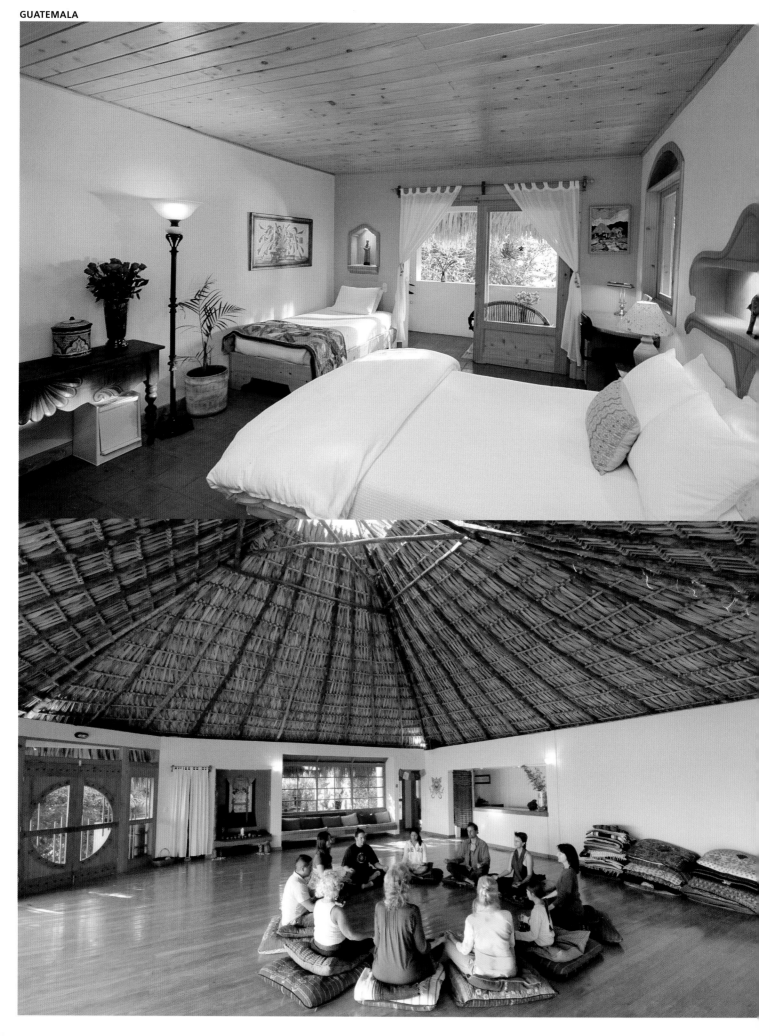

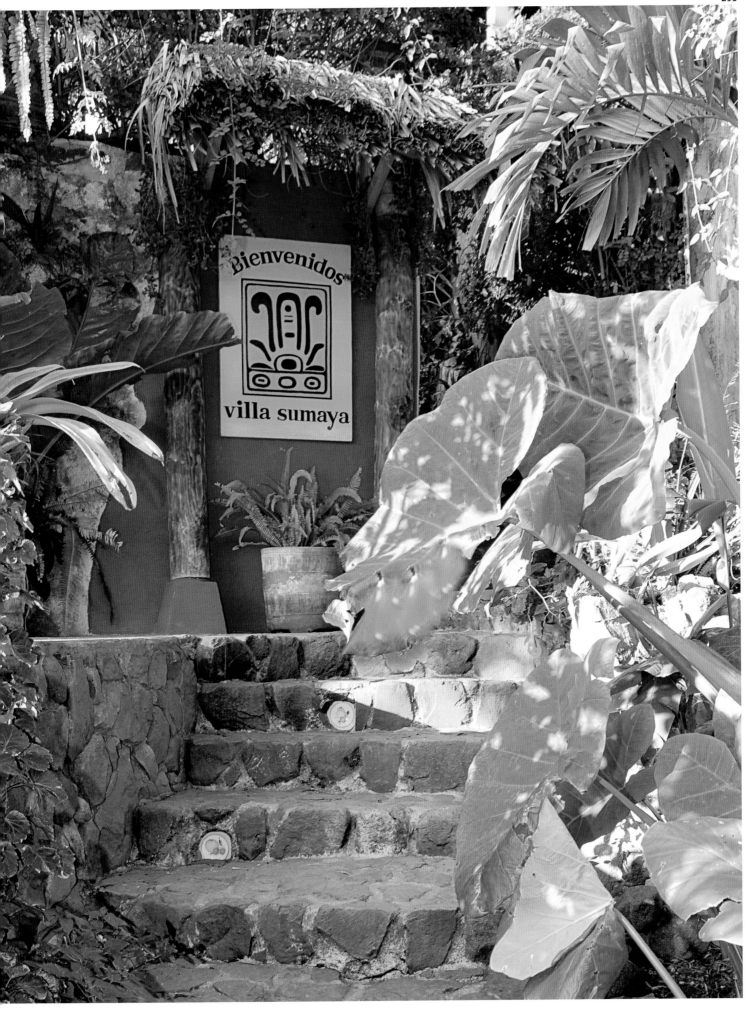

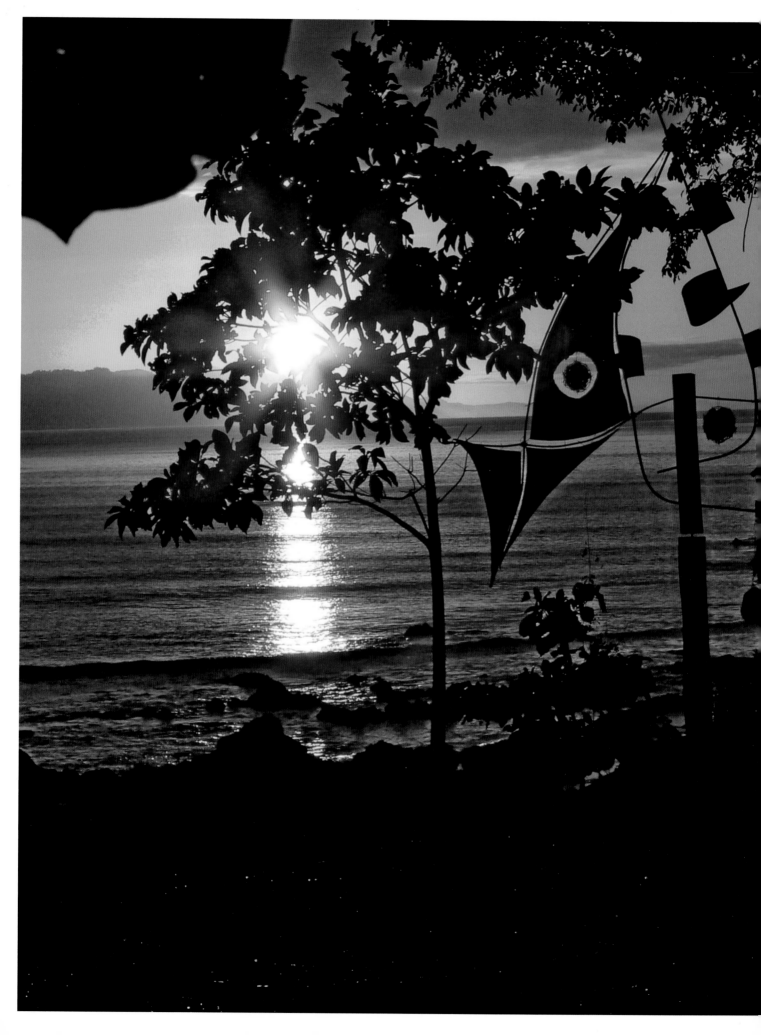

Let's not talk of paradise from the off; let's talk for the time being of a tiny country located between the Pacific and the Caribbean, of a couple of straw-covered huts in the midst of an enchanted botanical garden, of colourful hammocks woven for eternity and of a beach to whose flotsam and jetsam you would happily belong. Naturally, only the strongest in character and most flipped-out of New York's teachers ask their followers to come here. Nowhere else can monkeys, hanging casually from the auditorium's branches, see such intensive, imaginative Asana sessions as those that are held here on the spectacular yoga platform directly at the ocean's edge. They scrutinise their relations from the city and wonder why they are contorting themselves so. There is laughter and the chattering of a multitude of voices from the balcony. The birds in the giant trees have the answer: because they still have the urban jungle in their heads. But watch out: after the shortest time, on the most beautiful patch of this small country, the people, too, swing wildly and daringly through the day. They drink ice-cool guava juice and, as they do so, they become more and more beautiful.

Books to pack: "How to Be Wild" by Simon Barnes and "I Am That" by Sri Nisargadatta Maharaj

Tierra de Milagros

Rio Carbonera
Puerto Jimenez, Península de Osa
Costa Rica
Tel. +917 415 4846
info@tierrademilagros.com
www.tierrademilagros.com

Directions	Located directly on the Golfo Dulce. 50-min flight from San José, capital of Costa Rica
Yoga	Hatha, Ashtanga, Sivananda, Iyengar, Anusara
Teachers	Schuyler Grant, Alison Novie, Sianna Sherman, Douglas Brooks, Kenneth Graham
Rooms	15 rooms for max. 30 guests
Food	Organic vegetarian
Treatments	Facials, wraps, scrubs, massage, acupuncture
Leisure	Surfing, kayaking, horseback riding, hiking, swimming with dolphins

Reden wir nicht gleich vom Paradies, reden wir zunächst von einem winzigen Land, eingeklemmt zwischen Pazifik und Karibik, von ein paar strohgedeckten Hütten inmitten eines verwunschenen botanischen Gartens, von bunten Hängematten, die für die Ewigkeit geknüpft wurden, und von einem Strand, zu dessen Strandgut man gerne gehört. Logisch, dass hier die charakterstärksten und ausgeflipptesten Lehrer New Yorks ihre Anhänger herbestellen. So intensive, fantasievolle Asana-Stunden, wie sie hier auf der spektakulären Yoga-Plattform direkt am Ozean abgehalten werden, bekommen die Affen, die lässig an Ästen im Zuschauerraum hängen, woanders nicht zu sehen. Nachdenklich mustern sie ihre Verwandten aus der Stadt und fragen sich, warum die sich so verrenken. Gelächter und vielstimmiges Gezwitscher vom Balkon. Die Vögel in den Baumriesen haben die Antwort: weil sie noch den Großstadtdschungel im Kopf haben. Doch aufgepasst: Nach kürzester Zeit hangeln sich hier, am schönsten Fleck dieses kleinen Landes, auch die Menschen wild und wagemutig durch den Tag. Trinken eisgekühlten Guavensaft und werden dabei immer schöner.

Reisebegleiter: »How to be wild« von Simon Barnes und »Ich bin« (Teil 1, 2 und 3) von Sri Nisargadatta Maharaj

N'employons pas tout de suite le terme de paradis, parlons d'abord d'un minuscule pays coincé entre l'océan Pacifique et la mer des Caraïbes, de quelques cabanes aux toits de paille au cœur d'un jardin botanique ensorcelé, de hamacs multicolores fixés comme pour l'éternité et d'une plage sur laquelle on voudrait bien échouer à tout jamais. Il est donc logique que les professeurs les plus remarquables et les plus excentriques de New York fassent venir leurs adeptes ici. Nulle part ailleurs les singes qui, désinvoltes, se suspendent aux branches dans la salle, ne peuvent assister à des séances d'Âsana si intensives, si créatives qu'à celles qui se tiennent sur la spectaculaire plate-forme de yoga au bord de l'océan. D'un air pensif ils dévisagent leurs cousins de la ville en se demandant bien pourquoi ceux-ci se contorsionnent ainsi. Eclats de rire et babillages de mille et une voix résonnent du balcon. Les oiseaux nichés dans les arbres géants ont, eux, la réponse : c'est parce qu'ils ont encore dans la tête la jungle des métropoles. Mais attention : à peine installé ici dans le plus bel endroit de ce petit pays, les hommes aussi, farouches et intrépides, se déplacent du matin au soir à la force de leurs bras. Ils boivent du jus de goyave et n'en deviennent que plus beaux.

Livres à emporter : « How to be wild » de Simon Barnes et « Je suis » (tomes 1, 2 et 3) de Sri Nisargadatta Maharaj

Anreise	Direkt am Golfo Dulce gelegen, 50 min Flug von San José, Hauptstadt von Costa Rica
Yoga	Hatha, Ashtanga, Sivananda, Iyengar, Anusara
Lehrer	Schuyler Grant, Alison Novie, Sianna Sherman, Douglas Brooks, Kenneth Graham
Zimmer	15 Zimmer für max. 30 Gäste
Küche	Biologisch-vegetarisch
Anwendungen	Facials, Wraps, Scrubs, Massagen, Akupunktur
Aktivitäten	Surfen, Kajak, Reiten, Wandern, Schwimmen mit Delfinen

Accès	Situé directement sur le Golfo Dulce, à 50 min de vol de San José, capitale de Costa Rica
Yoga	Hatha, Ashtânga, Shivananda, Iyengar, Anusara
Professeurs	Schuyler Grant, Alison Novie, Sianna Sherman, Douglas Brooks, Kenneth Graham
Chambres	15 chambres pour 30 personnes max.
Restauration	Cuisine bio et végétarienne
Traitements	Soins du visage, enveloppements, gommages, massages, acuponcture
Activités	Surf, kayak, équitation, randonnées, nage avec les dauphins

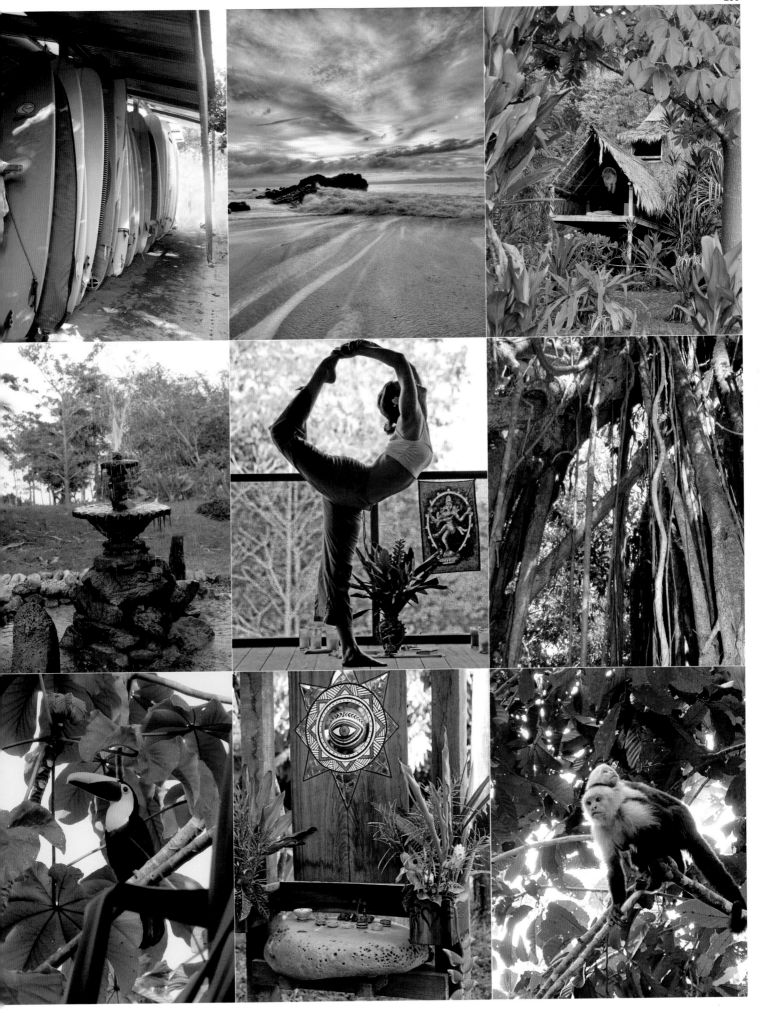

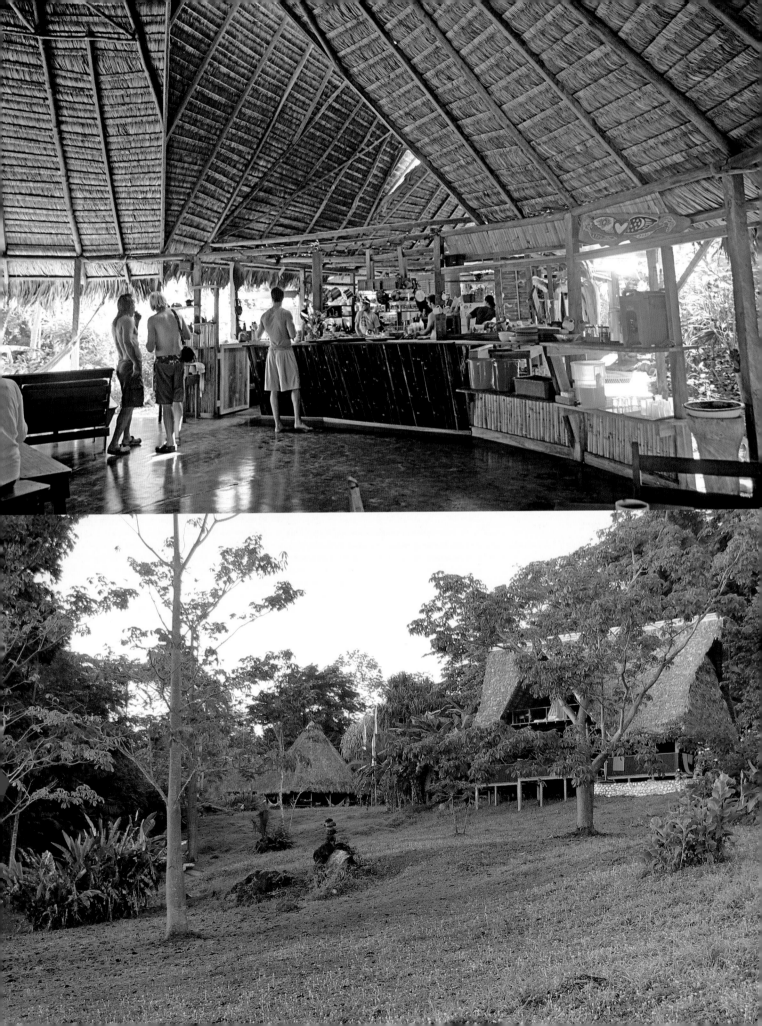

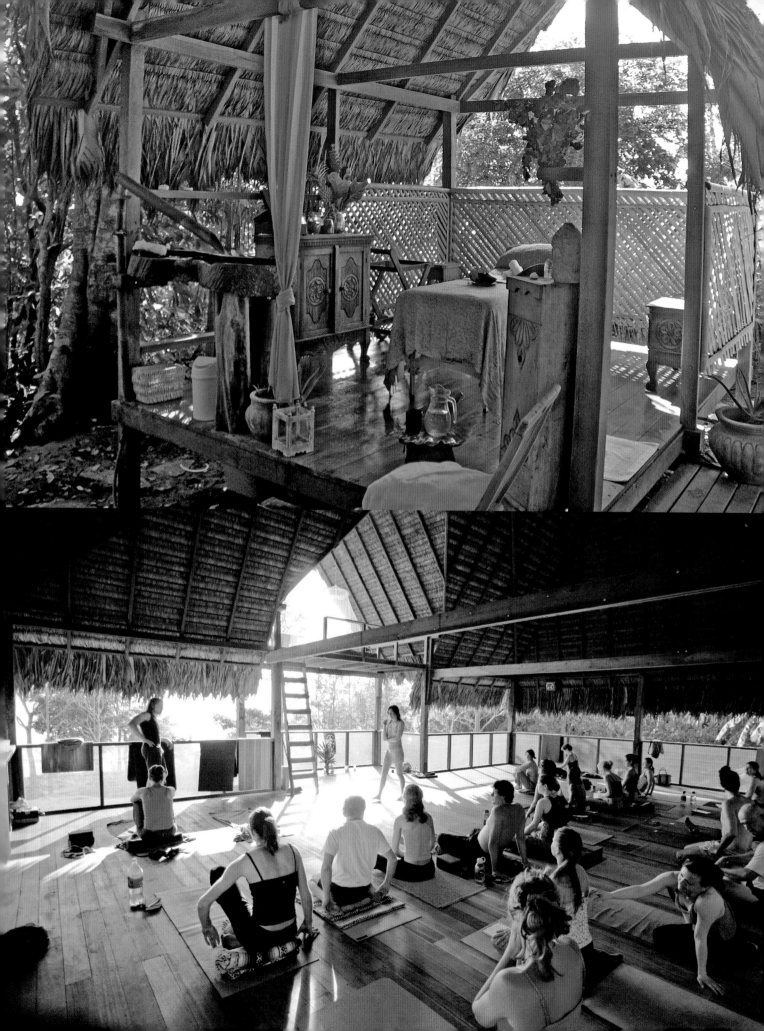

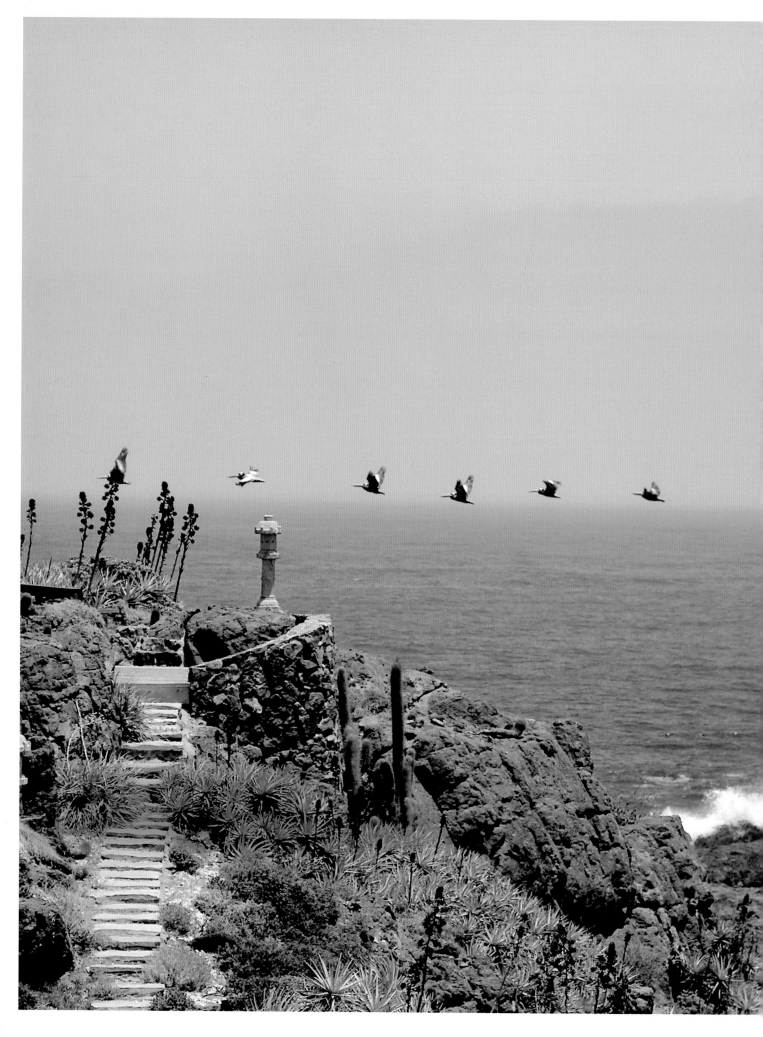

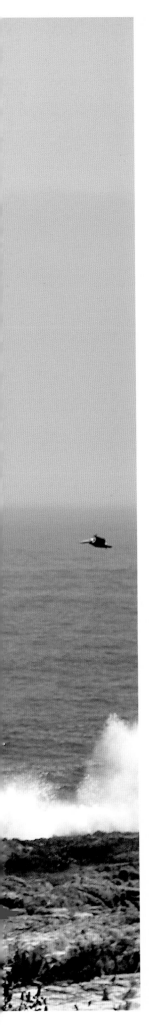

Practise the Primary Series with the Italian Ashtanga Yoga master Lino Miele here, and the breath still flows freely in the hundredth Chaturanga. Or do backbends with the exuberantly charming Anusara teacher Amy Ippoliti until the heart is as open as the ocean. It is as if a mountain had sunk in the sea, and only the summit still juts out—that is how surreal this place at the end of the world seems. Behind are the thousand-year-old glaciers, the Chilean highlands with their desert, the canyons and cacti; in front is the Pacific. No wonder that Gustavo Ponce, founder of Canal Om, himself developed a method for Dynamic Yoga, Sattva Yoga, which he also teaches here. At the end of a quiet day, after yoga, meditation, a long ride along the beach or a soothing bath in the saltwater pool heated to 100 degrees Fahrenheit, it is so peaceful that you can hear the stones talking. Come on, they whisper, they've lit the fire in the restaurant and a bottle of red is standing on the big table—called the monk's table here. Whoever has bagged the centrally heated comfortable single room with a view of the barren but beautiful garden should know that though Brahmacharya perhaps literally means abstinence, the word can also be translated—as the legendary yoga teacher Sharon Gannon has it—with "good sex".

Books to pack: "In Patagonia" by Bruce Chatwin and "House of the Spirits" by Isabel Allende

Canal Om

Wellness by the Sea
Km 213, Panamerican Highway, close to Los Vilos
Chile
Tel. +56 2 233 1524, +56 2 233 0409 and
+56 9 9258 9041
contacto@canalom.com
and oficina@yogashala.cl
www.canalom.com

Directions	132 miles north of Santiago, 10 miles away from Los Vilos. 2 hrs from Santiago Airport
Yoga	Iyengar, Ashtanga, Axis Sattva, Prana Shakti
Teachers	Gustavo Ponce and guest teachers
Rooms	3 double rooms, 7 twin rooms and 8 single rooms for max. 28 guests
Food	Vegetarian, Kundalini chef
Treatments	Massage, hydromassage, sauna, saltwater pool, thalassotherapy
Leisure	Tennis, horseback riding, day trips, swimming, archery

Hier mit dem italienischen Ashtanga-Altmeister Lino Miele die erste Serie des Sonnengrußes zu üben, lässt den Atem noch im 100. Chaturanga frei fließen. Oder mit der quirlig-charmanten Anusara-Lehrerin Amy Ippoliti Rückbeugen zu machen, bis das Herz so weit wie das Meer wird. Als sei ein Berg in der See versunken, und nur die Spitze ragt noch heraus, so surreal erscheint einem dieser Platz am Ende der Welt. Im Rücken die 1000-jährigen Gletscher, das chilenische Hochland mit seiner Wüste, den Schluchten und Kakteen, vor sich der Pazifische Ozean. Kein Wunder, dass Gustavo Ponce, Gründer von Canal Om, selbst eine Methode für dynamisches Yoga entwickelt hat, Sattva-Yoga, die er hier ebenfalls unterrichtet. Am Ende eines stillen Tages, nach Yoga, Meditation, einem langen Ritt am Strand oder einem tröstlichen Bad im auf 38 Grad erhitzten Salzwasserpool, ist es so ruhig, dass man die Steine sprechen hört. »Los komm«, flüstern sie, »im Restaurant haben sie Feuer im Kamin gemacht, und eine Flasche Rotwein steht auch auf dem großen Tisch, den sie hier Mönchstisch nennen.« Wer das zentral geheizte, gemütliche Einzelzimmer mit Blick in den kargschönen Garten erwischt hat, sollte wissen, dass Brahmacharya vielleicht wortwörtlich Enthaltsamkeit heißt, dass es aber ebenso wie von der legendären Yogalehrerin Sharon Gannon mit »guter Sex« übersetzt werden kann.

Reisebegleiter: »In Patagonien« von Bruce Chatwin und »Das Geisterhaus« von Isabel Allende

Ici, quand on effectue la série primaire avec Lino Miele, le maître italien incontesté d'Ashtânga, on parvient à respirer encore librement même après le centième Chaturanga. Ou bien avec Amy Ippoliti, charmante et pétulante professeur Anusara, on peut faire des exercices de flexion du dos jusqu'à ce que le cœur soit aussi vaste que la mer. Comme une montagne engloutie dans les flots et dont seulement la pointe dépasse encore, ainsi apparaît ce site du bout du monde, tel un cliché surréaliste. Derrière soi, les glaciers millénaires, le haut plateau chilien avec son désert, les gorges et les cactus et, devant soi, l'océan Pacifique. Il n'est guère étonnant que Gustavo Ponce, fondateur de Canal Om, ait conçu lui-même une méthode de yoga dynamique, le Sattva Yoga, qui est également enseignée ici. A la fin d'une journée tranquille, après le yoga, la méditation, une longue chevauchée sur la plage ou un bain réconfortant de 38 degrés dans la piscine à l'eau salée, tout est si calme que l'on entend parler les pierres. Viens donc, murmurent-elles, au restaurant un bon feu flambe dans la cheminée et une bouteille de vin rouge t'attend aussi sur la grande table qu'ils ont surnommée ici la table du moine. Celui à qui échoit la confortable chambre simple, raccordée au chauffage central, avec vue sur le jardin à la sobre beauté devrait savoir que si Brahmacharya signifie littéralement abstinence, il peut aussi bien être traduit par « good sex » comme le faisait Sharon Gannon, la légendaire professeur de yoga.

Livres à emporter : « En Patagonie » de Bruce Chatwin et « La Maison aux esprits » d'Isabel Allende

Anreise	213 km nördlich von Santiago, 16 km von Los Vilos. 2 Std. vom Flughafen Santiago entfernt
Yoga	Iyengar, Ashtanga, Dynamic, Axis Sattva, Prana Shakti
Lehrer	Gustavo Ponce und Gastlehrer
Zimmer	3 Doppelbettzimmer, 7 Zweibettzimmer und 8 Einzelzimmer für max. 28 Gäste
Küche	Vegetarisch, Kundalini-Koch
Anwendungen	Massagen, Hydromassagen, Sauna, Meerwasserpool, Thalasso-Therapie
Aktivitäten	Tennis, Reiten, Ausflüge, Schwimmen, Bogenschießen

Accès	Situé à 213 km au nord de Santiago, à 16 km de Los Vilos. A 2 h de l'aéroport de Santiago
Yoga	Iyengar, Ashtânga, Dynamic, Axis Sattva, Prana Shakti
Professeurs	Gustavo Ponce et enseignants invités
Chambres	3 chambres à lits doubles, 7 chambres à deux lits et 8 chambres simples pour 28 personnes max.
Restauration	Cuisine végétarienne, cuisinier Kundalini
Traitements	Massage, hydromassage, sauna, piscine à l'eau de mer, thalassothérapie
Activités	Tennis, équitation, excursions, natation, tir à l'arc

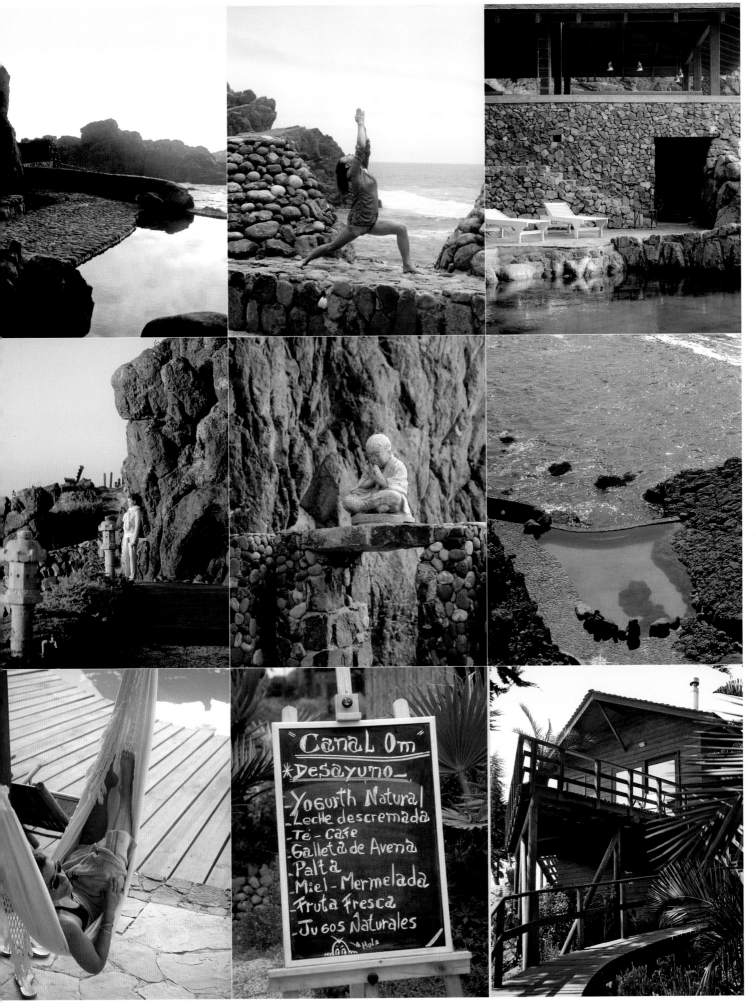

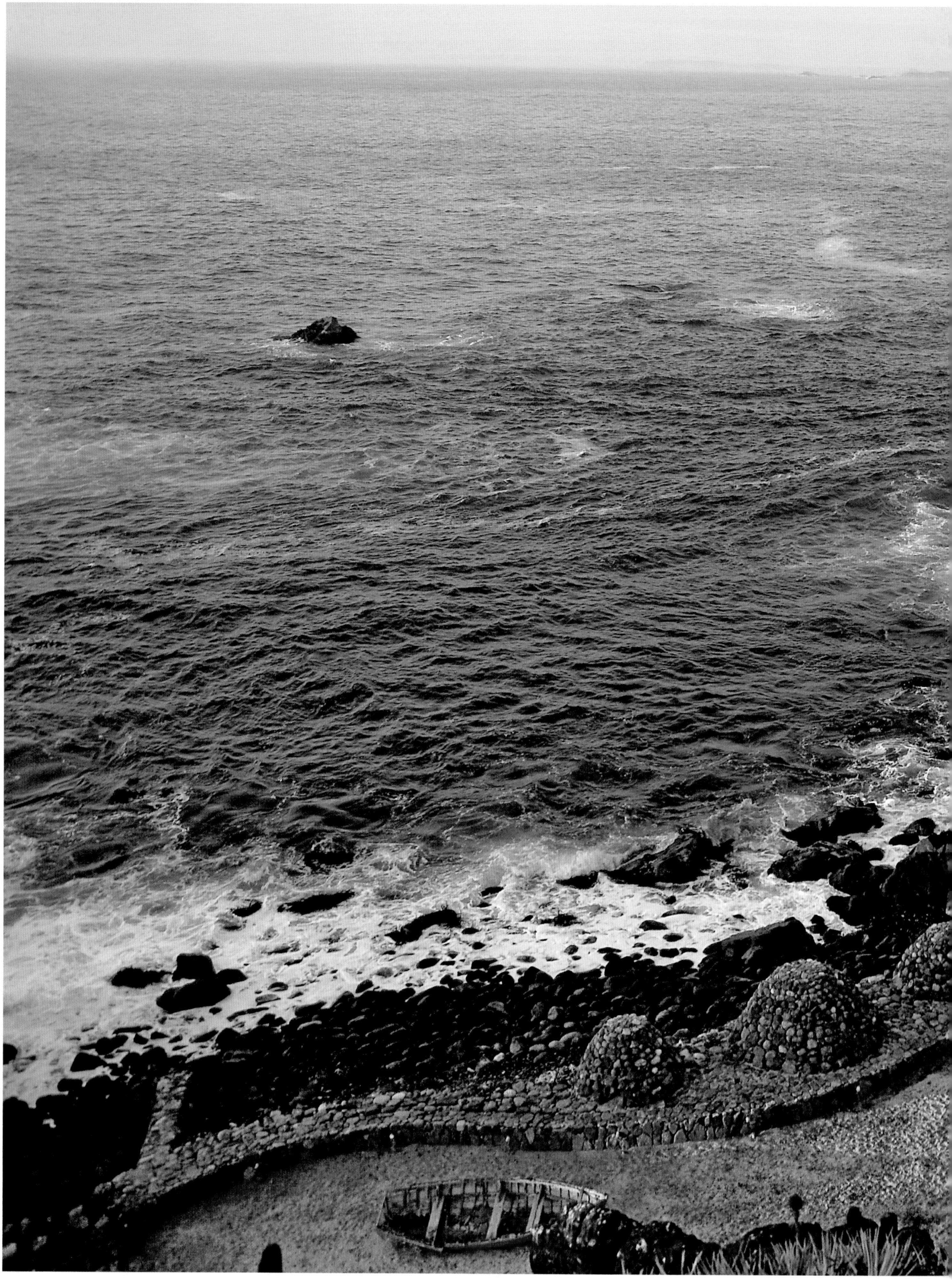

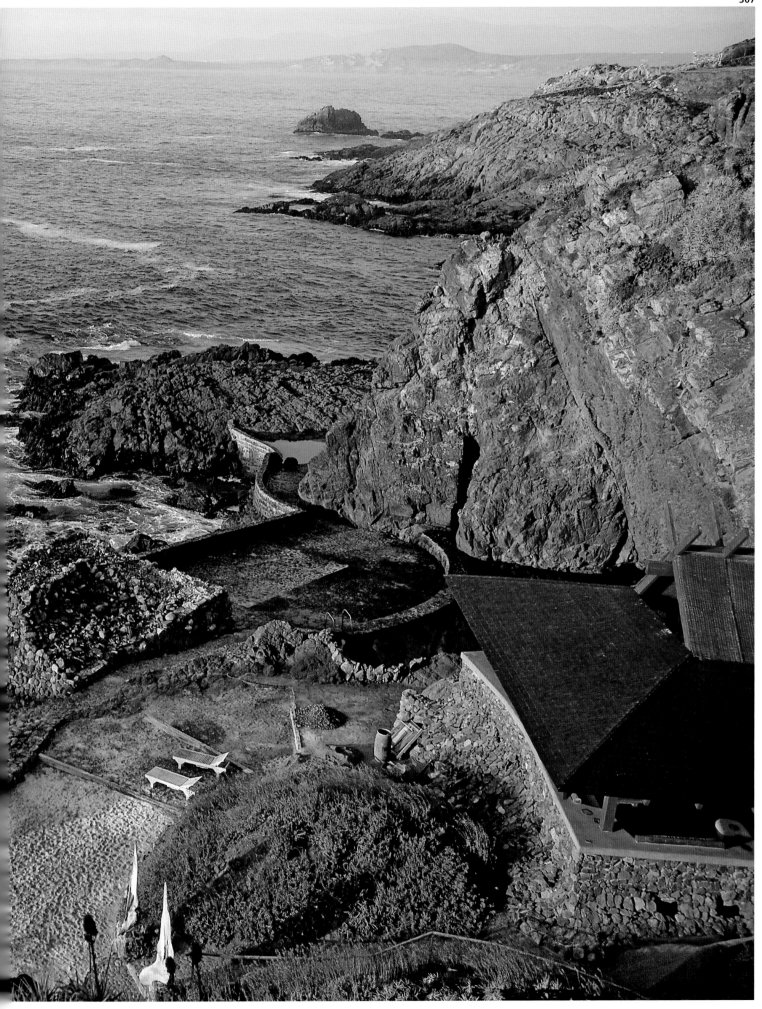

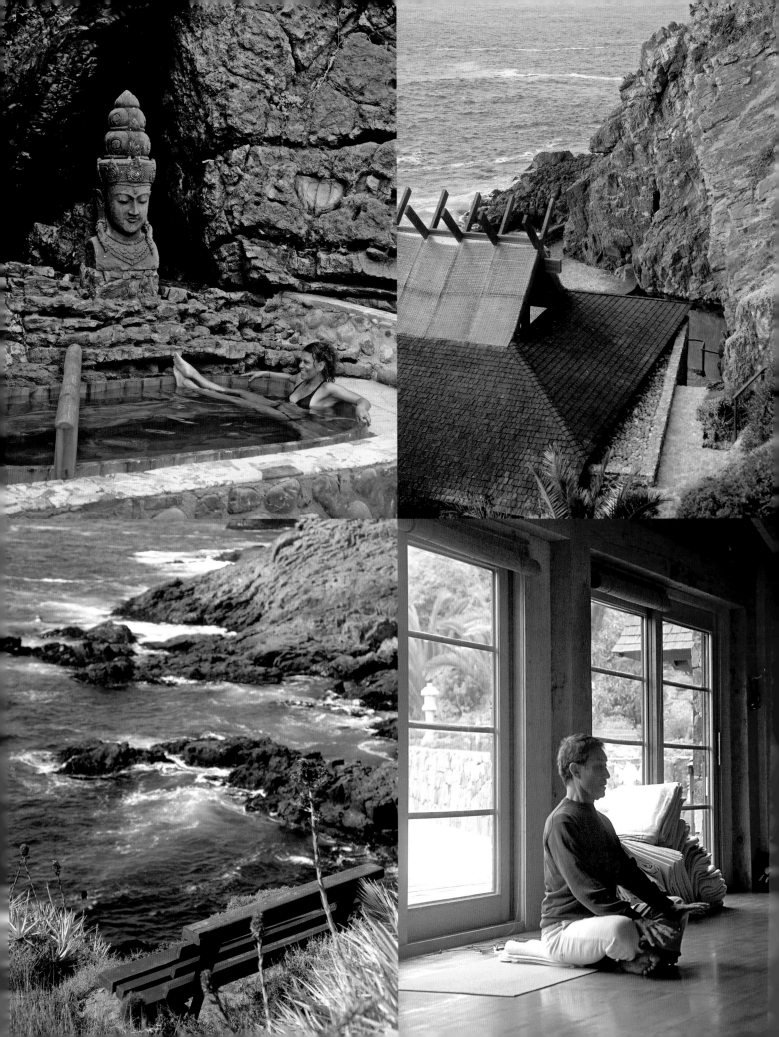

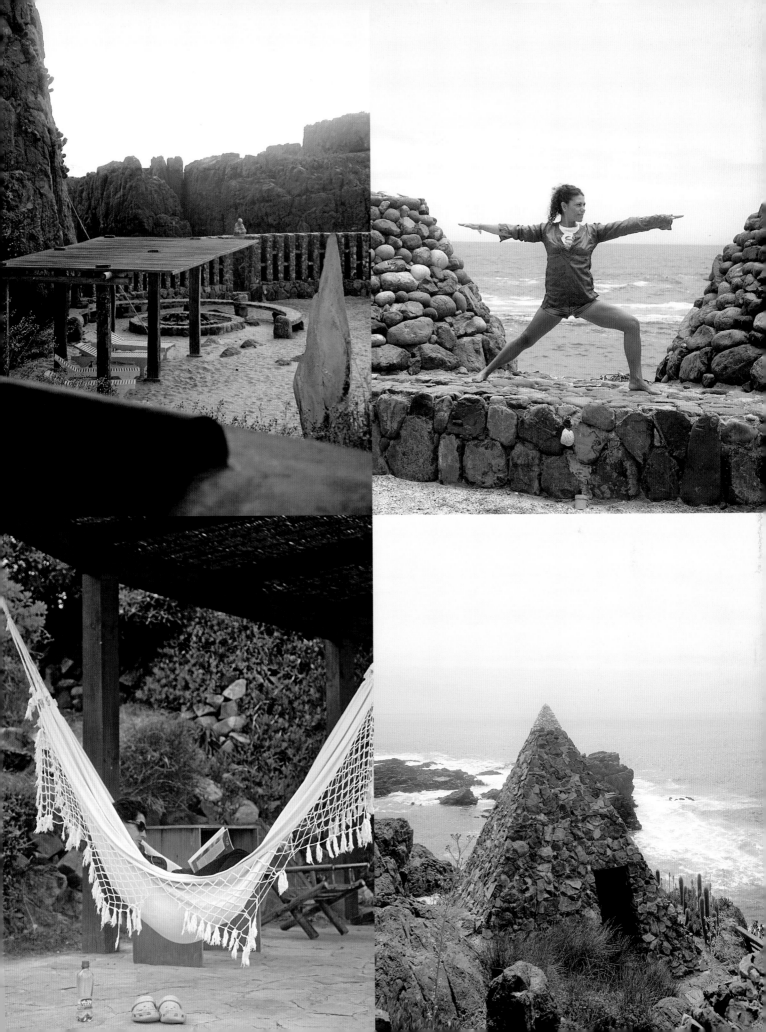

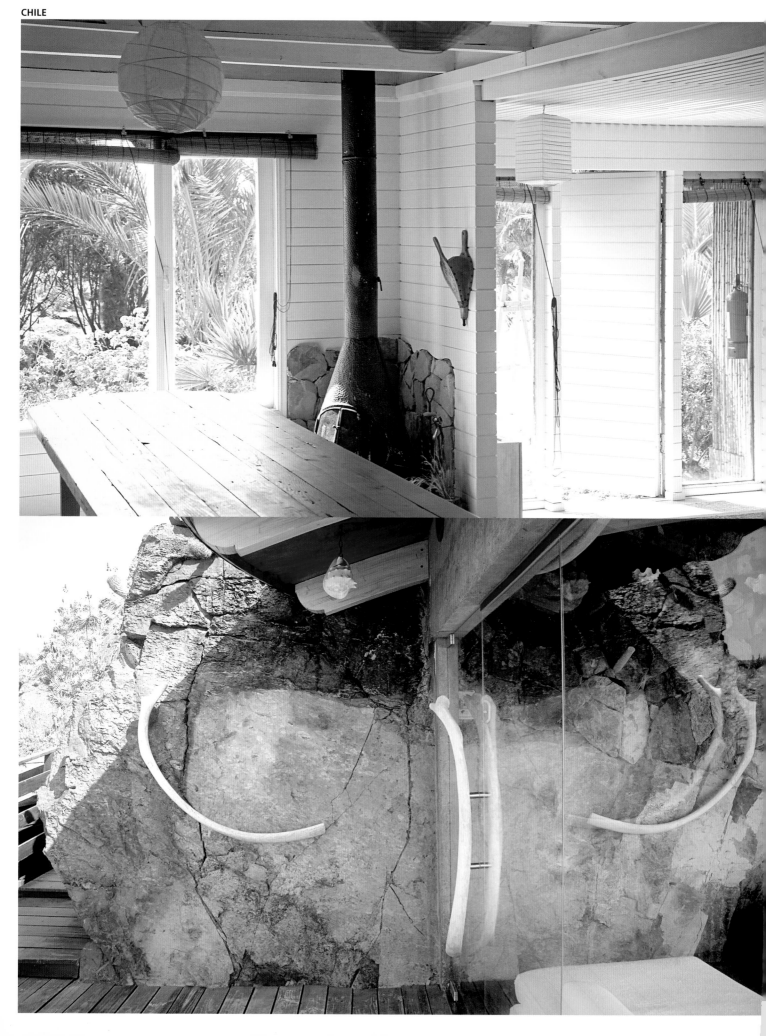

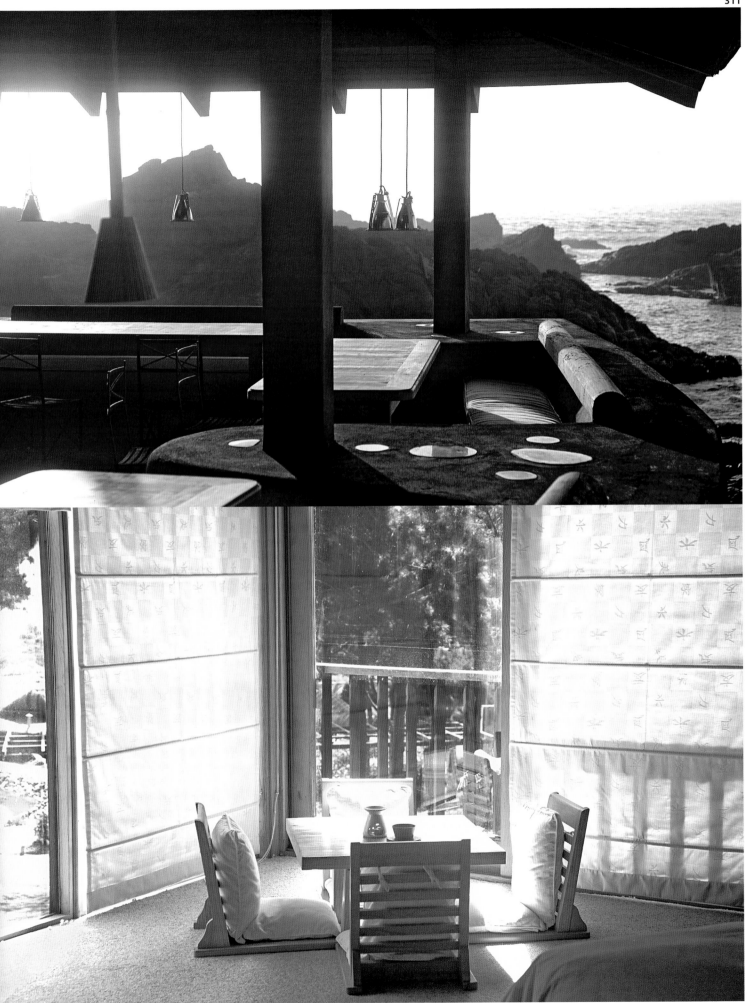

Yoga Styles by Kristin Rübesamen

Anusara

In this branch of Iyengar Yoga developed by the American John Friend, the ideas of tantric philosophy play a bigger role than in other forms of Hatha Yoga. The focus is on the three "A's"—attitude, alignment und action.

In der von dem Amerikaner John Friend entwickelten Unterart des Iyengar Yogas spielen tantrische Philosophiekonzepte eine stärkere Rolle als in anderen Formen von Hatha Yoga. Im Mittelpunkt stehen die drei „A's" – Attitude, Alignment und Action.

Dans cette branche de l'iyengar yoga développée par l'Américain John Friend, les concepts de la philosophie tantrique jouent un rôle plus important que dans les autres formes de l'hatha yoga. On s'y concentre sur les trois A : attitude, alignement et action.

Ashtanga

A contemporary form of classical Indian yoga. It consists of certain sequences of challenging asanas (body postures). Ashtanga yoga, developed by Shri K. Patthabis Jois, is one of the most successful methods in the West.

Zeitgemäße Form klassischen indischen Yogas. Es besteht aus bestimmten Sequenzen schwieriger Asanas (Körperhaltungen). Das von Shri K. Patthabis Jois entwickelte Ashtanga Yoga zählt zu den im Westen erfolgreichsten Methoden.

Une des formes contemporaines du yoage indien classique. Elle consiste en une succession d'asanas (postures) difficiles et dynamiques. L'ashtanga yoga, développé par Shri K. Patthabis Jois, est une des méthodes les plus populaires en Occident.

Bikram

A branch of hatha yoga that is also known "hot yoga". Bikram consists of a series of 26 asanas and two breathing exercises, which are carried out in a room heated to 35-40° Celsius. The high temperature permits a greater degree of stretching and at the same time promotes the reduction of stress.

Auch „Hot Yoga" genannte Unterart des Hatha Yoga. Bikram besteht aus einer Serie von 26 Asanas und zwei Atemübungen, die in einem 35-40° Celsius heißen Raum durchgeführt werden. Die hohe Temperatur erlaubt stärkere Dehnungen und fördert gleichzeitig den Stressabbau.

Branche de l'hatha yoga également appelée « yoga chaud ». Le bikram consiste en une série de 26 asanas et deux exercices de respiration, réalisée dans une pièce chauffée à une température comprise entre 35 et 40°C, qui permet de davantage étirer le corps tout en réduisant le stress.

Chinese Yoga (Qi Gong)

A Chinese system of health exercises that is thousands of years old. Chinese yoga consists of relaxed movements carried out slowly with great concentration. It is based on meditative body postures, but breathing exercises and meditation also play a part.

Ein tausende Jahre altes chinesisches System von Gesundheitsübungen. Chinese Yoga besteht aus entspannten Bewegungen, die langsam und sehr konzentriert ausgeführt werden. Seine Basis sind meditative Körperhaltungen. Doch auch Atemübungen und Meditation spielen eine Rolle.

Système chinois d'exercices de santé vieux de milliers d'années. Ce yoga chinois est composé de mouvements relâchés enchaînés avec lenteur et concentration. Il se fonde sur des postures corporelles méditatives, même si exercices de respiration et méditation jouent aussi un rôle important.

Dynamic Yoga

The fitness version of hatha yoga. Free of any spiritual superstructure, it concentrates on the functional aspects of the asanas and their sequence. The aims of dynamic yoga are above all physical: stamina, more stable joints, flexibility and coordination.

Die Fitness-Variante von Hatha Yoga. Frei von nahezu allem spirituellem Überbau stehen hier die funktionellen Aspekte der Asanas und ihrer Abfolgen im Vordergrund. Die Ziele von Dynamic Yoga sind vor allem körperlicher Art; es geht um Ausdauer, bessere Gelenkstabilität, Flexibilität und Koordination.

La version sportive de l'hatha yoga. Libre de toute superstructure spirituelle, elle se concentre sur les aspects fonctionnels des postures et de leur enchaînement. Les objectifs du yoga dynamique sont avant tout physiques : endurance, stabilisation des jointures, souplesse et coordination.

Freedom Style

Sit on the mat, listen within yourself and then move your body in the way that feels right: this is freedom-style yoga. This variety, developed by the American Erich Schiffmann, is based on intuition and demands a certain level of self-confidence.

Auf der Matte sitzen, in sich hineinhören und den Körper dann so bewegen, wie es sich richtig anfühlt – das ist Freedom Style Yoga. Die von dem Amerikaner Erich Schiffmann entwickelte Lehre basiert auf Intuition und erfordert ein gewisses Maß an Selbstvertrauen.

Vous asseoir sur le tapis, écouter en vous-même, puis bouger votre corps comme bon vous semble : voilà ce qu'est le yoga « libre ». Cette variété, développée par l'Américain Erich Schiffmann, est fondée sur l'intuition et exige un certain niveau de confiance en soi.

Hatha Yoga

This is what is generally understood in the West as "yoga", but has its historic roots in the Hatha Yoga Pradipika, written in the 14th century, which puts the emphasis on the cleansing of the physical body. Includes asanas and prayanama.

Das, was in der westlichen Welt gemeinhin unter „Yoga" verstanden wird, historisch aber auf die im 14. Jh. geschriebene Hathayogapradipika zurückgeht, die die Reinigung des physischen Körpers in den Vordergrund stellt. Umfasst Asanas und Prayanama.

Ce qu'on entend en général par « yoga » en Occident. Cette école puise ses racines dans l'Hatha Yoga Pradipika, rédigé au 14e siècle, qui insiste sur la purification du corps physique. Inclut asanas et prayanama.

Istha

A system of yoga devised by Mani Finger and oriented to the individual. Ishta combines the principles of hatha yoga, tantra and ayurveda into a comprehensive experience of consciousness. A session includes asanas and pranayama, meditation, massages and visualisation.

Von Mani Finger entwickeltes, auf das Individuum ausgerichtetes Yoga-System. Ishta verbindet die Prinzipien von Hatha Yoga, Tantra und Ayurveda zu einer umfassenden Bewusstseinserfahrung. Die Stunden beinhalten Asanas und Pranayama, Meditation, Massagen und Visualisierung.

Un système de yoga imaginé par Mani Finger et orienté vers l'individu. L'Ishta combine les principes de l'hatha yoga, du tantra et de l'ayurveda en une expérience complète de la conscience. Au cours d'une séance se succèdent asanas, pranayama, méditation, massages et visualisation.

Iyengar

A therapeutically effective version of hatha yoga developed by B.K.S Iyengar, in which correct posture and exact work during the asanas are at the centre of attention. Accessories such as belts and cushions are used in Iyengar Yoga.

Die von B.K.S Iyengar entwickelte und therapeutisch wirksame Version des Hatha Yoga, bei der die korrekte Körperhaltung und genaues Arbeiten während der Asanas im Mittelpunkt steht. Bei Iyengar Yoga werden auch Hilfsmittel wie Gurte oder Polster verwendet.

Une version thérapeutique efficace de l'hatha yoga développée par B.K.S Iyengar, dans laquelle on concentre son attention sur l'exactitude et la précision des postures pendant les asanas. Des accessoires comme des ceintures et des coussins sont utilisés dans cette discipline.

Jivamukti

Developed in New York in the 1980s from ashtanga yoga, this is a very athletic form of yoga in which the asanas flow into each other. A jivamukti class includes music, sung mantras, the study of ancient writings and meditation.

Eine in den 80er Jahren in New York entwickelte, sehr sportliche Weiterentwicklung von Ashtanga-Yoga, bei der die Asanas fließend ineinander übergehen. Zu Jivamukti-Stunden gehören Musik, gesungene Mantras, das Studium alter Schriften und Meditation.

Développée à New York dans les années 1980 à partir de l'ashtanga yoga, il s'agit d'une forme très athlétique de yoga dans laquelle les asanas s'enchaînent sans pause. Un cours de jivamukti se déroule en musique et inclut chant de mantras, étude des textes anciens et méditation.

Kirtan

This musical form of yoga (also known as "chanting") consists of singing Sanskrit mantras—an easy and highly effective way of calming the nerves and opening the heart and body. In kirtan the community repeat what a singer has first sung to them.

Diese musikalische Form von Yoga (auch „Chanten" genannt) besteht aus dem Singen von Sanskrit-Mantren – eine leichte, sehr wirksame Methode, um die Nerven zu beruhigen und Herz und Körper zu öffnen. Beim Kirtan singt die Gemeinschaft nach, was ein Sänger vorsingt.

Cette forme musicale du yoga (également appelée « psalmodie ») consiste à entonner des mantras en sanskrit – un moyen facile et très efficace de calmer les nerfs, d'ouvrir le cœur et le corps. Dans le kirtan, le groupe répète ce que le chanteur a entonné en premier.

Kriya Yoga

The "yoga of doing" is a variation on raja yoga; its most important element is to breathe evenly, which is intended to lead to deep inner peace and harmony. The exercises are not difficult, and are passed directly to the pupils by the master.

Das „Yoga des Tuns" ist eine Variante des Raja-Yoga; sein wichtigstes Element ist gleichmäßige Atmung, die den Menschen zu tiefer innerer Ruhe und Ausgeglichenheit führen soll. Die Übungen sind nicht schwierig und werden direkt vom Meister an den Schüler weitergegeben.

Le « yoga du faire » est une variante du raja yoga ; son élément le plus important est le maintien d'une respiration régulière, qui doit mener à une harmonie et une paix intérieures profondes. Les exercices ne sont pas difficiles, et sont transmis directement du maître aux élèves.

Kundalini

A branch of raja yoga with its roots in tantrism, aiming to make kundalini (an ethereal power) rise through the chakras (centres of energy). It includes asanas, pranayama, mantras, mudras (symbolic hand postures executed with concentration) and visualisations.

Eine im Tantrismus beheimatete Unterform von Raja Yoga, die das Aufsteigen des Kundalini (einer ätherischen Kraft) durch die Chakren (Energiezentren) zum Ziel hat. Elemente sind Asanas, Pranayama, Mantren, Mudras (konzentriert ausgeführte, symbolische Handstellungen) und Visualisierungen.

Une branche du raja yoga qui puise ses racines dans le tantrisme, dont le but est de faire surgir le kundalini (une puissance éthérée) des chakras (centres d'énergie). Elle enchaîne asanas, pranayama, mantras, mudras (postures symboliques des mains exécutée dans une grande concentration) et visualisations.

Meditation

Exercises in concentration to collect the spirit and extend consciousness. In yoga, meditation is supported by many bodily postures and exercises. Asanas held for a long time without movement are regarded as meditative in themselves. Meditation plays an important role in raja yoga.

Konzentrationsübungen zur Sammlung des Geistes und Erweiterung des Bewusstseins. Im Yoga unterstützen viele Körperhaltungen und -übungen die Meditation. Lange, bewegungslos gehaltene Asanas gelten selbst bereits als meditativ. Eine große Rolle spielt Meditation bei Raja Yoga.

Exercices de concentration visant à rassembler ses esprits et étendre sa zone de conscience. Dans le yoga, la méditation est soutenue par divers exercices et postures corporelles. Les asanas maintenus longtemps sans mouvement parasite sont considérés comme des exercices de méditation en tant que tels. La méditation joue un rôle important dans le raja yoga.

Nada Yoga

A type of yoga that focusses on the reciting of mantras, pranayama, sound meditation, kirtan chants and contemplative listening to music and natural sounds. This is intended to guide the practitioner to turn inwards in order to perceive inner tranquillity.

Yoga-Praxis, bei der das Rezitieren von Mantras, Pranayama, Klang-Meditation, Kirtan-Gesang und das kontemplative Lauschen auf Musik und (Natur-) Geräusche im Vordergrund stehen. Dadurch soll die Hinwendung nach innen zur Wahrnehmung innerer Ruhe erreicht werden.

Type de yoga qui se concentre sur la récitation de mantras, le pranayama, la méditation par le son, les chants kirtan et l'écoute contemplative de la musique et des sons de la nature. Celui qui le pratique apprend à regarder en lui-même pour percevoir sa paix intérieure.

Nidra Yoga

Not bodily exercises, but exercises to relax the body, for awareness of breathing, inner relaxation, visualisations etc are the characteristics of nidra yoga. The practitioner is taken to the borderline between waking and sleeping, which makes deep layers of consciousness accessible.

Keine Körperübungen, sondern Übungen zu Körperentspannung, Atemwahrnehmung, innerer Entspannung, Visualisierungen etc. zeichnen Nidra Yoga aus. Dabei gerät der Übende in einen Grenzbereich zwischen Wachen und Schlafen, der ihm tiefe Bewusstseinsebenen zugänglich macht.

Succession d'exercices visant à détendre le corps plutôt qu'à le muscler, caractérisée par la prise de conscience de la respiration, la relaxation intérieure, les visualisations, etc. Le pratiquant du nidra yoga est transporté dans une zone frontière entre l'éveil et le sommeil, qui rend accessibles les couches profondes de la conscience.

Power Yoga

A method that Bryan Kest in Los Angeles derived from ashtanga yoga, taking on knowledge from sports medicine. With its clear and uncomplicated exercises it is aimed at a clientele that is primarily seeking a workout rather than spiritual enlightenment.

Eine in Los Angeles von Bryan Kest entwickelte Ableitung von Ashtanga-Yoga, in die Erkenntnisse der Sportmedizin eingeflossen sind. Mit seinen klaren, unkomplizierten Übungen richtet es sich an ein „Fitness"-Publikum, das statt spiritueller Erleuchtung vor allem ein Workout sucht.

Méthode créée par Bryan Kest à Los Angeles à partir de l'ashtanga yoga, qui intègre des connaissances liées à la médecine du sport. Ses exercices clairs et simples visent une clientèle en quête d'une discipline physique que d'édification spirituelle.

Prana Shakti

A gentle form of yoga developed by the Chilean Gustavo Ponce. The aim is to give orientation to the centres of energy ("chakras"). The exercises and breathing techniques also strengthen the immune system. The hand movements of prana shakti yoga are similar to those of Japanese reiki.

Vom Chilenen Gustavo Ponce entwickeltes, sanftes Yoga, das die Energiezentren („Chakras") ausrichten soll. Übungen und Atemtechnik kräftigen überdies das Immunsystem. Die Handbewegungen von Prana Shakti Yoga ähneln denen der japanischen Reiki-Praxis.

Forme douce de yoga développée par le Chilien Gustavo Ponce dont l'objectif est de centrer les nœuds d'énergie, ou « chakras ». Les exercices et les techniques de respiration renforcent aussi le système immunitaire. Les mouvements des mains typiques du yoga prana shakti ressemblent à ceux du reiki japonais.

Pranayama

A Sanskrit word meaning "extension of the life force", and one of the five great principles of yoga. It refers to breathing exercises which have a harmonising, relaxing or vitalising effect. They can be practised separately or used to support asanas.

Sanskrit-Wort, das „Erweiterung der Lebensenergie" bedeutet und eines der fünf großen Yoga-Prinzipien ist. Gemeint sind Atemübungen, die harmonisierend, entspannend oder vitalisierend wirken. Sie können separat geübt oder zur Unterstützung von Asanas eingesetzt werden.

Mot sanskrit signifiant « extension de la force de vie » ; parmi les cinq grands principes du yoga. Il se réfère aux exercices de respiration qui ont un effet harmonisant, relaxant et vitalisant. Ils peuvent être pratiqués séparément ou en soutien aux asanas.

Prenatal

A gentle form of yoga to alleviate the typical complaints of pregnant women and as preparation for giving birth. The asanas leave the stomach area completely relaxed so that the base of the pelvis is not weakened. The breathing exercises are targeted above all at extending breathing capacity.

Sanftes Schwangeren-Yoga zur Linderung typischer Beschwerden wie auch zur Geburtsvorbereitung. Die Asanas lassen den Bauchraum völlig entspannt, damit der Beckenboden nicht geschwächt wird. Bei den Atemübungen wird vor allem auf die Ausdehnung der Atemkapazität hingearbeitet.

Forme douce de yoga visant à soulager les désagréments typiques de la grossesse et préparer les femmes à l'accouchement. Les asanas ne sollicitent jamais la zone ventrale afin de ne pas affaiblir le plancher pelvien. Les exercices de respiration ont pour principal objectif d'augmenter les capacités respiratoires.

Raja Yoga

A spiritual form of ashtanga yoga that aims at gaining mastery over the spirit and is regarded as the highest form of yoga, leading to union with God. The means to achieve this are meditation, awareness, visualisations and observing oneself.

Spirituelle Form des Ashtanga Yoga, die die Beherrschung des Geistes zum Hauptziel hat. Gilt als Königsweg des Yoga, auf dem man zur Vereinigung mit Gott gelangt. Mittel hierzu sind Meditation, Achtsamkeit, Visualisierungen und Selbstbeobachtung.

Forme spirituelle de l'ashtanga yoga visant à acquérir la maîtrise de l'esprit, considérée comme la variante la plus sophistiquée du yoga, qui permet l'union avec le Divin. Pour y parvenir, le pratiquant recourt à la méditation, à la prise de conscience, aux visualisations et à l'observation de soi.

Restorative

Also known as the "candlelight yoga" of gentle movements and lying postures. Light stretches, twists and relaxation exercises, which can also be done with accessories such as sandbags and cushions, enable body and soul to let loose.

Auch als „Candle Light Yoga" der sanften Bewegungen und liegenden Posen bekannt. Leichte Dehnungen, Twists und Entspannungsübungen, die auch mit Hilfsmitteln wie Sandsäcken und Kissen durchgeführt werden können, bringen Körper und Geist zum Loslassen.

Également connu sous le nom de « yoga à la bougie », consiste en un enchaînement doux de mouvements et de postures allongées. De légers étirements, torsions et exercices de relaxation peuvent aussi être réalisés avec des accessoires comme des sacs de sable et des coussins, afin d'aider le corps et l'esprit à se relâcher et se libérer.

Sattva Yoga

Sattva yoga combines elements of hatha yoga ("bodily yoga") and raja yoga ("spiritual yoga"), in order to bring the physical body into equilibrium and cleanse the energetic body. The process leads to the goals of clarity and enhanced consciousness.

Sattva Yoga verbindet Elemente von Hatha Yoga („körperlichem Yoga") und Raja Yoga („geistigem Yoga"), um den physischen Körper in Balance zu bringen und den Energiekörper zu reinigen. Am Ende des Prozesses stehen Klarheit und ein erhöhtes Bewusstsein.

Le sattva yoga combine des éléments de l'hatha yoga (« yoga du corps ») et du raja yoga (« yoga de l'esprit »), afin d'équilibrer le corps physique et de purifier le corps énergétique. Ce processus permet d'accéder à la clairvoyance et aux états supérieurs de conscience.

Satyananda

A method developed by Paramhamsa Satyananda and his Bihar School of Yoga, which alongside asanas, pranayama and meditation also provides guidance for leading a true yogi lifestyle in all areas of existence. The aim at all times is spiritual development.

Von Paramhamsa Satyananda und seiner Bihar School of Yoga entwickeltes Konzept, das neben Asanas, Pranayama und Meditation auch Anweisungen für einen echten Yogi-Lifestyle in sämtlichen Lebensbereichen enthält. Ziel ist stets die spirituelle Weiterentwicklung.

Méthode développée par Paramhamsa Satyananda et son école de yoga, la Bihar School of Yoga, qui recourt aux asanas, au pranayama et à la méditation mais guide aussi ceux qui la pratiquent vers un mode de vie fidèle aux enseignements du yoga dans tous les domaines de l'existence. À tout instant, l'objectif est le développement spirituel.

Scaravelli

The yoga of Vanda Scaravelli, a pupil of B.K.S. Iyengar, is characterised by gentle, flowing forms and the fundamental importance of breathing. The exercises are intended to relax the nervous system and spirit, and to set free new energies.

Das Yoga von Vanda Scaravelli, einer Schülerin von B.K.S. Iyengar, zeichnet sich durch sanfte, fließende Formen und die zentrale Bedeutung der Atmung aus. Durch die Übungen sollen Nervensystem und Geist entspannt und dadurch neue Energien freigesetzt werden.

Le yoga imaginé par Vanda Scaravelli, un disciple de B.K.S. Iyengar, se caractérise par des mouvements doux et fluides et l'importance fondamentale accordée à la respiration. Les exercices visent à détendre le système nerveux et l'esprit, et à libérer des énergies nouvelles.

Sivananda

A global network of ashrams and schools that teach classical yoga techniques. The five pillars taught are those of classical yoga: asanas, pranayama and deep relaxation, as well as meditation (including mantra meditation) and a correct diet.

Weltweites Netzwerk aus Ashrams und Schulen, die klassische Yogatechniken lehren. Die fünf Grundpfeiler sind die des klassischen Yoga: Asanas, Pranayama und Tiefenentspannung, aber auch Meditation (einschließlich Mantra-Meditation) und richtige Ernährung.

Réseau mondial des ashrams et des écoles qui enseignent les techniques du yoga classique. Les cinq piliers (ou membres) enseignés sont ceux du yoga classique : asanas, pranayama et relaxation profonde, ainsi que méditation (notamment par les mantras) et régime strict.

SUP (Stand Up Paddle) Yoga

To be carried into a meditative mood by water, to be "one's own island" and to enjoy the beauty of nature during the asanas—these are the aims of water yoga on a paddling board, a robust, oversize surfboard.

Sich vom Wasser in meditative Stimmung versetzen zu lassen, eine „eigene Insel" zu sein und während der Asanas die Schönheit der Natur zu genießen – darum geht es beim Wasser-Yoga auf dem „Paddling Board", einem stabilen, übergroßen Surfboard.

Être emporté dans une humeur méditative par l'eau, être « sa propre île » et jouir de la beauté de la nature pendant les asanas – tels sont les objectifs de ce yoga aquatique qui se pratique sur une planche de surf très large et longue.

Tantra

Tantric yoga, like kundalini yoga, tries to awaken the energy of consciousness and thus to overcome the artificial dualism between body and spirit, between the path and the goal. Meditation and breathing control are important instruments.

Tantrisches Yoga versucht ähnlich wie Kundalini-Yoga die Bewusstseins-Energie zu erwecken und darüber den künstlichen Dualismus zwischen Körper und Geist sowie Weg und Ziel aufzuheben. Wichtige Hilfsmittel sind Meditation und Atemkontrolle.

Le yoga tantrique, tout comme le yoga Kundalini, tente d'éveiller l'énergie de la conscience, et ainsi de surmonter la dichotomie artificielle entre corps et esprit, entre le chemin et le but. La méditation et le contrôle de la respiration sont des instruments importants de cette discipline.

Tibetan Buddhist Meditation

Tantric meditation, in which the participants identify with the virtues of a Buddha, in order to liberate the spirit from ignorance, jealousy, hate etc, and to reach a state of pure serenity through peace, love and empathy.

Tantrische Meditation, in der sich die Teilnehmer mit den Tugenden eines Buddhas identifizieren, um so den Geist von Ignoranz, Eifersucht, Hass etc. zu befreien und über Ruhe, Liebe, Mitgefühl den Zustand reiner Glückseligkeit zu erreichen.

Méditation tantrique dans laquelle le pratiquant s'identifie aux vertus de Bouddha, afin de libérer l'esprit de l'ignorance, de la convoitise, de la haine, etc. pour parvenir à un état de sérénité profonde et pure, par la paix, l'amour et l'empathie.

Traditional Hatha

Traditional hatha yoga encompasses not only physical exercises and breathing control, as is usual in the Western world, but also shatkriya (rituals of cleansing), mudras (positions of the hands) and meditation in a holistic scheme.

Traditionelles Hatha Yoga umfasst nicht nur, wie in der westlichen Welt üblich, körperliche Übungen und Atemkontrolle, sondern als ganzheitliches Konzept auch Shatkriya (Reinigungsritale), Mudras (Handstellungen) und Meditation.

Le hatha yoga traditionnel englobe des exercices physiques et de contrôle de la respiration, tels qu'enseignés en Occident, mais aussi le shatkriya (rites de purification), les mudras (postures des mains) et la méditation, dans un schéma holistique.

Undogmatic Yoga

As the name says: this is no specific school. Those who teach undogmatic yoga follow no particular philosophy or master, but combine various elements to make a suitable whole, usually seen in holistic terms.

Wie der Name schon sagt: keine bestimmte Schule. Wer undogmatisches Yoga anbietet, folgt keiner bestimmten Philosophie und keinem Meister, sondern verbindet unterschiedliche Elemente zu einem sinnvollen, in der Regel holistischen Ganzen.

Comme son nom l'indique, il ne s'agit pas d'une école spécifique. Ceux qui enseignent le yoga non dogmatique ne suivent aucune philosophie particulière ni aucun maître, mais combinent des éléments d'origines variées pour constituer un ensemble cohérent de pratiques, généralement abordé de façon holistique.

Vedanta Philosophy

One of the six schools of Hindu philosophy, which arose from the Vedas, religious writings that are about 4000 years old—the Samhitas, Brahmanas, Aranyakas and Upanishads. Vedanta equates the human self with God.

Eine der sechs philosophischen Schulen des Hinduismus, die aus den Veden, etwa 4000 Jahre alten religiösen Überlieferungen, entstanden ist – den Samhitas, den Brahmanas, den Aranyakas und den Upanishaden. Der Vedanta setzt das menschliche Selbst mit Gott gleich.

Une des six écoles de la philosophie hindoue, née des Vedas, textes religieux vieux de quelque 4000 ans – Samhitas, Brahmanas, Aranyakas et Upanishads. Vedanta établit le lien entre humain et divin.

Vijnana Yoga

A type of yoga that combines physical exercises (asanas) with the integration of inner tranquillity. Dhyana (sitting still to improve inner collectedness and awareness) and svadhyaya (reading traditional yoga texts) are therefore important elements.

Yoga-Richtung, die physische Übungen (Asanas) mit der Integration innerer Ruhe verbindet. Wichtige Elemente sind daher auch Dhyana (stilles Sitzen zur Verbesserung von innerer Sammlung und Achtsamkeit) und Svadhyaya (Lesen traditioneller Yogatexte).

Type de yoga qui combine exercices physiques (asanas) et travail sur la tranquillité intérieure. Parmi les éléments importants figurent par conséquent le dhyana (rester assis, immobile, afin d'améliorer la capacité de recueillement et la prise de conscience) et le svadhyaya (lecture des textes de yoga traditionnels).

Vinyasa/ Vinyasa Flow

A very popular, dynamic school of yoga that combines movements with flowing breathing, releases tension and creates space for new life force in this release. In its practice it is important to build up the right tension.

Sehr populäre, dynamische Yoga-Schule, die Bewegungen mit fließender Atmung verbindet, Spannung behebt und in der Gelöstheit Raum für neue Lebenskraft schafft. In dieser Praxis ist das Aufbauen des richtigen Spannungsbogens von Bedeutung.

École de yoga dynamique très populaire qui combine mouvements, respiration libre et relâchement des tensions afin de créer de l'espace pour une nouvelle force de vie. Dans cette discipline, il est important d'atteindre une tension juste.

Yin Yoga

An extremely quiet, passive style of yoga in which seated or lying positions are held for a long time without muscular activity. The aim is to relax larger or smaller areas of the body and thus to achieve spiritual release.

Sehr ruhiger, passiver Yogastil, in dem Positionen in sitzender oder liegender Haltung ausgeführt und lange Zeit ohne Muskelaktivität gehalten werden. Ziel ist die Entspannung großer und kleiner Körperregionen und damit auch das geistige Loslassen.

Style de yoga extrêmement paisible et passif dans lequel les postures assises ou allongées sont maintenues longtemps, sans activité musculaire. L'objectif est de détendre les diverses parties du corps, petites et grandes, afin de parvenir à une profonde détente spirituelle.